PRAISE FOR
THE RESOLUTION ZONE

"*The Resolution Zone* is a must read. Dr. Sears' vision is clearly presented building on fundamental new discoveries from experimental medicine. I highly recommend this book and hope you'll embrace its very valuable messages."

—*Professor Charles N. Serhan, PhD, DSc., Endowed Professor Harvard Medical School, Distinguished Scientist and Director, Center for Experimental Therapeutics at Brigham and Women's Hospital*

"*The Resolution Zone* represents another masterpiece, emerging from Dr. Sears' decades of work to understand the role of diet in controlling inflammation and the resulting disease conditions it is associated with. The reader will find easy to follow dietary guidelines that will be of assistance to maintain wellness not only to reduce inflammation, but also to promote resolution of chronic inflammation, while promoting repair of the tissue injured by the silent inflammatory process."

—*Camillo Ricordi, MD, Stacy Joy Goodman Professor of Surgery, Distinguished Professor of Medicine, Professor of Biomedical Engineering, Microbiology and Immunology, Director, Diabetes Research Institute and Cell Transplant Center, University of Miami*

"*The Resolution Zone* illuminates the complex connection between diet, metabolic health, and wellness. Dr. Sears wisely places their complicated interactions in the appendices to spare the non-scientific reader these details, yet provides the research scientist with detailed biochemistry to support his defined dietary system. Any reader will be empowered to utilize food as medicine by reading this book."

—*Carol Johnston, PhD, RD, Professor and Associate Director, Nutrition Program, School of Nutrition and Health Promotion, Arizona State University*

"*The Resolution Zone* explains how unresolved inflammation is responsible for most of the chronic diseases we currently struggle with as well as aging itself. This book is highly recommended not only for all those seeking optimal health but also for all physicians desirous of learning why and how these dietary measures work."

—*Joseph C. Maroon, MD., Professor and Vice Chairman, Department of Neurological Surgery, Heindl Scholar in Neuroscience, University of Pittsburgh, and team neurosurgeon, Pittsburgh Steelers*

"In *The Resolution Zone*, we see the culmination of decades of his research and experience which begin with Dr. Sears' first book in 1995, *The Zone*. He convincingly shows us how our diet can be effectively used as our most effective drug."

—*Julian E. Bailes, MD., Bennett Tarkington Chairman of the Department of Neurosurgery NorthShore University HealthSystem, Co-Director, NorthShore Neurological Institute, and Clinical Professor of Neurosurgery University of Chicago Pritzker School of Medicine*

"*The Resolution Zone* leads you step by step from the very basic concepts on inflammation to the more practical aspects related to fight inflammation and disease disorders by simply using a healthy diet to boost your own pro-resolution capacities."

—*Joan Clària, PhD, Professor, Hospital Clinic of Barcelona and Barcelona University School of Medicine, Barcelona, Spain*

"I can strongly recommend *The Resolution Zone* to any reader who is interested in nutrition-related inflammation and willing to change his or her dietary lifestyle for their well-being."

—*Thomas Stulnig, MD, Associate Professor, Head of the Christian Doppler Laboratory for Cardio-Metabolic Immunotherapy and Clinical Division of Endocrinology and Metabolism and Clinical Division of Endocrinology and Metabolism, Department of Medicine, Medical University of Vienna, Austria*

"*The Resolution Zone* discusses one of the most prevalent causes of chronic disease, depression, and dementia—is the blockage of the resolution of inflammation. He shows you how this blockage develops and how you can reverse it. I highly recommend it."

—*Daniel G. Amen, MD, Founder Amen Clinics and author of* Feel Better Fast and Make It Last

BOOKS BY DR. BARRY SEARS

The Zone

Mastering the Zone

Zone Perfect Meals in Minutes

The Anti-Aging Zone

The Soy Zone

The OmegaRx Zone

What to Eat in the Zone

The Top 100 Zone Foods

A Week in the Zone

Zone Meals in Seconds

The Anti-Inflammation Zone

Il Bello Della Zona

Toxic Fat

La Zona del Futuro

The Mediterranean Zone

Positive Nutrition

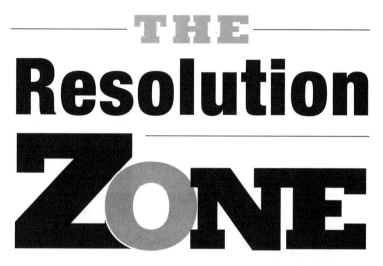

THE
Resolution
ZONE

The Science of the
Resolution Response

BARRY SEARS, PH.D.

ZONE
Press

Zone Press
Zone Enterprises, Inc.
2646 SW Mapp Road
Palm City, FL 34990

First Paperback Edition: 2019
10 9 8 7 6 5 4 3 2 1

Zone Press is an imprint of Zone Enterprises, Inc.

Library of Congress Cataloging-in-Publication Data

Sears, Barry, 1947-
    The Resolution Zone: The Science of the Resolution Response.
    ISBN 978-1-68245-125-0

    1. Inflammation and resolution. 2. Zone Pro-Resolution Nutrition. 3. Omega-3 fatty acids and inflammation. 4. Polyphenols and metabolism

Text Design by Neuwirth & Associates, Inc.

CONTENTS

Prologue

MY JOURNEY TO UNDERSTAND CHRONIC DISEASE

MORE THAN FORTY years ago, I had a hunch that could possibly change the course of medicine. That idea began with trying to understand the underlying cause of my family's history of heart disease. It's been a personal journey with many twists and turns as I have come to understand the intricate dance between our diet, inflammation, and its eventual resolution leading to healing.

The medical definition of healing is "the process of getting well." That description doesn't seem to be very high-tech in this day and age. On the contrary, the molecular basis of healing is characterized by a highly organized series of events that I term the "Resolution Response." This Resolution Response represents the dynamic balance of the hormonal and genetic factors that orchestrate the highly programmed responses that promote the healing of any internal or external injury to your body. The Zone represents the physiological state measured by simple clinical markers indicating you have optimized your internal Resolution Response to work at full efficiency. Reaching the Zone and thus optimizing how your Resolution Response is controlled by your diet and specific nutrients is the central theme of this book.

My journey to understand the Zone began with my research in the mid-1970s at the Boston University School of Medicine that focused on the role of dietary fats in the development of heart disease. With time, my research moved toward developing intravenous drug delivery technology using fats to reduce the toxicity of cancer drugs. My interest in inflammation heightened when the 1982 Nobel Prize in Medicine was awarded for the early studies into how a certain class of dietary fats could be transformed into a unique group of hormones known as eicosanoids that were key players in the inflammatory process. I reasoned that if the underlying cause of all chronic disease (including heart disease) involved inflammation, and if inflammation could be manipulated with diet, then that might possibly hold the key to controlling the future of medicine. Nothing like dreaming big.

Since eicosanoids are derived from certain dietary fatty fats, I felt it might be possible to control their synthesis using the diet as opposed to using anti-inflammatory drugs. That decision led me from the high-tech world of developing intravenous cancer drug delivery systems to the definitely low-tech world of health foods in the 1980s. My seemingly abrupt change was perceived by my academic colleagues as a fool-hardy choice since I was going from the leading edge of cancer drug delivery technology to the very low-tech health food industry populated by numerous charlatans and snake-oil salesmen.

My research ultimately led to my first book on inflammation, *The Zone*, published in 1995. It was a complex work written primarily for physicians to demonstrate how the dietary manipulation of insulin and the right balance of essential fatty acids was critical for the control of inflammation. To the surprise of everyone (including myself and my publisher), the book sold millions of copies. As to why *The Zone* was so successful, no one is quite sure. Maybe it was because it offered a new viewpoint on our growing obesity epidemic that had started to explode starting in 1980. At the time when *The Zone* was published, you had Robert Atkins shouting that carbs make you fat, and his equally vocal opponent Dean Ornish responding that it was fat that makes you fat. This was like the old Miller Lite commercials featuring ex-NFL players shouting, "More taste, less filling" at each other.

My insights described in *The Zone* were very different and far more complex. My contention was that diet-induced inflammation makes you fat, as well as increasing the likelihood of developing chronic diseases and aging at a faster rate. I used the term "Zone" to describe a physiological state where you could consistently control the intensity of diet-induced inflammation and thus better manage any type of chronic disease. However, reaching the Zone required a highly integrated dietary system to reduce inflammation throughout the body. Not exactly your typical cocktail conversation.

With time, I began to suspect stronger biological forces were at play than simply reducing the levels of eicosanoids necessary to ultimately reach the full potential of the Zone. I explored that concept in my book, *The OmegaRx Zone*, published in 2002. I realized that it wasn't just the reduction of inflammation that was important, but also the need to resolve it. Resolution is a totally separate process than turning on inflammation. In essence, you have to turn inflammation on, but you must also be able to turn it off. Fortunately, both phases of inflammation could be controlled by dietary fats. The hormones (eicosanoids) generated from one group of fats known as omega-6 fatty acids turn on inflammation, and other group of hormones (resolvins) derived from omega-3 fatty acids turn off inflammation.

Understanding the complexity of how resolvins are made and how they work can be traced to one person, Charlie Serhan at Harvard Medical School. Just as I felt like a voice in the wilderness discussing the growing role of diet-induced inflammation to the lay public in the 1990s, Charlie was in somewhat the same situation advocating the importance of the resolution of inflammation as he began introducing the concept of resolvins to the academic medicine community at the turn of the 21st century.

But even turning off inflammation using high-dose omega-3 fatty acids would not necessarily repair the damage. With my book, *The Mediterranean Zone*, published in 2014, I began to explore the role of polyphenols as dietary agents acting as gene activators to increase tissue repair in the body as well as well as maintaining gut health to further reduce the intensity of diet-induced inflammation. In the same book I also began to discuss the activation of specific genes by polyphenols that completes the healing process.

What I have tried to do in this book is to synthesize the complex interaction of the three dietary components I have described in the past (the Zone Diet, omega-3 fatty acids, and polyphenols) into an orchestrated dietary system that I term the "Zone Pro-Resolution Nutrition" system. This dietary system allows you to optimize the body's natural healing process because their orchestration also controls the effectiveness of your internal Resolution Response.

The first part of this book starts with a short overview of the Zone, why it is important to spend your life in the Zone, and how to get there.

The second part of this book details what constitutes the Resolution Response and how diet-induced inflammation has become the driving force for many of the health problems we experience at various stages of life. In this section, I discuss the individual dietary components of the Zone Pro-Resolution Nutrition system in greater detail and how they can be organized into a personalized dietary program to keep you in the Zone for a lifetime.

Next, I explore the reasons you want to use the Zone Pro-Resolution Nutrition system as a systems-based approach to address the various problems caused by unresolved inflammation that prevent you from reaching your goals at various stages in your life. Although your goals may change with time, the dietary pathway to reach those goals remains the same.

Finally, in the last section, I discuss my vision on the future of medicine. The way medicine is practiced today (treating the symptoms of chronic disease with increasingly expensive drugs) is simply unsustainable for the future. However, I firmly believe that the Zone Pro-Resolution Nutrition system and its ability to optimize the Resolution Response offers a new view of the future of medicine. Following the Zone Pro-Resolution Nutrition dietary system, you have the ability to control the hormones and the expression of key genes that allows you to maintain wellness as long as possible by optimizing the body's natural Resolution Response we commonly refer to as healing. This type of "medicine" is not only sustainable, but can immediately be put into practice in your own kitchen.

Some of the terms you will be reading in this book will probably be new to you. That's why I have a glossary in Appendix B that makes it easier to quickly understand how each concept is an integral part of the healing process.

I welcome you to *The Resolution Zone*.

1

What Is the Zone?

ALTHOUGH I HAVE been writing about the Zone and its implications for the future of medicine for more than twenty years, I am still constantly asked, "What is the Zone?"

The concept of the Zone is based on understanding the complexities of inflammation and its resolution. The popular media would lead you to believe that inflammation is the bane of our existence. In reality, without a strong inflammatory response we couldn't exist because we would be sitting targets for microbial invasion and our injuries would never heal. However, if the same inflammation that initially protects us is not turned off, then it begins to attack our own bodies. The technical term that describes the turning off of the initial inflammation response and repairing tissue damaged by it is called resolution. It's not inflammation per se, but *unresolved inflammation* that is the problem.

Inflammation remains a very complex topic. That's why it is constantly misunderstood. To make it simpler to comprehend, consider the following relationship:

Inflammation = Damage
Resolution = Healing

Inflammation is the result of injury either external or internal to our body. We need some inflammation to protect us against microbial invaders or to heal physical injuries, but we also need to resolve that initial inflammation and then begin to repair the damage it has caused in order to heal to maintain wellness. Both responses are generated on demand because you never know when an injury might occur. However, it is only when these two distinct phases of inflammation are continually balanced, that you are in the Zone where you can maintain wellness for a lifetime. If not, your life is likely to be far more challenging than it should be.

Today much of the inflammation in your body is a consequence of the foods you eat causing diet-induced inflammation that amplifies any existing unresolved inflammation.

2

Why Do You Want to Be in the Zone?

THE SIMPLE ANSWER is to achieve a meaningful lifestyle and health goals with greater ease. Some of these would include the following:

- Better weight management with loss of excess body fat
- Improved physical and mental performance
- Maintaining mental and physical wellness for a longer period of time

As I will address later in this book, they might also include many of the problems we struggle with at various stages of our life, ranging from improved fetal nutrition for your children to improving the management of any chronic disease in order to maintain healthy aging for as long as possible. All of these outcomes are possible by being in the Zone.

However, maintaining wellness is the primary reason you want to be in the Zone. You don't realize how priceless wellness is until you begin to lose it by developing a chronic disease. The best way to treat a chronic disease is not to develop it in the first place. We often mistakenly believe if we don't have a chronic disease that is the same as being well. That is simply not true. Unfortunately, most chronic diseases take years, if not decades, to develop before their symptoms begin to manifest themselves. That disease might be diabetes, heart disease, cancer, or even Alzheimer's. None of these conditions develop overnight. It is only after years of constant tissue damage caused by unresolved cellular inflammation that a particular organ becomes less efficient resulting in loss of function. It would be nice to know years ahead of time that your levels of unresolved cellular inflammation were increasing so you could correct the underlying problem at an earlier stage well before the development of some chronic disease. So, perhaps a better definition of wellness might be your ability to continuously balance the "turning on" and "turning off" of inflammation. In other words, being in the Zone.

Being in the Zone doesn't mean you will never develop a chronic disease. However, it does mean that you can dramatically reduce that likelihood. Furthermore, if you have a chronic disease, you should be able to manage it more effectively with fewer drugs. In either case, your healthspan (longevity minus years of disability) will likely increase the longer you are in the Zone.

As I will discuss later, there are easily validated clinical markers that define the Zone. These are also the same markers that can define your true current state of wellness. These markers allow you to see into your future and gives you the opportunity to correct the underlying problem of increasing cellular inflammation before it develops into a chronic disease. This is the foundation of what I call "evidence-based wellness."

Bringing all the markers of the Zone into their appropriate ranges can be accomplished in a relatively short period of time using the correct dietary strategy, and in particular the Zone Pro-Resolution Nutrition system. Staying in the Zone requires consistently maintaining that same dietary strategy.

Being in the Zone is like being pregnant—either you are, or you aren't. My best estimate is that fewer than 1 percent of Americans are currently in the Zone. This goes a long way to explain why we pay more for health care than any country in the world. It also means that there is a great upside potential to radically improve health care in America. The only way to get to the Zone is through the diet, and in particular following a comprehensive dietary system that produces rapid hormonal and genetic changes that can be maintained for a lifetime. If you don't, then your life may likely be more difficult than it should be. Thus, avoiding future health difficulties that arise from chronic unresolved cellular inflammation and maintaining your wellness are the real reasons you want to be in the Zone.

3

How Do You Get in the Zone?

THE BEST WAY to maintain the dynamic balance of inflammation and it resolution is by using a comprehensive dietary system that I term the Zone Pro-Resolution Nutrition system. This dietary technology consists of three distinct dietary strategies working together as a synergistic team.

1. The Zone Diet to *reduce* diet-induced inflammation.
2. Omega-3 fatty acids to *resolve* residual cellular inflammation.
3. Polyphenols to *repair* the damaged tissue once residual cellular inflammation is sufficiently reduced.

Consider *reduction, resolution,* and *repair* to be the 3R's of wellness. No single dietary intervention is sufficient for getting you to the Zone; you need all three working together as synergistic team. Consider the Zone Pro-Resolution Nutrition system as a highly orchestrated combination of dietary hormonal and genetic control therapy required to get you to the Zone.

Although the science behind the Zone is complex and robust, the consistent use of the Zone Pro-Resolution Nutrition system is actually quite simple to implement for a lifetime once you know the rules of the game.

Here is a quick summary of the dietary rules to reach the Zone:

1. Calories do count. Don't kid yourself. Whether you are looking to lose excess body fat or live longer, the fewer calories you consume the more likely you are going to achieve your personal health and performance goals. However, the hormonal responses generated by those calories count even more. The secret is to consume the least number of calories without hunger and fatigue by generating the correct hormonal responses at each meal that you eat. It seems like a tall order, but it is easily accomplished using the Zone Pro-Resolution Nutrition system.

2. There is no magic nutritional bullet. Forget about the addition of "super-foods" or removal of "evil" food ingredients like dairy, gluten, or lectins. Such topics make for bestselling books, television news, or internet blogs that require a limited attention span, but they have nothing to do with the lifelong hormonal and genetic control necessary to reduce unresolved cellular inflammation.

3. Consistency counts. The more consistent you are in your food choices, the easier it is to see the benefits. Try to think of your meals as drugs. They don't have to taste like drugs, but their hormonal and genetic benefits are short-lived, meaning you have to follow a consistent dietary lifestyle if your goal is to maintain your wellness.

4. You are only a few meals from getting back on track. One bad meal can take you out of the Zone because of its rapid hormonal consequences, but the right dietary choices over the next few meals can easily bring you back to the Zone by balancing the hormones in the blood and changing the expression of key genes.

Maintaining wellness requires a system. The next chapter gives you an overview of the Zone Pro-Resolution Nutrition system which is your dietary pathway to reach the Zone and thus optimize your internal Resolution Response.

4

Overview of the Zone Pro-Resolution Nutrition System

A DEFINED DIETARY PATHWAY TO THE ZONE

THE ZONE PRO-RESOLUTION Nutrition system is a comprehensive dietary strategy that provides a powerful approach to reversing the adverse consequences of unresolved cellular inflammation. It does this by regulating the hormones and the expression of key genes that can be controlled by the diet to maintain the appropriate balance between the intensity of inflammation with its resolution, and finally by orchestrating its ultimate repair of any damage caused by inflammation. This is how healing works.

The Zone Pro-Resolution Nutrition system is a systems-based approach to maintain wellness by optimizing your Resolution Response. No single one of the three dietary components of the Zone Pro-Resolution Nutrition system is sufficient alone to achieve healing of injuries since it requires a constant orchestration of hormonal and genetic responses. Likewise, the interactions of the dietary components of the Zone Pro-Resolution Nutrition system are far more complex than the "drug A inhibiting enzyme B" thinking that currently dominates current pharmaceutical thinking.

The three dietary pillars necessary for the Zone Pro-Resolution Nutrition system to be successful are:

- Zone Diet
- Omega-3 Fatty Acids
- Polyphenols

Each of these dietary tools have unique benefits and are synergistic. This means the more of these dietary strategies you use correctly, the greater your ability to decrease unresolved cellular inflammation.

ZONE DIET

We must eat to survive. But to survive well, you must eat less. That seemingly paradoxical statement is the foundation of calorie restriction. The definition of calorie restriction is far more complex than simply reducing calories because at the same time you have to maintain, if not increase, your intake of essential nutrients. For human cells, essential nutrients include essential amino acids, essential fatty acids, and vitamins. For the bacteria in your gut, you need fermentable fiber and polyphenols. Anything less is malnutrition. The Zone Diet was developed to optimize all of the above factors for the increased intake of essential nutrients with the least number of total calories without hunger or fatigue as more fully explained in Chapter 8.

The Zone Diet is the foundation of the Zone Pro-Resolution Nutrition system because it reduces the intensity of diet-induced inflammation that amplifies any existing cellular inflammation. Thus, the Zone Diet should be considered as an anti-inflammatory diet. But unlike anti-inflammatory drugs, the Zone Diet doesn't reduce your ability to mount an inflammatory response when needed, but it does reduce the intensity of that response therefore making it easier to eventually resolve.

Inherent within the Zone Diet is the need to consume adequate levels of fermentable fiber. Currently gut health is all the rage and for good reason. The trillions of bacteria in your gut should be considered a separate body organ that is critical for the control of diet-induced inflammation in your body. But the bacteria in your gut must be fed to meet that goal. Their primary food source is fermentable fiber. But not all dietary fiber is fermentable, meaning that much of it can't be used as nutrients by the bacteria in your gut. Although the definition of fermentable fiber is relatively vague, your best source with the best impact on hormonal response will usually come from non-starchy vegetables. Without adequate levels of fermentable fiber in the Zone Diet, the thin barrier between the alien world of the bacteria in our gut and the cells in our body is likely to start breaking down resulting in another source of inflammation that ultimately must be resolved to have an optimal Resolution Response.

OMEGA-3 FATTY ACIDS

Although the Zone Diet is the ideal dietary intervention to reduce the intensity of diet-induced inflammation, it will have little effect reducing unresolved cellular inflammation. Reaching that goal requires the adequate intake of omega-3 fatty acids. Only if you have adequate levels of omega-3 fatty acids in the blood can you begin to generate the hormones (i.e., resolvins) necessary to resolve inflammation as described in Chapter 10. How much do you need? It depends on how closely you follow the Zone Diet. The more closely you follow the Zone Diet, the fewer omega-3 fatty acids you will need to stay in the Zone. On the other hand, the less closely you follow the Zone Diet to reduce diet-induced inflammation, the more omega-3 fatty acids you will need to resolve cellular inflammation.

POLYPHENOLS

Only after you have resolved cellular inflammation, can you begin the process of repairing the damaged tissue to complete the Resolution Response. This is the job of polyphenols to continuously activate the key gene transcription factor that is responsible for generating the repair of damaged tissue after residual cellular inflammation is resolved and, in the process, slow down your rate of aging as I will describe in Chapter 11.

To understand how these dietary components function together as a system, you need some knowledge of how nutrition affects the control of your hormones and your genes.

YOUR BIOLOGICAL INTERNET

We like to think of the internet as the ultimate expression of today's technology because millions of individuals can stay in real time contact and access information from the greatest libraries of the world, but it is also a technology that can also provide misinformation. However, our bodies contain a far more sophisticated internet-like communication system (which I term the Biological Internet) that allows trillions of cells in your body to communicate with each other virtually in real time to fine-tune your metabolism leading to better control of your cognitive, physical, and emotional responses. When your Biological Internet is working correctly the result is continued wellness, but it also has the ability to provide mis-information to your cells.

Unlike the electrons that drive the internet, hormones (hundreds of them and potentially far more yet to be discovered) drive our Biological Internet. This gives the human body far greater nuances than anything envisioned in Silicon Valley. Yet if your hormones are not interacting correctly, then your Biological Internet can rapidly become dysfunc-tional. The hormones that ultimately control the levels of unresolved cel-lular inflammation are the consequence of the dynamic balance of eicosanoids derived from omega-6 fatty acids and resolvins derived from omega-3 fatty acids. Eicosanoids increase cellular inflammation and re-solvins reduce it. It is the hormonal balance of these two powerful hor-monal groups that is one of the keys to using the Zone Pro-Resolution Nutrition system to optimize your Resolution Response.

THE ROLE OF GENE TRANSCRIPTION FACTORS

The other key to the Zone Pro-Resolution Nutrition system is its ability to control certain critical gene transcription factors. We also constantly hear that genetic engineering represents the future of medicine. After nearly twenty years of research on our decoded DNA, we don't seem to have that many genes in the first place. Corn and wheat have far more genes than we do, and they don't rule the world. Furthermore, our DNA is virtually identical to that of a chimpanzee. The difference between us, chimpanzees, corn, and wheat are that we have far more gene transcrip-tion factors. These complex proteins act as short-cuts to allow us to re-spond faster to outside stimuli by turning on selected DNA sequences to make specialized proteins. There are hundreds of known gene transcrip-tion factors, and undoubtedly far more yet to be discovered. However, the two key gene transcription factors that can be affected by the Zone Pro-Resolution Nutrition system are nuclear factor kappaB (NF-κB) and AMP kinase. NF-κB turns on inflammation that causes tissue damage, and AMP kinase is the key for repairing tissue damaged by cellular inflammation. The Zone Pro-Resolution Nutrition system provides the dietary pathway to control these two critical gene transcription factors. This dietary gene therapy is the other key for understanding how the Zone Pro-Resolution Nutrition system works to repair damaged tissue to maintain wellness.

PUTTING IT ALL TOGETHER

Consider being in the Zone like a biological gyroscope that must be constantly balanced by hormonal and genetic effects using the Zone Pro-Resolution Nutrition system. This can be visualized by the following graphic.

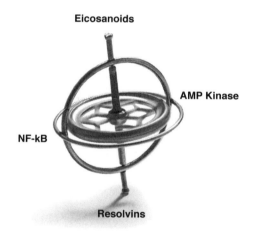

Not only do you constantly need to balance both eicosanoids and resolvins, but you also have to balance the master genetic switches of inflammation (NF-κB) and metabolism (AMP kinase). If these hormones and gene transcription factors are maintained in dynamic equilibrium, then your Resolution Response is optimized and the rate of healing from any injury is dramatically accelerated.

5

How Inflammation Keeps You Alive and the Resolution Response Keeps You Well

WE OFTEN THINK of inflammation as something dangerous to our health. In reality, the opposite is true. You need some inflammation to stay alive otherwise you would always be an easy target for microbial invasion and physical injuries would never heal. But the injury that caused the initial inflammation must be resolved completely for the healing process to be successful.

A SHORT HISTORY OF INFLAMMATION

Studying inflammation is not new. The ancient Greeks tried to describe it as the internal fire. The ancient Romans tried to describe it as heat, pain, swelling, and redness. In the 19th century the German physician, Rudolf Virchow, added loss of function to the ancient Roman description. Today, loss of function can be interpreted as organ damage which is the foundation of virtually every chronic disease.

On the other hand, the concept of resolution was first discussed in the *Cannon of Medicine* written by the Persian philosopher, Avicenna, in 1025. Yet our knowledge of the molecular basis of resolution began only 20 years ago and continues to evolve.

UNDERSTANDING THE RESOLUTION RESPONSE

If inflammation is complex, then the Resolution Response required to repair the damage caused by inflammation is even more so. To make it simpler to understand, consider the following relationship:

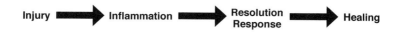

Any injury (external or internal) to the body creates inflammation. Your ability to completely heal that injury is governed by a complex series of highly orchestrated sequential steps that constitute the Resolution Response. If your internal Resolution Response is robust, the injury is healed completely. However, complete healing only occurs if the intensity of the inflammatory response caused by an injury is balanced by an equivalent strength of the Resolution Response. Since these injuries occur continuously in every organ, you must ensure that your Resolution Response remains at optimal efficiency if you want successful healing of that injury to take place.

Thus, wellness can be defined as the constant on-demand balancing of any inflammation generated by any injury (external or internal) with an appropriate Resolution Response. If you are in the Zone, you have done everything possible using your diet to optimize the Resolution Response to maintain wellness for a lifetime. This is why the medical definition of healing is "the process of getting well."

What happens if the Resolution Response is inhibited or blocked? Then the consequence of that injury-induced inflammation follows a very different pathway.

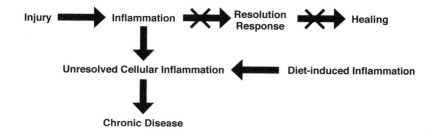

If the Resolution Response is inhibited, then inflammation caused by a random injury cannot be healed completely. As a result, the levels of unresolved cellular inflammation begin to increase, but it is still below the perception of pain. More ominously, this unresolved cellular inflammation can be further amplified by your diet (i.e., diet-induced inflammation). Eventually, the compounding levels of unresolved cellular inflammation (whatever its initial cause) will cause your organs to begin losing function because of increased inflammatory damage. When enough organ function is lost, you develop a chronic disease.

Development of chronic disease doesn't happen overnight. It is the result of a continued inhibition of the body's natural Resolution Response that sets the stage for the eventual development of chronic disease. If the initial injury has not completely healed, then constant reinjury to it can be constantly amplified by diet-induced inflammation and a continuing blockage of an adequate Resolution Response. This combination accelerates the rate at which a chronic disease begins to develop. This could include diabetes, heart disease, cancer, or Alzheimer's. The ultimate cause of any chronic disease is not inflammation per se, but the lack of a strong Resolution Response in your body to resolve and repair the tissue damage caused by inflammation.

Injuries are random, but the Resolution Response is not. It is a highly orchestrated system of timed molecular events controlled by hormonal and genetic factors. Yet as complex as the Resolution Response is, it is completely under dietary control. Your diet can either improve the Resolution Response or continue to inhibit it. When you are in the Zone, you have done everything possible to optimize the Resolution Response.

Think of the relationship between inflammation and the Resolution Response like a continuous cycle of yin and yang. Scientifically this means a continuing cycle beginning with the initiation of inflammation caused by an injury to the final resolution of the inflammatory response by your Resolution Response that results in healing. This brings you back to equilibrium to await the next random injury to your body. A good example is cutting your hand with a knife. Initially it hurts producing a combination of heat, pain, swelling, and redness (the initial signs of inflammation). Yet within a few days, the cut has healed completely (both internally and externally) if you have a robust Resolution Response.

A more detailed description of inflammation and its relevance to understanding the Resolution Response can be found in Appendix C.

CONSEQUENCES OF UNRESOLVED INFLAMMATION

In an ideal world, the intensity of the inflammatory response initiated by an injury would ideally be balanced by the Resolution Response and the damaged tissue is repaired and returns to normal function, just like the analogy of healing the cut hand.

Unfortunately, we don't live in such an ideal world. Either the initiation phase is too strong, the Resolution Response is too weak or in the worst-case scenario, both phases of inflammation are moving in the wrong directions at the same time. Now you have a mismatch of both phases of inflammation, and the end result is growing levels of unresolved cellular inflammation in the target organ that continues to inhibit the Resolution Response. A typical example of this would be the development of Alzheimer's disease, which is an inflammatory disease that progresses without any perception of pain.

PLAN B: FIBROSIS

If cellular inflammation is not sufficiently resolved by the Resolution Response, the body often reverts to Plan B to curtail the continuing cellular damage. This process is known as fibrosis, which is simply the formation of internal scar tissue to stop the spread of any unresolved cellular inflammation. If the scar tissue is in the walls of the heart vessels, it is called an atherosclerotic plaque. In the liver, it is called cirrhosis. In the lung, it is called chronic obstructive pulmonary disease, or COPD. Scar tissue can even form in your fat cells. All of these untoward consequences are the result of unresolved cellular inflammation. Eventually when enough scar tissue accumulates, the organ begins to lose function. Increased fibrosis in various organs is also the central hallmark of accelerated aging. In fact, it is estimated that 45 percent of all deaths are associated with significant fibrosis.

However, fibrosis can be significantly mitigated by optimizing the Resolution Response using the Zone Pro-Resolution Nutrition system to prevent the body from resorting to Plan B to deal with unresolved cellular inflammation.

SUMMARY ▶

Although inflammation is designed to protect you from microbial invasions and physical injuries, you always require a robust and constant Resolution Response to maintain wellness. Both responses have evolved to work together over hundreds of millions of years of evolution because if your injuries would never heal, life as we know it would be impossible. Being in the Zone means that you have optimized your Resolution Response to random injuries that can strike at any time.

6

Diet-Induced Inflammation

IN THE LAST chapter I briefly discussed the finely tuned orchestration of the inflammation response that has evolved to protect us against microbial invasion and physical injuries that is coupled with the body's internal Resolution Response to maintain wellness. Unfortunately, this finely tuned system is not prepared to protect us from diet-induced inflammation.

Radical changes in our diet within the past fifty years have introduced a new source of inflammation: diet-induced inflammation. This type of inflammation is just as inflammatory as any injury and can continually amplify the levels of any existing unresolved cellular inflammation. In the constant presence of diet-induced inflammation, a seemingly mild (but incompletely healed) injury becomes a starting point to keep increasing the levels of cellular inflammation leading to the more rapid development of a chronic disease.

Diet-induced inflammation hijacks normal precise balance between injury-induced inflammation and the Resolution Response. The result has been the creation of a worldwide epidemic of chronic unresolved cellular inflammation. Many of these dietary changes first started in America, where food industrialization was first developed, and then via globalization it has spread to the rest of the world. It's a story of not only what we have added to the human diet, but also what we have taken out of the human diet. It almost seems like a bad script for a B-grade science fiction movie about a virus implanted in our bodies by an alien race so they can more easily take over the planet. Unfortunately, this is now a reality not a movie script.

DIETARY CHANGES THAT HAVE INCREASED CELLULAR INFLAMMATION

Let's start with the foods we have recently added to the human diet. The foremost of these are the overconsumption of omega-6 fatty acids. Omega-6 fatty acids are the molecular building block necessary to generate the eicosanoids needed to initiate the inflammatory response. Omega-6 fatty acids constituted a minor component of the human diet until the early part of the 20th century, when we learned how to extract these fatty acids in greater abundance from vegetables sources (corn, soy, sunflower, and safflower) using chemical solvents such as hexane. As a result, the levels of omega-6 fatty acids in the diet have dramatically increased. Today, omega-6 fatty acids are the second least expensive source of calories known (only refined table sugar is slightly less expensive) and are a central component of all processed foods and primary ingredients for the restaurant industry. However, not all omega-6 fatty acids are directly involved in the production of eicosanoids. Arachidonic acid (AA) is the primary omega-6 fatty acid that can be transformed into the eicosanoids necessary for the initiation of inflammation. However, the greater the levels of omega-6 fatty acids in the diet, the greater the potential they will be converted into excessive levels of AA in the body. In fact, in 1974 it was shown that injecting high levels of AA into rabbits caused death within three minutes. The moral of the story is that you need some AA to start the inflammatory process, but not too much that can cause adverse effects. Furthermore, the more omega-6 fatty acids you consume, the more likely you will produce too much AA.

The eicosanoids derived from AA also activate the gene transcription factor NF-κB, the master switch for turning on inflammation that I described in the previous chapter. You need some AA for an appropriate inflammatory response. However, too much AA in your body will generate excess cellular inflammation in every cell.

What speeds up the transformation of omega-6 fatty acids into AA is the hormone insulin. Insulin is secreted in response to the rate that blood glucose levels rise after eating a meal. This leads to the other recent addition to the human diet: refined carbohydrates. Refined carbohydrates have removed most of the fermentable fiber and vitamins to make processed foods easier to manufacture and to digest. In fact, products made with refined carbohydrates (like white bread) are so easy to digest that the glucose in them enters into the blood at a faster rate than does table sugar. This rapid rise in blood glucose (known as the glycemic load of a meal) increases insulin levels in the blood which in turn greatly accelerates the formation of AA. This process is described in greater detail in Appendix C.

Another unexpected consequence of the increased levels of refined carbohydrates in our diet has been the simultaneous reduction of the fermentable fiber content. The need for this unique type of fiber (described in Chapter 8) is the key for gut health, especially for maintaining a strong barrier between the bacteria in the gut and the blood. If this barrier is compromised, it is known as a "leaky gut." This occurs when bacterial fragments and large protein fragments enter into the blood and generate increased inflammation.

INSULIN RESISTANCE AND INFLAMMATION

The rise in insulin levels with a diet rich in refined carbohydrates is a transitory event until you develop a condition known as insulin resistance. Once you develop insulin resistance, insulin levels remain constantly elevated, further accelerating the production of AA from omega-6 fatty acids by activating the key enzymes in that process. The result is the creation of even more eicosanoids.

What actually causes insulin resistance? It's the increased levels of cellular inflammation that disrupts the signaling process from the insulin receptor to the interior of the cell. This is why the combination of omega-6 fatty acids and refined carbohydrates can be a deadly duo as each component reinforces the other into making more AA. This increases the intensity of diet-induced inflammation, thus making it very difficult to fully activate the Resolution Response, thereby creating increased levels of chronic unresolved cellular inflammation.

UNDERSTANDING INSULIN RESISTANCE

If there was a clear indication of the existence of cellular inflammation in your body, it would be the presence of insulin resistance. Since reducing insulin resistance is one of the key benefits of the Zone Pro-Resolution Nutrition system, it makes sense to learn something about this condition.

The vast majority of hormones work in a three-step process. First, they are released from their appropriate gland, then travel through the bloodstream searching for their target cells. Next the hormone has to interact with a specific receptor on the surface of the target cell. Finally, the initial message carried by the hormone is transmitted into the interior of the target cell by activation of second messengers inside the cell to accomplish its final task. It sounds complicated, and it is. If anything goes wrong in this complex relay race, it is as if the hormone was never released in the first place and the elegant hormonal communication system that runs your Biological Internet no longer functions well.

Hormone resistance occurs when any of these steps become less efficient. This is especially true for the hormone insulin because it acts as the central hub for controlling the storage and release of nutrients such as fat and glucose, the transport of amino acids into cells for rebuilding tissue, modification of enzyme activity, control of satiety in the hypothalamus, enhanced memory and learning in the brain, and other metabolic functions requiring insulin signaling.

The most likely suspect that causes insulin resistance is the third step of hormonal action, which is the increased level of cellular inflammation inside the cell blocking hormonal communication. It's as if insulin is talking, but the target cell isn't listening. Considering all the things that insulin is supposed to do, you can see that your metabolism can quickly become dysfunctional if you develop increased levels of insulin resistance. The body tries to correct this problem by secreting higher and higher amounts of insulin, so instead of simply speaking, insulin is now shouting at the target cell to do something. This leads to constantly elevated levels of insulin in the blood (i.e., hyperinsulinemia) and in the presence of excess dietary omega-6 fatty acids resulting in an even further increase in AA production.

If insulin levels rise in the blood due to insulin resistance, then more of the dietary fat you consume will be driven into storage in your adipose tissue. At the same time, elevated insulin in the blood prevents the release of stored body fat for energy production in your muscle cells. That's why the first sign of insulin resistance is often increased weight gain as well as physical fatigue.

In addition, insulin resistance increases the levels of glucose in the blood so that it is more likely to cross-link with circulating proteins. These glycosylated proteins (Advanced Glycosylated End products or AGE) can bind to the receptors (known as Receptor for AGE or RAGE) on the surface of every cell that activate the master genetic switch (NF-κB) for inflammation that further increases cellular inflammation. Increased glucose levels in the blood also inhibits the activation of AMP kinase which is the final step of the Resolution Response necessary for healing to take place. This is why there is a strong association of insulin resistance with virtually every chronic condition ranging from obesity, to metabolic syndrome (pre-diabetes) and diabetes, hypertension, heart disease, cancer, and even Alzheimer's.

HOW DO YOU KNOW IF YOU HAVE INSULIN RESISTANCE?

At the clinical level, the severity of insulin resistance requires a specialized blood test (i.e., a hyperinsulinemic-euglycemic clamp) that is only performed under research conditions. However, if your fasting blood glucose level on your annual physical is greater than 100 mg/dL, you probably have the beginnings of insulin resistance. As I will discuss in the next chapter, your TG/HDL ratio from your annual physical provides even an even better clinical marker of your level of insulin resistance. If you have diabetes or pre-diabetes (i.e., metabolic syndrome), then you are certain to have severe insulin resistance. The American Diabetes Association estimates that approximately 30 million Americans have type 1 and type 2 diabetes and 86 million Americans have prediabetes, so among these two populations there are more than 110 million Americans with severe insulin resistance. If you are obese, then you are likely to have severe insulin resistance. In studies using the highly sophisticated hyperinsulinemia euglycemic clamp testing, it has been shown that even 16 percent of normal weight Americans have severe insulin resistance.

DIETARY CHANGES THAT ARE DECREASING RESOLUTION AND REPAIR

If the growing intensity of diet-induced inflammation caused by changes in our diet (the increased consumption of both omega-6 fatty acids and refined carbohydrates) as well as removing fermentable fiber wasn't bad enough, we have also simultaneously been reducing the intake of two other essential dietary ingredients critical for the optimization of the Resolution Response. These missing nutrients are omega-3 fatty acids and polyphenols.

Omega-3 fatty acids are also essential fatty acids, but the hormones (resolvins) generated from these fatty acids are critical for resolving cellular inflammation and will be discussed in greater detail in Chapter 10. While the levels of omega-6 fatty acids have dramatically increased in the last fifty years, the levels of omega-3 fatty acids have decreased even more so. This has greatly inhibited the Resolution Response by reducing the potential generation of resolvins thus explaining why unresolved cellular inflammation is increasing so rapidly.

Another food group in significant decline are polyphenols. These are complex phytochemicals found in fruits and vegetables, and to a lesser extent, whole grains. Polyphenols are now known to be activators of certain gene transcription factors that activate AMP kinase, but only if consumed in adequate amounts. Once AMP kinase is activated, among the wide variety of other genes it controls include those responsible for generating anti-oxidative enzymes that reduce excessive levels of free radicals. This is critical because free radicals are known activators of NF-κB, so as dietary polyphenols decrease, free radicals remain elevated and unresolved cellular inflammation increases. Activating AMP kinase, the master gene transcription factor that controls your metabolism is the critical final step to complete the Resolution Response and for that you need adequate levels of dietary polyphenols.

SUMMARY ▶

Diet-induced inflammation is having a negative impact on worldwide health. The growth of industrialized food has been like opening Pandora's box and unleashing a tsunami of cellular inflammation by inhibiting the body's internal Resolution Response. The result is increasingly higher levels of unresolved cellular inflammation that is definitively driving up health care costs globally as well as decreasing the healthspan of Americans. But once you know the causes of chronic unresolved cellular inflammation, you can begin to put together a cogent dietary plan to reverse it. That plan is the Zone Pro-Resolution Nutrition system.

7

Markers of the Zone

YOU CAN'T CONTROL what you can't measure. The Resolution Response is controlled by hormonal and genetic factors that are exceptionally difficult to measure because they either don't circulate in the blood (like NF-κB or AMP kinase) or because of an extremely short lifetime at vanishingly low levels (such as eicosanoids and resolvins). However, there are blood markers that are easily measured in the blood that indicate whether or not your Resolution Response is optimized. These blood markers define the Zone.

Being in the Zone indicates that you have done your best to optimize your Resolution Response. Since the markers of the Zone can be easily measured in the blood, this enables you to optimize your Resolution Response using the Zone Pro-Resolution Nutrition system with great precision.

Coming from a pharmacological and academic background, I know it is essential to have clinical markers to support your statements no matter how effectively any potential drug or dietary intervention may be working. Otherwise, you are simply fooling yourself.

My basic contention is that virtually all chronic diseases are the consequence of increased levels of chronic unresolved cellular inflammation leading to loss of function. The extent of that unresolved inflammation can be easily determined by the clinical markers that also define the Zone. Thus, your ability to maintain a robust Resolution Response to reduce unresolved cellular inflammation can also be used to define your current state of wellness and ultimately increasing your healthspan. This is why the markers of the Zone are also ultimately markers of your true extent of wellness.

RULES FOR USEFUL CLINICAL MARKERS

For a clinical marker to be useful, it must be validated. That means it must be reproducible from lab to lab. The more complex the marker (and that usually means the more expensive the equipment used to measure it), the less likely the probability it can be validated from one lab to another. In other words, any clinical result is relatively useless unless it can be replicated by someone else. This doesn't mean someone is lying to you, but the complexity of the sample preparation and the sophistication of instrumentation often makes the interpretation of the results non-reproducible in the hands of someone else who is equally qualified to do the test.

Furthermore, any clinical test used to define the Zone should come from the blood. The blood doesn't lie. In addition, the meaning of the test must be easily understood by yourself without a lot of hand waving by someone else. Finally, the results of the blood test should give you a clear direction of what dietary steps you have to undertake to optimize your Resolution Response.

MARKERS OF THE ZONE

Over the years, I have developed three blood markers for the Zone that meet all of the above criteria. Each one looks at each of the different components (reduction, resolution, and repair) that constitute the Resolution Response. Furthermore, all three markers must be within their appropriate ranges needed to keep you in the Zone. Each marker measures a different aspect of the Resolution Response. If all three tests are not in their optimal ranges, then you are simply not in the Zone and can't optimally heal the damage created by an injury. Finally, if you are not in the Zone, then you can't be considered well. If you are not in the Zone, this means that unresolved cellular inflammation is building up in your body that will continue to block your Resolution

Response. So, let's look at each of the markers of the Zone in greater detail.

TG/HDL ratio: Measuring your ability to reduce diet-induced inflammation

How well you reduce diet-induced inflammation is best measured by the TG/HDL ratio. This marker is a surrogate marker of insulin resistance, primarily in the liver but also in other insulin-sensitive organs (muscles, adipose tissue, and the brain).

The liver is the body's central assembly plant where dietary fatty acids are transported from the gut and then metabolized into lipoproteins which are then sent back out into the blood to transport the fatty acids to the other organs. Insulin is the hormone that controls much of the metabolism that takes place in liver. One of the first consequences of diet-induced inflammation in the liver is the development of insulin resistance in that organ. This results in a dysfunctional processing of lipoproteins resulting in triglycerides (TG) levels rising and HDL cholesterol levels falling.

The TG/HDL ratio is easily calculated from results you get in most standard annual physicals, although you may have to do a little simple math to determine the TG/HDL ratio.

The following table shows the ranges of TG/HDL ratios and how they correspond to the level of diet-induced inflammation in the liver, and probably every other insulin-sensitive organ in the body.

TG/HDL ratio	Degree of insulin resistance
Greater than 3	High
2-3	Moderate
1-2	Low
Less than 1	Ideal

You want your TG/HDL ratio to be less than one. The optimal dietary intervention to lower your TG/HDL ratio is to follow the Zone Diet. The Zone Diet will lower your TG/HDL ratio significantly within 30 days due to the rapid reduction of insulin resistance.

AA/EPA ratio: Measuring your ability to resolve cellular inflammation

The best indication of your ability to resolve residual cellular inflammation is the AA/EPA ratio. The AA/EPA ratio also correlates very well with the levels of various cytokines (inflammatory proteins produced by activation of NF-κB) in the blood. As you lower the AA/EPA ratio, the levels of the inflammatory cytokines are also lowered. Remember cytokines are the pro-inflammatory proteins released from your cells if unresolved cellular inflammation remains elevated.

Arachidonic acid (AA) is the molecular building block for eicosanoids and eicosapentaenoic acid (EPA) is the molecular building block for resolvins. The better their balance in your blood, the greater your ability to resolve residual cellular inflammation.

The first use of the AA/EPA ratio to demonstrate its correlation with the reduction of inflammatory cytokines appeared in the *New England Journal of Medicine* in 1989. Its use in clinical research has been extremely robust over the years demonstrating that as you lower the AA/EPA ratio, there is a significant clinical improvement of various chronic disease conditions including cardiovascular, autoimmune diseases, and neurological diseases. Most importantly, recently published research demonstrates that the lower your AA/EPA ratio, the longer you live.

The following table indicates the AA/EPA ratio ranges you want to achieve to maintain your wellness.

AA/EPA ratio	Risk of developing a future chronic disease
Greater than 15	High
10-15	Concern
6-10	Moderate
3-6	Good
1.5-3	Ideal
Less than 1	Moderate

The higher the AA/EPA ratio, the lower your potential to resolve any existing residual cellular inflammation in your body. The ideal ratio is similar to that found in the Japanese population who have the greatest longevity, greatest healthspan (i.e., longevity minus years of disability), lowest rates of heart disease as well as the lowest rates of depression in the industrialized world. Can your AA/EPA ratio be too low? Possibly because you might increase the risk of bleeding or not be able to initiate an adequate inflammatory response once the AA/EPA ratio drops below 1.

So how do various populations rank in their AA/EPA ratios? The Japanese are usually between 1.5 and 3. Italians are between 10-15, and Americans are 20 or greater. This marker indicates that Americans are one of the most inflamed populations in the world and goes a long way toward explaining the rapidly growing cost of health care in America.

The best way to reduce the AA/EPA ratio is to supplement your diet with increased levels of omega-3 fatty acids while simultaneously reducing your intake of omega-6 fatty acids.

HbA_{1c}: Measuring your ability to repair damaged tissue caused by unresolved cellular inflammation

A very good clinical marker that defines your ability to repair the tissue damaged by cellular inflammation is the level of glycosylated hemoglobin also known as HbA_{1c}. Although this blood marker is usually used to confirm the presence of diabetes, it is also a good marker of oxidative stress. Oxidative stress is usually a consequence of the overproduction of free radicals indicating that less energy is being produced by your cells to repair tissue damage. Also, the higher the HbA_{1c}, the more you inhibit the activity of AMP kinase. This is why diabetics have lower AMP kinase activity than non-diabetics. AMP kinase must be operating at peak efficiency to complete the last critical step necessary to optimize the Resolution Response.

The following table of HbA_{1c} levels estimates the levels of oxidative stress in your body.

HbA_{1c}	Degree of Oxidative Stress
Greater than 6.5%	Very High
5.7 to 6.4%	High
5.2 to 5.6%	Moderate
4.9-5.1%	Ideal
Less than 4.9%	Moderate

The reason that having a HbA$_{1c}$ level of less than 4.9% is less than ideal is because this may indicate the body is increasing cortisol secretion to maintain blood glucose levels by a process known as neo-glucogenesis. This often happens when following ketogenic diets as discussed later in this book. It should be noted that increased cortisol generates insulin resistance (this makes you fat) as well as lowering your immune response (this makes you sick).

The best way to decrease oxidative stress is supplementation with high-dose polyphenol extracts. They not only activate genes that reduce oxidative stress, but also increase the efficiency of energy production needed to repair damaged tissue by their activation of AMP kinase. If your level of HbA$_{1c}$ is higher than the ideal range, then the fastest way to increase your ability to repair tissue damaged by cellular inflammation is to increase your intake of polyphenols.

Each of these three markers needs to be in their ideal range for you to be considered well because only then will your Resolution Response be optimized. In other words, you want to be in the Zone. If any of the three markers is outside their ideal range, you have the appropriate dietary intervention to bring each of these markers back into their appropriate target ranges. Consider these markers of the Zone as your navigational buoys of wellness.

Subjective markers of the Zone

People still hate to give blood, let alone pay for a blood test. Are there any subjective markers that might indicate you are moving toward the Zone? Actually, there are several.

The first is the lack of hunger or fatigue for four to five hours after a meal. This indicates you are controlling the hormones in the blood and the gut that generate satiety signals to the brain. As demonstrated by Harvard researchers in 1999, the hormonal changes induced by any meal are rapid, but will usually last no more than five hours. The goal of the Zone Diet is the generation of the appropriate hormonal changes to prevent hunger and mental fatigue for the next four to five hours. Think of how many meals you typically consume that provide that level of satiety? The lower that number, the more you should consider following the Zone Diet.

Another marker that you can do on your own is determining your body fat percentage. The accumulation of excess body fat is a potential reservoir for unresolved cellular inflammation to spread to other organs as I explained in my book, *Toxic Fat*. Subjectively, you can determine if you have excess body fat by simply standing stark naked and look at yourself in the mirror. You can be even more precise by measuring your level of body fat using some simple measurements requiring only a tape measure. At www.zonediet.com/resources/body-fat-calculator you can find such a free body fat calculator to determine your levels of body fat.

Whatever method you use, the more excess body fat you have, the more likely you are generating more unresolved cellular inflammation. Ideally, your percent body fat should be no greater than 15 percent (for males) or 25 percent (for females) according to the American Council of Exercise. If your percent body fat is greater than 25 percent for males or 32 percent for females, then you are considered obese. Population studies conducted from 1999 to 2003 suggested that 70 percent of Americans would be considered obese based on their percentage of body fat whereas only 31 percent would be considered obese using the standard measurement of BMI. As I will discuss later, losing excess body fat is difficult, but any reduction of excess body fat indicates you are moving closer to the Zone.

Measuring appetite suppression with a watch or determining your percent body fat may sound a little simplistic. However, there are more precise subjective markers to indicate your progress toward reaching the Zone thus optimizing your Resolution Response.

Metabolic changes

Daily performance: Increase in daily physical performance (especially increased energy) is indicative that you are producing more energy (in the form of ATP) with fewer calories. This will be reflected in both physical and mental performance as you stabilize blood sugar levels and reduce cellular inflammation in your fat cells, making it easier to release stored body fat for energy production. This is also an indication that AMP kinase activity is increasing.

Reduction in desire for carbohydrates: Your craving for carbohydrates will significantly decrease, if not be eliminated, as you stabilize blood sugar levels. If blood sugar levels are stable, then the brain has adequate levels of its optimal fuel to maintain peak energy production and thus maintain mental acuity. If blood sugar levels are too low (i.e., hypoglycemia), then you will have a constant desire for more dietary carbohydrates to help raise blood sugar levels for the brain's energy needs.

Neurological changes

Sleep: The need for sleep is determined by the amount of time required to re-establish neurotransmitter equilibrium. This process speeds up as you reduce inflammation in the brain.

Less grogginess upon waking: Grogginess upon waking is indicative of disturbances in your circadian rhythms that start the release of hormones to bring you out of deep sleep early in the morning. In other words, you won't need that cup of caffeinated coffee in the morning to get you out of your morning stupor.

Sense of well-being: Another consequence of reducing neuro-inflammation is an improved state of constant well-being as opposed to being depressed, anxious, or constantly irritable.

Mental concentration: This is controlled by stabilizing blood sugar levels. One of the first signs of reduced insulin resistance is increased mental concentration with greater focus.

Reduction of headaches: Improving blood flow will reduce vasoconstriction, which is the underlying cause of most headaches. With adequate oxygen transfer to the brain, headache pain is reduced. An added benefit of getting more oxygen to the brain is to enhance your ability to think more clearly since you are producing higher levels of ATP.

Skin condition

Fingernail strength: The structural protein keratin is under strong dietary control. The Zone Pro-Resolution Nutrition system leads to rapid fingernail growth with improved strength.

Hair strength: Keratin is also the principal structural component of the hair. Hair texture and thickness of the hair fiber itself can be used as an indicator similar to fingernail strength.

Wrinkles and skin color: Reduction of cellular inflammation in the skin will also reduce degradation of collagen and elastin that causes the skin to form wrinkles. In addition, you will see better blood flow in the skin caused by the increased vasodilation of blood vessels located in the dermis thus improving facial color in the skin. As you move closer to the Zone, you will notice that wrinkles are decreasing in magnitude due to the accelerated rebuilding of collagen and elastin structure in the skin that comes with an improved Resolution Response.

Gut health

Stool quality: The Zone Pro-Resolution Nutrition system will also improve gut nutrition with a corresponding increase in mucus production improving the speed at which food moves through your gut. The result is better stool quality and greater ease of exit from the colon.

Flatulence: Flatulence or gas is caused by the metabolism of anaerobic bacteria in the lower part of the intestine. This is your indication that adequate levels of fermentable fiber are reaching the bacteria in the colon. Better stool quality and increased movement of the stool through the colon, will significantly reduce bloating which is usually caused by a build-up of fermentation gases that can't easily escape because of poor stool quality.

SUMMARY ▶

The physiological changes generated as you get closer to the Zone by using the Zone Pro-Resolution Nutrition system can be rapid. Some of these changes occur within hours, others within days, and most within a month. These benefits can easily be quantified in the blood and confirmed by a wide variety of subjective markers. However, as quickly as positive changes can be observed or measured, those same benefits can rapidly disappear because the hormonal and genetic changes induced by the Zone Pro-Resolution Nutrition system are short term. That's why following the Zone Pro-Resolution Nutrition system is a lifetime dietary program designed to keep your Resolution Response working at optimal efficiency.

8

Zone Diet

REDUCING DIET-INDUCED INFLAMMATION

WHEN PEOPLE HEAR the word diet, the first thought that springs into mind is a short period of time filled with hunger and deprivation so they can fit into a swimsuit and then go back to their old eating habits.

Actually, the word diet comes from the ancient Greek root that means "way of life." Diet is a lifelong dietary pattern for some hopefully noble purpose like enjoying a longer healthspan. Diet also generally means discipline, but only if the longer-term purpose is worth it. The goal of the Zone Diet is to reduce the intensity of diet-induced inflammation by attenuating the hormonal factors that increase the intensity of the inflammatory response. That results in a longer healthspan.

Controlling diet-induced inflammation significantly reduces the amplification of existing unresolved cellular inflammation, thus reducing the likelihood of the development of chronic disease. This is why the Zone Diet is the necessary first step of optimizing your Resolution Response. Without a consistent dietary strategy to reduce diet-induced inflammation, you are entrusting your future to genetic good luck (it sometimes happens) or abdicating your future to the drug companies to manage symptoms of some future chronic disease. Unfortunately, drugs will become increasingly more expensive (even those that are generic) as well as making it more likely that you will become a walking polypharmacy taking even more drugs to counteract the side effects of the original drugs.

MOLECULAR BASIS OF THE ZONE DIET

The Zone Diet is primarily based on hormonal control theory. The body works best on the concept of homeostasis. Think of this concept as a biological thermostat keeping the levels of hormones in the blood within certain operating limits (i.e., a zone). The Zone Diet was developed to keep these hormones in such a zone if you are willing to treat your diet *as if* it were a drug taken at the right dose and at the right time.

In the 1990s the diet debate centered on eliminating so-called "evil" foods. For some like Dean Ornish, it was fat. For others, like Robert Atkins, it was carbs. Neither one understood the impact of the diet on the hormonal balance that affected the generation of pro-inflammatory eicosanoids that caused inflammation, which in turn results in insulin resistance.

In reality, both were partially right and partially wrong. Ornish was partially correct that the wrong types of fat (omega-6 fats and palmitic acid) were very pro-inflammatory. But that was no excuse to throw the baby out with the bathwater by eliminating almost all fat and all animal protein because it also contained fat.

Likewise, Atkins was partially correct that consuming too many carbohydrates (especially high glycemic ones like grains and starches) relative to protein would disturb the protein-to-carbohydrate ratio necessary to stabilize blood glucose levels. But by removing most of the dietary carbohydrates, Atkins had also removed the fermentable fiber and polyphenols needed for gut health thereby increasing the likelihood of gut-derived inflammation caused by a leaky gut. At the same time, he was advocating all the benefits of ketosis by eating more fat (especially butter) unaware of the pro-inflammatory properties of saturated fatty acids such as palmitic acid, which is the primary saturated fatty acid in butter. The Atkins diet also perturbs the protein-to-carbohydrate ratio to induce ketosis. One hormonal consequence of ketosis is to induce the production of excess cortisol that would break down muscle to convert it into glucose for maintaining brain function. The increase in cortisol not only increases insulin resistance but also depresses the immune system.

The Zone Diet was ideally suited to moderate the hormonal extremes advocated by either Ornish or Atkins as shown below.

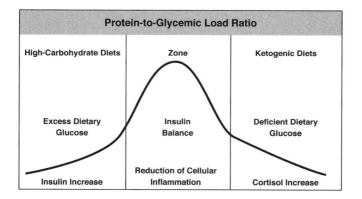

You need some carbohydrates, but not too much to maintain a balance of insulin. You also need some protein at every meal, but not too much to maintain glucagon levels that help maintain blood glucose levels. Finally, you also need some non-inflammatory fat at each meal, but not too much, to help release one of the satiety hormones (CKK) from the gut to help maintain satiety as well as provide taste.

However, the ultimate controlling factor for insulin levels in the blood is not the levels of carbohydrates in an individual meal, but the degree of insulin resistance a person currently has. That is determined by their levels of cellular inflammation in insulin-sensitive tissues like the muscle, liver, fat cells, and hypothalamus in the brain. It is insulin resistance that keeps blood insulin levels constantly elevated. This is known as hyperinsulinemia. This same insulin resistance also makes it difficult for the hypothalamus in the brain to correctly receive satiety signals that tell you to stop eating. It is not insulin per se that makes you fat and keeps you fat, but *insulin resistance* that makes you fat and keeps you fat. Thus, the primary goal of the Zone Diet is to first reduce insulin resistance, and then prevent it from returning. To accomplish both goals you have to maintain a relatively constant protein-to-glycemic load ratio at each meal while restricting calories without hunger or fatigue.

Notice from the diagram that describes the Zone Diet that the shape of the protein-to-glycemic load ratio is a bell-shaped curve simply because not everyone is genetically the same. But on the other hand, they aren't that genetically different either.

PROBLEMS WITH DIET STUDIES

One of the reasons there is so much confusion with diet studies is they are often poorly controlled. Well-controlled diet studies require that you provide all the food to the subjects so that they don't have to think. Such studies are difficult to do as well as being very costly. As a result, very few are ever done. Most diet studies just give their subjects some simple written instructions with limited education and hope that they will follow them. Such an approach rarely works for any long-term studies because people tend to revert to their old dietary habits, such as, trying to follow four different diets over a two-year period as shown by Harvard in 2009.

Even more confusing results come from epidemiological studies of populations that make dietary assumptions that best fit the gathered data. In reality, epidemiological studies are only useful in generating a hypothesis to be clinically tested. It's much easier to take the mass of data from epidemiological studies and put it into the computer and see what comes out. Consider this to be the "wisdom of the crowd." As an example, epidemiological studies were done at Harvard that indicated women who took birth control pills appeared to live longer. On the basis of those studies, over $260 million was spent on a 10-year study to confirm their hypothesis. Unfortunately, the clinical trial based on their positive epidemiological studies found that those who were using birth control pills had higher levels of cancer.

However, the worse trials may be meta-analysis diet studies that take a lot of different studies with different protocols and try to analyze the resulting mix. It's like making scientific sausage.

Even well-controlled diet studies are far more complex than drug studies as you have four variables to control: protein, carbohydrate, fat, and calories. At least two of these diet variables must be held constant to compare the impact of the other two dietary variables. As an example, you can keep the total calories and protein intake constant, and then compare the effects of varying the fat and carbohydrate intakes. And then you need to do it again for the next two variables, and again and again, until you have conducted eight separate long-term studies. Furthermore, you have to supply much, if not all the food, to ensure compliance.

My first book, *The Zone*, put many nutritional academics' elegant epidemiological constructs in doubt, and thus created a firestorm within the scientific community. But unlike most popular book authors who haven't done any academic research, I had a solid publication record and strong patent portfolio. In other words, I knew a thing or two about research.

Soon after *The Zone* was published, David Ludwig at Harvard Medical School asked me to give a talk at the department of pediatric endocrinology because he had read the book and found the scientific concepts behind the Zone interesting, although highly controversial.

After my lecture they were intrigued, because if I was right, then everyone else in nutrition might be wrong. So, David and a group of those Harvard researchers wrote a government grant to do a study to determine if my predictions of the effect of the Zone Diet on hormone responses might be correct. The proposed grant to the government was promptly turned down because the concept was considered too outlandish by the reviewers. Undaunted, they reached into their internal slush funds and did the study themselves. It was a well-crafted and very clever study. Their subjects were obese adolescents brought to Harvard on three separate occasions over a two-month period to test the effect of three different meal combinations on their hormonal responses. On each visit, the child was provided a Zone meal for dinner and stayed overnight in the metabolic ward. They were awakened at 6 a.m. the next day and had catheters put into their arms to monitor their blood levels to determine how each meal affected their hormones. Then they received one of three different meals on each visit for breakfast. All of the meals contained the same number of calories (about 400), but had different ratios of protein-to-carbohydrate. One of them was a Zone meal consisting of an egg white omelet with some low-fat cheese and a bowl of slow-cooked oatmeal. On the other two other visits, they were given meals that were higher in carbohydrates and lower in protein than the Zone meal, but with different glycemic loads. Then they measured the hormone levels in the blood of each child for the next five hours. The results confirmed the predictions I had made earlier at my seminar about the hormonal effects of the protein-to-the glycemic load ratio of the meal. Five hours after eating each test breakfast meal, the catheters were removed from their arms and then the children were given the same meal for lunch that they had for breakfast on that particular visit. Then they brought the children into a conference room with TVs and comic books where they sat for the next five hours. The room's conference table was covered with foods like sandwiches, doughnuts, and chips, and the children were told they could help themselves to any of these food items if they got hungry. When the Harvard researchers tallied up the resulting food intake, they found those who had consumed two Zone meals back-to-back consumed 46 percent fewer calories compared to when they had eaten the two high-glycemic-load meals with less protein but the same number of calories. The children simply were not hungry after eating the two consecutive Zone meals. After that study, the glycemic load became a hot topic at Harvard. Later they performed a similar study with obese adults and found that the Zone Diet reduced inflammation nine times more effectively than the then-standard diet currently being recommended by the USDA.

There have been more than thirty published studies on the Zone Diet where it has been compared to either high-carbohydrate diets or ketogenic diets. Each study came to the same conclusion that the Zone Diet is superior in hormonal control, blood sugar control, blood lipid control, appetite control, fat loss, and most importantly, the reduction of cellular inflammation.

ZONE DIET: CALORIE RESTRICTION WITHOUT HUNGER OR FATIGUE

One of the problems the nutritional community had with the concept of the Zone Diet is they apparently never completely read any of my books. When they saw my recommendation that 30 percent of the calories on the Zone Diet should come from low-fat protein, their immediate response was that the Zone Diet was a high-protein, ketogenic diet that would damage the kidneys and immediately stopped reading the book. If they continued reading just a little further, they would have seen that on the Zone Diet you were actually consuming more carbohydrates than protein, so it couldn't be considered a high-protein diet nor could it generate ketosis. Furthermore, they didn't realize that the Zone Diet was also a calorie-restricted diet so that the absolute amount of protein was no more than what Americans were currently eating but spread out more evenly through the day like the intravenous delivery of a cancer drug.

Calorie restriction is not a new concept, but it usually entails constant hunger and fatigue. What was unique about the Zone Diet was the potential that calorie restriction could be practiced for a lifetime without hunger or mental fatigue because the hormonal effects generated by the balance of the protein-to-the glycemic load would stabilize blood sugar levels between meals.

HISTORY OF CALORIE RESTRICTION

The oldest form of calorie restriction is fasting. It was mentioned by Hippocrates and practiced by many religious sects. Fasting is the most extreme version of calorie restriction because it forces the body to cannibalize itself. Initially fasting has some beneficial actions such as activating the gene transcription factor, AMP kinase, that controls our metabolism to provide the energy needed for the repair of damaged tissue. One of the first consequences of initial fasting is that the activation of AMP kinase accelerates a process called autophagy in which your cell's damaged molecules are recycled into new materials required for cellular repair. It's like taking out the garbage. But after all the garbage is cleaned up, if you continue fasting, your body starts digesting protein from healthy tissue to supply glucose for the brain. This happens through a process known as neo-glucogenesis mediated by increasing the levels of the hormone cortisol. Initially during neo-glucogenesis, you lose non-essential protein such as hair and facial muscle. Eventually, the process extends to digesting essential muscle tissue like the heart. (This is why you can't fast for more than 50 days—eventually you will die of heart failure.)

Dying due to complete fasting is not a desired outcome for achieving optimal health. Perhaps a less severe method of calorie reduction other than fasting might work. The goal of calorie restriction is to consume the least number of calories while supplying the adequate essential nutrients we need to survive including protein, essential fats, as well as vitamins and minerals.

The first recorded evidence of the long-term benefits of a calorie-restricted diet came from Luigi Cornaro, a 15th-century Venetian nobleman. By his late 30s Luigi Cornaro was near death due to his lavish lifestyle of excess food, drink, and the good life. He started a rigorous calorie-restriction program consuming only about twelve ounces of food per day consisting of coarse grain bread, meat broth with a little protein and an egg yolk, vegetable soups, and about three glasses of unaged (new) wine. It worked. He wrote his first diet book (*Discourses on the Temperate Life*) at age 83 and managed to write two more books on calorie restriction and longevity before dying at 102.

Now we can fast forward to 1935 when Clive McCay demonstrated that restricting calories (but not nutrition) in rats resulted in a significant increase in their lifespans. His experiments have been repeated in a large number of species, including monkeys that are the most genetically similar to humans. Although the increase in lifespan is not as great as with less evolved organisms, the increase in healthspan is significant because of the delay in the development of a wide variety of chronic diseases.

What about humans? Here the clinical data is much more limited. Much of it comes from the CALERIE (Comprehensive Assessment of Long-Term Effects of Reducing Intake of Energy) trials in which either overweight or normal-weight individuals were asked to reduce their calorie intake by 25 percent over a two-year period. By the end of two years, only about half that calorie restriction goal (about a 12 percent reduction in calories) was actually reached. While they lost body fat (as well as muscle mass), interestingly their levels of insulin-like growth factor (IGF-1) did not decrease. This is the opposite effect found in all the animal experiments suggesting that humans are probably metabolically different than rats.

One likely reason the subjects couldn't achieve the projected level of calorie restriction was they were probably always hungry because of an unbalanced ratio of the protein-to-glycemic load used in those studies. Frankly, who wants to be hungry for two years, let alone the rest of their life? The Zone Diet solves that problem because as I will show you shortly, it is actually difficult to eat all the food on the Zone Diet even when restricting calories. I call it the Zone Paradox.

THE ZONE PARADOX

One of the reasons the nutritional community has such a hard time in understanding the Zone Diet is because its starting point is not the number of calories you need, but the amount of protein required to maintain your muscle mass. You have plenty of calories already stored as excess body fat that can be released for your energy needs, but only if you can reduce the insulin resistance that keeps those fatty acids trapped in your fat cells.

When you lose muscle, you not only lose strength, but you also lose the primary depot in the body to dispose of excess glucose in the blood. The amount of protein you need on a daily basis to maintain your current muscle mass depends on two factors: (1) the amount of muscle mass you have, and (2) how physically active you are. Neither of these factors come from a bathroom scale, but you can easily calculate them using tables I have published in my earlier books or using a simple calculator found at www.zonediet.com/resources/body-fat-calculator.

Not surprisingly males need more protein than females to maintain their higher levels of muscle mass. Also, as you might expect, athletes have more muscle mass than their sedentary peers and require more dietary protein to maintain their higher level of existing muscle mass. Furthermore, they require additional dietary protein to replace the muscle protein damaged during intense exercise. In other words, the amount of protein you need on a daily basis to maintain your muscle mass is unique to you.

Once you determine the amount of protein you need on a daily basis to maintain your existing muscle mass, then you simply divide that amount of protein evenly at every meal like you would when taking a drug. For most females that will be about 3 ounces of low-fat protein at a meal and for most males that will be about 4 ounces of low-fat protein at each meal (this is essentially the size and thickness of the palm of your hand). In either case, these are not excessive amounts of protein. In fact, this is exactly the same recommendation of every dietician in the world who states that you should never consume more low-fat protein at any meal than you can fit on the palm of your hand. I totally agree. I only add that you should never consume any less low-fat protein than that at any meal otherwise you will not consume enough protein to induce satiety for the next five hours. It should be noted that male or female athletes will need slightly more protein than the average person, but not that much as I will discuss in Chapter 17.

Frankly, I don't care where the protein comes from as long as it is low-fat protein because your goal is to set the hormonal balance to increase the release of excess stored body fat to be used for energy. This also ensures you are consuming protein that is low in saturated fat, especially palmitic acid that is the most pro-inflammatory of the saturated fats. That low-fat protein could be chicken, fish, very lean red meat, egg whites, dairy, tofu, or plant-based meat substitutes.

Thus, the first step of constructing a Zone meal is based on the amount of protein you need. The next step for making a Zone meal is you have to balance the protein at each meal with the right amount of carbohydrates. That's about a third more carbohydrates than protein in terms of grams. The types of carbohydrates for the best hormonal response is determined by your current level of insulin resistance. For most individuals that will be about three to four servings of non-starchy vegetables at each meal and adding a little fruit like a half-cup of berries or a very small piece of fruit, such as half a small apple. Both types of carbohydrates are known as low-glycemic carbohydrates because the glucose in them doesn't enter the blood at a rapid rate. Such a meal will automatically be rich in fermentable fiber and polyphenols that are essential for gut health as explained in the next chapter.

Finally, to complete your Zone meal, you add a dash (that's a small amount) of monounsaturated fat like olive oil, guacamole, or slivered nuts. A dash can be considered a teaspoon of olive oil, a tablespoon of guacamole, or 1/3 ounce of nuts. That's it for a Zone meal. Now just repeat the same template meal after meal and you are following the Zone Diet.

The Zone Diet is a calorie-restricted diet that is protein-adequate, carbohydrate-moderate (but rich in fermentable fiber and polyphenols), and low in fat, It is also very difficult to eat all the food because you would be eating ten servings of vegetables and fruits per day. At the same time, you are stabilizing blood glucose levels for the brain as well as sending satiety signals (by consuming adequate protein at each meal) from the gut to the brain directly via the vagus nerve that tells you to stop eating. Who could argue with that? Apparently every "expert" in nutrition.

DOING THE MATH

I have come to conclude that one of the reasons nutritional science is in such a morass is that no one ever does the simple math for different diets. First, the only way you are going to lose excess body fat is to restrict calories. That can only be achieved if you stabilize blood glucose levels, send the correct satiety signals from the gut to the brain to stop eating, and reduce insulin resistance so that stored fat can easily be released between meals to provide high-octane fuel for your body.

I have already stated that the appropriate protein-to-glycemic load balance for the Zone Diet is about 1/3 more low-glycemic load carbs than low-fat protein at each meal. And if you want about 30 percent of calories as fat in that meal, then the number of calories coming from protein and carbohydrate in a meal would be 70 percent of the rest of the calories (all three macronutrients must equal 100 percent). So, if you want about 1/3 more calories as low-glycemic carbohydrates relative to protein at the meal, then the total carbohydrate-protein-fat composition of a Zone meal is about 40 percent low-glycemic load carbohydrates, 30 percent low-fat protein, and 30 percent fat, but primarily as monounsaturated fat. But caloric percentages are meaningless unless you look at the absolute level of each macronutrient because it is the balance of protein and carbohydrates in grams at each meal that determines the appropriate hormonal responses for the next five hours.

Let's see what the Zone Diet looks like on a daily basis, remembering that protein and carbohydrates contain four calories per gram and fat contains nine calories per gram.

	Typical Female	Typical Male
Carbohydrates per day	120 grams	150 grams
Protein per day	90 grams	112 grams
Fat per day	40 grams	50 grams

Let's look at calories per day. If you are consuming 1,200 calories per day (typical for the average female) that would be three meals each consisting of a little less than 400 calories per meal and one Zone snack. At 1,500 calories per day (typical for the average male), that would be three meals consisting of 400 calories per meal plus one or two Zone snacks.

Your brain needs about 130 grams of glucose per day, meaning your carbohydrate intake should be an adequate amount to keep the brain happy with its optimal fuel (which is glucose, not ketones) throughout the day. On the other hand, consuming too much carbohydrate at any meal will cause an over-secretion of insulin leading to a reduction in blood glucose levels within a few hours leading to hypoglycemia causing increased hunger and mental fatigue.

The amounts of protein consumed on the Zone Diet are pretty close to what the average American (female or male) is already eating, but now evenly split throughout the day. Finally, the Zone Diet would qualify as a low-fat diet by any standard.

You'd think you would starve on 1,200 calories per day. But let me show you how much food would be required to achieve that calorie level:

CARBOHYDRATES (120 GRAMS) PER DAY

8 servings (4 cups) of cooked non-starchy vegetables requires
  about two pounds of raw vegetables
2 servings (1 cup) of fresh fruit
1 serving of either legumes (3 oz.) or slow-cooked oatmeal (3 oz.)
This amount of carbohydrates would also provide more than 40
  grams of total fiber and lot of polyphenols

PROTEIN (90 GRAMS)

3 servings of 3 oz. of low-fat protein at each meal

FAT (40 GRAMS)

2 tablespoons of extra virgin olive oil per day that translates into
  2 teaspoons per meal

Most women would have a hard time consuming that amount of food even when consumed evenly throughout the day. At 1,500 calories per day for the average male, the amounts of food to be consumed are correspondingly greater. You can find hundreds of Zone meals as well as a protein calculator to determine your own unique protein requirements at www.zoneliving.com.

Besides never being hungry or mentally fatigued following the Zone Diet, a recent study published in 2017 indicated there are some significant health benefits from eating ten servings of vegetables and fruits per day like a 33 percent reduction in stroke, a 24 percent reduction in heart disease, a 13 percent reduction in cancer, and finally a 31 percent reduction in all-cause mortality. I am eagerly waiting for any drug to deliver similar performance results.

SUMMARY ▷

The Zone Diet is an anti-inflammatory diet because it reduces the intensity of diet-induced inflammation. This is accomplished by reducing the intake of omega-6 and saturated fatty acids that are pro-inflammatory. It also reduces the activation of the gene transcription factor, NF-κB, which is the genetic master switch that turns on the inflammatory response as well as improving gut health to reduce the entry of bacterial fragments into the blood (explained in the next chapter) and reducing the formation of glycosylated proteins, both of which can activate NF-κB. This is why following the Zone Diet is the obligatory first stage for optimizing your Resolution Response because it is your best dietary tool to reduce the overall intensity of diet-induced inflammation. Mastering this stage of the Zone Pro-Resolution Nutrition system makes it much easier to initiate to the next stages of the Resolution Response which are the resolution of residual cellular inflammation and then repairing the tissue damage caused by that inflammation.

9

Fermentable Fiber

THE KEY TO MAINTAINING
GUT HEALTH

AS DISCUSSED IN the last chapter, by following the Zone Diet you will consume a lot of non-starchy vegetables. I made this recommendation several decades ago based on the hormonal benefits of using very low glycemic load carbohydrates to stabilize blood sugar levels by controlling the balance of hormones in the blood.

At the time of my initial carbohydrate recommendations, very little was known about the molecular biology of the gut. Now, more than 20 years since the publication of *The Zone*, we know both the gut as an organ and the bacteria that reside in the gut operate together in a very complex interplay that has a significant impact on keeping inflammation under control. Outside of the brain, our gut may be the most complex organ in the body that I describe in greater detail in Appendix G. What controls this complex interaction between the trillions of bacteria in the gut and the gut itself is the level of fermentable fiber in your diet. That's why in this chapter I want to outline how the Zone Diet also reduces the potential of bacterial fragments from generating gut-induced inflammation.

There has been a lot of talk about gut health recently, but most people do not know what that means exactly. A healthy gut, in short, requires a unique source of nutrition, which is called fermentable fiber. Fermentable fiber is the key dietary component to maintain an incredibly thin barrier that acts as a defense between you and the trillions of "friendly" bacteria in your gut waiting for the opportunity to invade the blood and cause significant inflammatory damage.

Make no mistake about it, you are in a constant battle with bacteria for your survival. It is estimated that there are 5,000 different species of mammals, more than 40,000 species of fish, approximately 5,000,000 species of insects and potentially 1,000,000,000,000 (1 trillion) species of bacteria. Bacteria have been around for more than 3 billion years, whereas humans have been in existence for less than 200,000 years.

Furthermore, relatively few bacteria found in the gut have been cultured in laboratories, so they represent a biological black hole that we know very little about. One of the few things we do know is that bacteria are more successful as a species (in terms of longevity) than humans and are more likely to kill us before we kill them. They can mutate their genetic code rapidly, we can't. They can reproduce in 20 minutes. It's doesn't seem like a fair fight.

The primary weapon we have at our disposal to maintain our biological coexistence with bacteria are the barriers in the gut that separate their world from ours. Consider these biological barriers in the gut an inner skin that lines your digestive tract as your primary defense system against constant bacterial invasion. But it is not a static wall. It also must allow digested nutrients (amino acids, carbohydrates, and fatty acids as well as vitamins and minerals) into the body so we can survive. This inner skin is also constantly moving ingested food through the gut, allowing the nutrients from digested food into the blood, and sending information on nutrient status to your primary brain via hormones. At the same time, it protects you from pathogenic microbes (including fungi, parasites, viruses, and other "unfriendly" bacteria) just waiting for the opportunity to invade our bodies. Finally, it is an incredibly effective barrier that separates two seemingly alien worlds. One world consists of your human cells that requires oxygen to survive, whereas gut bacteria thrive best in a world without oxygen. If that inner skin is breached, these two worlds collide. The common name for this is called a "leaky gut." Whatever it is called, the result is a potential constant flow of a new source inflammation from the gut into our world. Just like diet-induced inflammation, gut-induced inflammation can lead to obesity, diabetes, autoimmune disorders, and a wide range of neurological conditions.

DETAILS OF YOUR INNER SKIN

Your inner skin is far more complex than your outer skin. Your inner skin has three primary defense components to protect you. The first is your mucus barrier. Mucus is composed of carbohydrate polymers synthesized by the goblet cells located in your gut wall. The thicker the mucus barrier, the less likely that microbes or large protein fragments can get close to the gut wall to cause a negative immunological response. The second defensive barrier is the quality of the tight junctions of your gut wall. The greater the integrity of these tight junctions at the face of the gut wall, the less leaky the gut becomes. This is explained in greater detail in Appendix G. Finally, your third and final defense is the vast array of immune cells lined up just behind the gut wall to attack and neutralize any protein or microbial fragments before they can enter into the body to cause significant inflammatory damage leading to systemic cellular inflammation. It is not the fermentable fiber per se that is important to maintain these defense systems, but the metabolites that are formed by its digestion by the resident bacteria in your gut. In particular, it is the very-short-chain fatty acids (especially butyric acid) that are essential for maintaining gut health.

WHEN THE GUT MALFUNCTIONS

You hear a lot about a leaky gut, but what does that really mean? The most likely suspect for a leaky gut is a reduction in the width of the mucus barrier. The mucus barrier is essentially a "no man's land" that not only blocks bacteria but also prevents proteins or large fragments of proteins from coming near the surface of the gut wall. If they come in direct contact with the outer cells of the gut the wall and the immune cells directly behind those cells, they will generate an immunological response. This is why most of the major food allergens are proteins. These are known as the Big 8 and include milk, eggs, fish, shellfish, nuts, peanuts, wheat, and soy. We can now add another protein to the traditional Big 8: gluten. A strong case can be made that "gluten sensitivity" is really a consequence of a leaky gut. A functional and robust mucus barrier would prevent the protein fragments from those foods from getting near the immunological cells located just inside your inner skin.

Perhaps the primary bacterial player for maintaining the mucus barrier is a recently discovered microbe known as *Akkermansia muciniphila*. It also appears that the more *Akkermansia* you have in your gut, the fewer inflammatory attacks you will be exposed to since its increased presence is associated with a decreased leaky gut. So, what's the connection?

Although there are 1,000 to 1,500 distinct bacteria species (these are considered your friendly bacteria) that reside in the gut, it appears that *Akkermansia muciniphila* may be the "best of the best." This is because this particular bacteria resides mainly in the outer layer of the mucus barrier and prevents more pathological microbes from getting close to the gut wall. Unfortunately, if you don't provide the gut with enough dietary fermentable fiber, *Akkermansia* gets hungry and its primary alternative food source now becomes the carbohydrate polymers that make up the mucus barrier. This degrades your primary barrier to prevent entry of microbes or large protein fragments from reaching the gut wall where they can cause an immunological response.

So, how do you make more of *Akkermansia* and keep that bacterial species nourished so they don't start digesting your mucus barrier? First you have to eat adequate amounts of fermentable fiber to nourish the bacteria in your gut. Next you have to consume optimal amounts of polyphenols as the "fertilizer" to enhance their growth. The primary dietary source of polyphenols are low-glycemic carbohydrates like non-starchy vegetables. What the polyphenols do is to activate AMP kinase in the gut wall to increase the production of mucus. Finally, you have to reduce the levels of oxygen in the gut to allow *Akkermansia* to survive because oxygen is toxic for these anaerobic bacteria. This reduction of oxygen in the gut is achieved with an adequate intake of omega-3 fatty acids that will activate another gene transcription factor (PPARα) that causes the gut cells to increase the oxidization of fatty acids consuming any residual oxygen in the gut thus maintaining an oxygen-free gut environment. The best indication that you have adequate levels of all three dietary components needed to maintain a healthy gut is to be in the Zone.

Besides maintaining a functional mucus barrier, you also have to maintain a tight barrier between the cells that line the gut wall. These are called tight junctions because they contain high levels of specialized proteins (occludins) that hold these surface cells together. The synthesis of occludins are also stimulated by the short-chain fatty acids that are the primary metabolites coming from the metabolism of the fermentable fiber in your diet. However, the assembly of the occludins into the gut wall is under the direction of AMP kinase.

These occludin proteins are not only important in maintaining the integrity of the gut wall, but also in other organs like the brain. In the brain, these cells form a tight blood-brain-barrier (BBB) that keeps virtually everything circulating in the blood out of the brain. As bad as a leaky gut is, a leaky brain is even worse. Unfortunately, these barriers in the gut, the brain, lungs, etc. can be disrupted very easily by the overproduction of pro-inflammatory eicosanoids (especially leukotrienes) derived from AA. Therefore, keeping your levels of pro-inflammatory eicosanoids low as well as consuming adequate levels of fermentable fiber necessary to produce short-chain fatty acids is one of your best ways to prevent a leaky gut as well as a leaky brain. Following the Zone Diet accomplishes both tasks.

OTHER CAUSES OF A LEAKY GUT

Obviously, the primary dietary contributor to a leaky gut is the lack of fermentable fiber as outlined above. As the amounts and diversity of fermentable fiber in your diet decreases, so does the diversity of the bacteria in your gut. Eventually, certain species of your gut bacteria go extinct. But lack of fermentable fiber is not the only factor that can lead to a leaky gut. There are a wide number of other factors including other components in your diet like alcohol and food additives as well as drugs and stress.

Other Dietary Factors

One dietary factor leading to a leaky gut is alcohol intake. Increased alcohol consumption will speed the development of both a leaky gut and eventually a leaky brain. Another new potential dietary culprit are artificial sweeteners. This occurs because of the greater genetic diversity of gut bacteria which are able to produce unique enzymes that can breakdown the artificial sweeteners (especially sucralose commonly known as Splenda) into toxic compounds that can decrease the levels of the necessary friendly bacterial diversity in the gut just like an antibiotic. Finally, a high-fat diet (especially if it rich in saturated fats like the Atkins diet or a ketogenic diet) can accelerate the transport agent of bacterial fragments (primary lipopolysaccharides or LPS) through the gut wall that generate inflammatory responses in the blood.

Drugs

Cancer chemotherapy drugs are among the most potent agents for inducing a leaky gut because they can't distinguish between killing a rapidly dividing cancer cell or killing a rapidly dividing cell that lines the interior of the gut.

Likewise, consistent use of standard antibiotics in even small amounts will also decrease diversity of the bacterial colonies in the gut and result in an increased permeability of the gut wall. This is because current antibiotics are broad-spectrum, indiscriminate killers of bacteria. In nature, bacteria will secrete specific antibiotics to protect their space from other bacterial intruders. On the other hand, broad-spectrum antibiotics usually come from a completely different microbial kingdom. As a result, their toxins are meant to destroy bacterial competitors, but not attack themselves or other members of their kingdom. As an example, penicillin is derived from a fungus to destroy other bacteria without much specificity but with no adverse effects on other fungi. Although it is possible to make specific narrow-spectrum antibiotics directed at only one type of offending bacteria, the cost for such targeted antibiotics is incredibly high as would be the cost for their drug approval. That's why we continue with using broad-spectrum antibiotics.

Anti-inflammatory drugs also provide a problem for gut health. Besides inhibiting resolution of inflammation (as explained in more detail in Appendix D), anti-inflammatory drugs can ironically produce more inflammation in the body by inducing a leaky gut.

Stress

The role of physiological stress through the activation of stress-induced hormones such as corticotropin-releasing hormone (CRH) is another factor that can impact gut permeability. The more stress you are under, the more CRH is produced in the brain that can travel via the vagus nerve to the gut and accelerate the formation of a leaky gut. The vagus nerve is a bidirectional transport highway between the brain and the gut. This is why many mind-body disorders that have neurological effects appear to start in the gut as I will explain later in the book.

THE ROLE OF THE ZONE PRO-RESOLUTION NUTRITION SYSTEM TO REPAIR A LEAKY GUT

Fortunately, there are number of dietary factors that can restore a functional gut barrier. All of these dietary factors are inherent in the Zone Pro-Resolution Nutrition system. As usual, it starts with the Zone Diet. The Zone Diet is rich in non-starchy vegetables as its primary carbohydrate source, thus it supplies adequate levels of a wide variety of dietary fermentable fibers critical for gut health. In addition, the Zone Diet reduces the production of pro-inflammatory eicosanoids (such as leukotrienes) that promote a leaky gut. The Zone Diet is also rich in polyphenols that promote the growth of key bacteria such as *Akkermansia* as well as reduce the likelihood of the development of a leaky gut. Another component of the Zone Pro-Resolution Nutrition system is supplementation with high-dose omega-3 fatty acids that will not only reduce inflammation in the gut wall, but also activate the fatty acid oxidation in the gut cells to remove residual oxygen in the interior of the gut to promote the growth of *Akkermansia*. Finally, the Zone Pro-Resolution Nutrition system uses supplemental polyphenols to further activate AMP kinase in the gut wall that is critical to preventing the formation of a leaky gut wall.

METABOLIC ENDOTOXEMIA

Your body has a unique way of recognizing the invasion of microbes from the gut. These are sensors known as toll-like receptors (TLR) that are located on every living cell and explained in greater detail in Appendix C. If a microbial fragment interacts with any of these TLR receptors on the surface of a cell, then a signal is immediately transferred to the gene transcription factor NF-κB inside the cell, which in turn causes the increased production of inflammatory proteins (cytokines) to combat the invasion. If the breach is significant, then a leaky gut becomes a superhighway for microbes from the gut to enter into the body and cause the equivalent of a five-alarm inflammatory fire. This condition is called sepsis and the mortality rates are about 50 percent. At lesser levels of increased gut permeability, the number of bacteria or their fragments (both will activate TLRs) that enter the blood is much lower and now they simply make you fat and far more likely to develop chronic metabolic diseases (such as obesity and diabetes) at an earlier age because of increased inflammation mediated by their interaction with the TLR system. This is called metabolic endotoxemia. The reason metabolic endotoxemia is so insidious is because you can't feel it and it is very difficult to measure. Nonetheless, you simply won't feel right in both the gut and the brain, as well as causing the accumulation of excess body fat.

A high-fat diet can accelerate metabolic endotoxemia for three reasons. First, a typical high-fat diet is also low in fermentable fiber. The second reason is that a high saturated fat diet (like a ketogenic diet) can also speed up the entry rate of bacterial fragments (lipopolysaccharide or LPS) into the blood by piggybacking with other fats (especially saturated fats like palmitic acid) that are assembled into lipoproteins known as chylomicrons that travel directly to the blood. Finally, the higher the levels of saturated fats (especially palmitic acid) in your diet, the more likely they can bind to the TLR receptors and fool them into thinking you are under bacterial attack.

How metabolic endotoxemia makes you fat is complex. Once microbial fragments breach both your primary defense barriers (the mucus barrier and an intact gut wall that has become leaky), they can enter the blood and then interact with the TLR system on every cell surface to generate inflammatory responses. Activation of the TLR receptors increases the activity of your genetic master switch of inflammation (i.e., NF-κB) resulting in cellular inflammation and its fellow traveler, insulin resistance, but now via a different molecular pathway. This is why there is a difference between diet-induced and gut-induced inflammation. Diet-induced inflammation is the result of an imbalance of nutrients entering the blood via the small intestine to generate an excess of pro-inflammatory eicosanoids that can activate NF-κB, whereas gut-induced inflammation is the result of microbial fragments entering the blood via the large intestine (i.e., colon) to activate NF-κB. The results are the same, just the pathways are different. Following the Zone Diet is the most effective way for reducing both types of dietary-induced inflammation.

The TLR receptor system on the surface of human cells is set up as a sensor system to detect microbial fragments. Once any microbial fragment (such as LPS) is detected, there is a rapid activation of NF-κB to increase the production of pro-inflammatory protein products such as inflammatory cytokines and the COX-2 enzyme required for the production of pro-inflammatory eicosanoids. Therefore, any leakage of microbes or microbial fragments into the blood from the gut can represent a significant source of potential systematic inflammation. As the levels of LPS rise in the blood, metabolic endotoxemia begins to increase. This added inflammatory burden appears to be a significant contributing factor to the development of obesity, metabolic syndrome (i.e., pre-diabetes), and diabetes. It should be noted that the levels of microbial fragments in the blood needed to induce metabolic endotoxemia are perhaps 50-100 times lower than the levels associated with the more severe inflammatory conditions (such as sepsis) that can potentially cause death.

PROBIOTICS

Throughout this chapter there has been little mention of probiotics. Probiotics are live bacteria. Most bacteria that exist outside those in the gut are generally pathogenic. However, a few live bacteria have been used for thousands of years to make the first biotechnology products (yogurt and fermented foods). These bacteria are not native to our gut, but at least they aren't trying to kill us.

Probiotics do have some benefits for gut health although far more limited than fermentable fiber and other prebiotics. Although probiotics don't colonize the gut, they can serve as target practice for the immune cells that line the gut. Just as soldiers in peace continually practice on the firing range to maintain their shooting skills, probiotics serve the same purpose, assuming they get to the gut. This is because like all live microbes they have to pass through the stomach's vat of acid that kills nearly all bacteria. Even those few that virtually enter into the small intestine and colon don't colonize the gut, but they provide non-pathological targets for your immune cells to refine their recognition skills to seek out microbes that are *persona non-gratia* and then destroy them.

On a scale of 1 to 10 for gut health benefits I give probiotics a 2, whereas I give adequate levels of fermentable fiber an 8. This means making sure you have adequate levels of fermentable fiber in your diet will have a far greater return on your gut health before you should consider adding probiotics to your diet. This might explain why the Federal Trade Commission fined Dannon more than $20 million in 2010 for making false advertising claims on the health benefits of the probiotics in their yogurt products.

SUMMARY ▶

As Hippocrates said 2,500 years ago, "all disease begins in the gut." We now have a far better understanding of why that statement is true if we consider that both diet- and gut-induced inflammation as ultimately coming from the diet. This is why reducing diet-induced inflammation and maintaining gut health following the Zone Diet is your obligatory first step to reach the Zone. Our growing knowledge of the molecular biology of the gut has shown us that the fermentable fiber found in the non-starchy vegetables (as well as fruits) plays a critical role in reducing gut-derived inflammation. These are the primary carbohydrates that you will be consuming on the Zone Diet. This is why the Zone Diet is the foundation for the Zone Pro-Resolution Nutrition system and is your primary dietary tool to not only reduce the intensity of diet-induced inflammation in the blood, but also reduce gut-induced inflammation at the same time.

10

Omega-3 Fatty Acids
AGENTS OF RESOLUTION

THE ZONE DIET is the foundation of the Zone Pro-Resolution Nutrition system for optimizing the Resolution Response because it reduces diet-inflammation that otherwise amplifies existing chronic unresolved cellular inflammation. That amplification factor can overwhelm the natural mechanisms of resolution and repair that are needed to lead to complete healing of any injury. To use an analogy, consider diet-induced inflammation like a burning house. First you must reduce the intensity of the existing fire before you can completely extinguish it, and only then can you begin to repair the damage.

In other words, the Zone Diet reduces the intensity of inflammatory fire, but it will not completely put it out. For that critical task you need high-dose omega-3 fatty acids to increase the generation of resolvins needed to resolve the remaining residual cellular inflammation in order to complete the Resolution Response by activating AMP kinase with adequate levels of polyphenols to repair the damage.

EICOSANOIDS VERSUS RESOLVINS

Eicosanoids are hormones derived from arachidonic acid (AA), which is an omega-6 fatty acid that turns on and determines the intensity of the inflammatory response. The vast majority of eicosanoids are pro-inflammatory, although there are a few that have anti-inflammatory properties as described in Appendix D. Technically, turning on inflammation is known as initiation. The higher the levels of eicosanoids in your body, the greater the intensity of cellular inflammation. The Zone Diet does an excellent job of reducing the formation of AA, thus lowering the levels of the eicosanoids that can amplify the intensity of cellular inflammation without compromising your initial inflammatory response to any injury (external or internal). Therefore, you can consider the Zone Diet to be an anti-inflammatory diet.

On the other hand, the long-chain omega-3 fatty acids eicosapentaenoic acid (EPA) and docosahexaenoic acid (DHA) are the molecular building blocks for the generation of resolvins necessary to turn off the inflammation response. Technically, this turning off of the inflammation process is known as resolution. Without adequate levels of EPA and DHA in your body, your body can't resolve the remaining residual cellular inflammation caused by some injury that has been amplified by diet-induced inflammation. This is why you need omega-3 fatty acids work in tandem with the Zone Diet because the initiation of inflammation must be in a constant working balance with its resolution if your goal is to reach the Zone and optimize the Resolution Response.

The vast majority of your omega-3 and omega-6 fatty acids in your diet consist of the shorter-chain omega-6 fatty acids (such as linoleic acid) or omega-3 fatty acids (such as alpha-linolenic acid). These fatty acids must be further metabolized into their longer-chain cousins that are the true building blocks for the eventual generation of both eicosanoids and resolvins. The metabolic pathways that lead to eicosanoids and resolvins are tedious and complex, and that is why I put them in Appendix D. However, here are key points to remember.

First, the enzymes in those metabolic pathways are the same for each group of essential fatty acids. This means if you have an excess of short-chain omega-6 fatty acids (like linoleic acid) in your diet, they will inhibit the further metabolism of short-chain omega-3 fatty acids into EPA and DHA. As a result, this means you will potentially generate many more eicosanoids and fewer resolvins. This alone virtually ensures you will be in a constant state of cellular inflammation.

Second, the activity of the key enzymes that are the "gate-keepers" for the generation of AA generation are controlled by the balance of the hormones (insulin and glucagon) generated by the Zone Diet. Insulin speeds up their activity, and glucagon inhibits their activity. This is why the balance of these two hormones controlled by the Zone Diet is key for reducing cellular inflammation. It is the balance of carbohydrates (that stimulate insulin) and protein (that stimulate glucagon) at every meal that determines the rate that AA is formed. Furthermore, if you develop insulin resistance (a predictable consequence of increased cellular inflammation), then your insulin levels are always elevated. If you are consuming a lot of omega-6 fatty acids as most Americans do primarily via vegetable-based cooking oils, then you are virtually guaranteed you will be making excessive levels of AA that generate increased levels of eicosanoids and maintain you in a state of constant cellular inflammation. This is shown below.

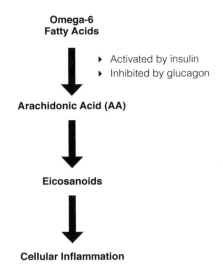

Once I understood the importance of maintaining the dynamic balance of insulin and glucagon to ultimately control the levels of AA, it became the driving force for developing the Zone Diet. The Zone Diet provided me the dietary tool I needed to reduce the intensity of diet-induced inflammation. In essence, the Zone Diet became the traffic cop critical for controlling the balance of hormones (insulin and glucagon) generated at each meal to decrease the production of AA that can ultimately increase cellular inflammation that in turn damages our organs.

However, when I wrote *The Zone*, virtually nothing was known about the resolution of inflammation. It was only later when I become aware of the importance of high-dose omega-3 fatty acids to turn off or resolve inflammation, did I realize that using high-dose omega-3 fatty acids would be critical. That's why my book *The OmegaRx Zone* was subtitled *The Miracle of the New High-Dose Fish Oil.*

Resolvins derived from omega-3 fatty acids represent a broad class of newly discovered hormones that include resolvins, protectins, maresins, and others. These hormones are derived from long-chain omega-3 fatty acids such as EPA and DHA and are essential to resolve the inflammatory process. But how much supplementation of omega-3 fatty acids will you need to generate an adequate resolution of residual cellular inflammation? That can be determined by the AA/EPA ratio in your blood that I discussed earlier as one of the three clinical markers that defines the Zone.

RESOLVIN PATHWAYS

Our current knowledge of the molecular pathways leading to resolution can easily be traced to one person—Charles Serhan at Harvard Medical School. Charlie started his research career in inflammation the same time that I became interested in eicosanoids. Charlie realized that while eicosanoids turned on inflammation, something had to turn it off. That led to his more than thirty-year journey into the mysterious world of resolvins. It has been Charlie's leadership in the discovery, synthesis, detection, and use of resolvins for disease treatment that has almost single-handedly driven this entire field.

I use the term "resolvins" to broadly describe the vast array of newly discovered hormones involved in resolution. Technically these hormones are known as specialized pro-resolving mediators (SPM). Frankly, that's a mouthful, so I simply lump them all together as resolvins to keep your focus on the resolution of cellular inflammation. Optimal resolution requires that adequate levels of both EPA and DHA be maintained as a reservoir in the body since resolvins are made on demand. Furthermore, you need adequate levels of both EPA and DHA because each omega-3 fatty acid generates different types of resolvins that have unique functions in the resolution process.

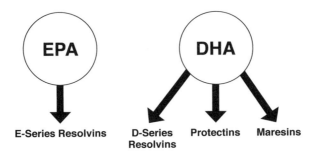

A brief overview of the different classes of resolvins that can be generated is shown below and is explained in more detail in Appendix D.

HOW MUCH EPA AND DHA DO YOU NEED?

Reaching an optimal AA/EPA ratio between 1.5 and 3 that is required for the resolution of residual cellular inflammation will usually require supplementation with highly purified omega-3 fatty concentrates for most individuals. How much supplementation depends on your current state of health as shown in the following chart.

Health Condition	Grams of EPA and DHA needed per day	Category of Supplementation
Currently Well	2.5	Minimum Dose
Obesity, Diabetes, or Heart Disease	5	Moderate Dose
Chronic Pain	7.5	High Dose
Neurological Disease	Greater than 10	Very-High Dose

To put these suggested levels of daily intake of EPA and DHA in perspective, the average American consumes about 150 mg (0.15 g) of EPA and DHA per day. That's why their AA/EPA ratio is about 20. The more you reduce AA by following the Zone Diet, the less supplementation with omega-3 fatty acids you will require to reach the ideal AA/EPA ratio necessary to enhance the resolution of residual cellular inflammation.

Let's look into that table with a little more detail. I consider 2.5 grams of EPA and DHA to be a minimum daily intake of omega-3 fatty acids. This is about the amount of EPA and DHA found in a tablespoon of cod liver oil—something that nearly every child took before leaving the house in the first half of the 20th century. You can quickly calculate that the current American intake of 150 mg of EPA and DHA per day represents a 95 percent reduction in my recommended minimum dose needed for the resolution of cellular inflammation.

OK, maybe you are not so healthy. Maybe you are obese (as defined by percent body fat, not BMI), have a high AA/EPA ratio (like most Americans), have a chronic disease like diabetes or heart disease, or have severe insulin resistance. You are definitely more inflamed. Now you will need about 5 grams of omega-3 fatty acids per day to bring your AA/EPA ratio into its appropriate range for resolution of unresolved cellular inflammation.

But what if your inflammation is no longer silent as might be the case in individuals with rheumatoid arthritis and other autoimmune conditions or those with cancer pain? Then you would need to take a higher dose of about 7.5 grams of omega-3 fatty acids per day. This is also true for elite athletes who live in a world of constant inflammation caused by the intensity of their exercise. Finally, what if the cellular inflammation is concentrated in the brain like various neurological conditions such as multiple sclerosis, depression, attention deficit disorder, Parkinson's, or Alzheimer's. Then you will likely need at least 10 grams of omega-3 fatty acids per day to reduce the AA/EPA ratio in the blood to an optimal range of 1.5 to 3. This would be considered a very high dose, but it is also a therapeutic dose required to reduce the AA/EPA ratio for the successful management of those neurological conditions.

The primary reason that omega-3 fatty supplementation is considered controversial is because the vast majority of human studies have used such a low dose of omega-3 fatty acids that the AA/EPA ratio is rarely reduced below 3, let alone even reaching an ideal level of 1.5. This is why you routinely hear news reports that omega-3 fatty acids have no benefits. If you use a placebo dose of omega-3 fatty acids, you should expect placebo results. This has been confirmed by two recent studies published in the same issue of the *New England Journal of Medicine* in which a dose 0.8 grams per day of omega-3 fatty acids had no cardiovascular benefits, but a dose of 3.9 grams of omega-3 fatty acids per day had significant cardiovascular benefits.

THE FAT-1 MOUSE

The benefits of achieving an appropriate AA/EPA ratio in the blood can be demonstrated in the fat-1 mouse. The fat-1 mouse is a genetically engineered animal containing genes from a worm that can now allow it to make the enzymes that convert much of the omega-6 fatty acids in every organ to omega-3 fatty acids, thus maintaining their AA/EPA ratio in their blood close to 1. When you cross-breed the fat-1 mouse to other mice that are genetically predisposed to develop a wide variety of chronic diseases, you find that the cross-bred fat-1 mouse is virtually resistant to developing conditions ranging from obesity, diabetes, autoimmune conditions, and neurological conditions found in the in-bred mice. The most likely reason is because of their lower AA/EPA ratio.

Obviously genetic engineering is not the most desirable way to lower your AA/EPA ratio, but you can do it via dietary supplementation. In animal models, it usually requires 100-200 mg EPA and DHA per kilogram body weight. For a 70 kg (154 pound) individual that would be about 7 to 14 grams of EPA and DHA per day. Those are also the same levels I have used in some of my clinical studies to better manage brain trauma, macular degeneration, and type 1 diabetes that I will describe later in this chapter.

WHY NOT JUST EAT MORE FISH?

Rather than taking omega-3 fatty acid supplements, why not simply eat more fish rich in omega-3 fatty acids? The Japanese are able to maintain a low AA/EPA ratio only because they are the largest consumers of fatty fish in the world. So why can't Americans? The problem is that the most popular types of fish consumed in America are lean, and therefore low in omega-3 fatty acids. This means you can't reach the necessary blood levels of omega-3 fatty acids you need for generating the necessary levels of resolvins required for optimal resolution of residual cellular inflammation.

Let's assume you wanted to consume 5 grams of omega-3 fatty acids, which was the amount used in the study published in the *New England Journal of Medicine* in 1989 to lower the levels of inflammatory proteins known as cytokines. So how much more fish would you need to eat? It depends on the fish. In the following table are commonly eaten fish and the amounts you would need to get 5 grams of EPA and DHA per day.

Fish	Grams of omega-3 fatty acids per 3.5 oz. filet	Oz. required for 5 grams of EPA and DHA per day
Tilapia	0.075	230
Grouper	0.100	175
Tuna, yellowfin	0.150	90
Cod	0.200	70
Swordfish	0.8	22
Salmon, wild chinook	1.1	16

Okay, maybe consuming one pound (16 oz.) of wild chinook salmon every day is not that difficult (although expensive), but trying to consume 14 pounds of tilapia to get the same level of EPA and DHA is simply impossible. Furthermore, if you have a chronic disease, the levels of EPA and DHA you must consume to get your AA/EPA ratio in its optimal range may require even significantly higher levels of fish consumption.

While eating enough fish to obtain adequate levels of EPA and DHA for resolution is possible, there are other significant problems caused by consuming more fish. In particular, heavy metal and chemical toxin contamination. Larger fish such as tuna and swordfish are predators, meaning they accumulate the heavy metals (primarily mercury) found in the smaller fish they consume. The larger the predator fish the more mercury it will contain. This is why there are warnings for pregnant mothers not to eat too much tuna or swordfish during pregnancy. However, a more insidious threat is that all fish contain chemical toxins such as polychlorinated biphenyls (PCBs). These industrial chemicals once thought to be inert are now known to be neurotoxins, carcinogens, and endocrine disruptors. That's why the worldwide production of PCBs was banned in 2001. Unfortunately, PCBs are highly persistent in the environment. In other words, they are going to be around for a long time. The higher the levels of the omega-3 fatty acids in a fish, the higher the levels of accumulated PCBs they contain since these toxins are fat-soluble and concentrate in the fat deposits of the fish.

The solution to both problems of high levels of mercury or PCBs and still getting adequate levels of EPA and DHA to promote resolution is the supplementation with ultra-refined omega-3 fatty acid concentrates.

OMEGA-3 FATTY ACID PURITY

The unfortunate fact is that all fish are contaminated by either environmental toxins like heavy metals (like mercury coming from coal burning) and industrial chemicals (like PCBs). You can run, but you can't hide from the fact. When you purchase concentrated omega-3 fatty acids in a supplement form, these problems remain. Regardless of how the omega-3 fatty acid supplements are made, their purity must be constantly tested relative to toxin levels (especially PCBs) and the rancidity of the final product.

Toxins

Although it is relatively easy to remove heavy metals such as mercury from any fish oil product, it is nearly impossible to completely remove PCBs from any omega-3 fatty acid concentrate. However, they can be reduced to exceptionally low levels using new manufacturing technologies, especially super critical fluid and low-temperature thermal purification technologies which have only recently been introduced.

Rancidity

Omega-3 fatty acids are also extremely prone to oxidation. This is why fish smells if it is not fresh. These oxidation products include aldehydes and ketones that are highly reactive chemicals that can cause damage to proteins and your DNA. You can measure the levels of these reactive chemicals using a standard test known as Total Oxidation or Totox.

SHOW ME THE DATA

Since prescription-grade omega-3 fatty acid concentrates developed in the 1990s are now generic products, their published standards by the FDA can be compared to fish oil products sold in the mass market (health food grade) and also the newer omega-3 fatty acid concentrates (such as the ultra-refined grade) using more advanced technologies such as super-critical fluids or low-temperature thermal fractionation that are now available. The comparison of these general standards that govern oil quality is shown in Table 1.

TABLE 1. PURITY STANDARDS FOR OMEGA-3 FATTY ACID CONCENTRATES

Type of oil	Upper PCB levels (ng/g)	Upper Totox Levels (meq/kg)
Health food grade	90	26
Generic prescription	50	26
Ultra-refined grade	5	20

It can be seen from Table 1 that omega-3 fatty acid concentrates sold by prescription are not all that different in terms of PCB purity and rancidity specifications from what is sold in a supermarket. Reducing the levels of PCBs in an omega-3 fatty acid product becomes critically important when giving high doses of omega-3 fatty acids. This is because PCB levels can build up in the blood, even when giving a prescription omega-3 fatty acid concentrate. It has been shown that if the daily intake of PCB levels increases by only 180 nanograms (0.00000018 gram) per day, that can increase the risk of cardiovascular disease by 60 percent. Those PCB levels are not very much. It is similar to adding one drop of water into the equivalent of three Olympic size swimming pools.

This is a problem in using high-dose omega-3 fatty acid concentrates to increase resolvin formation. According to the specifications in Table 1, a typical one-gram capsule of fish oil sold in the supermarket could potentially contain 90 nanograms of PCBs. Taking more than two capsules a day of such a product could increase your daily PCB intake by 180 nanograms and potentially increase the risk of heart disease. Taking four one-gram capsules of a prescription omega-3 product may possibly contain 200 nanograms of PCBs and still meet the FDA standards for a prescription drug. On the other hand, you could take 40 one-gram capsules of an ultra-refined omega-3 product before you would reach the same levels of PCB intake.

Using the new manufacturing technologies I described above, it is now possible to produce non-prescription omega-3 fatty acid concentrates of even higher purity (approximately one nanogram of PCBs in one-gram capsule) with nearly equal omega-3 fatty acid concentrations than the current FDA specification for prescription drug omega-3 fatty acid products. This is critical for long-term, high-dose applications necessary to maintain adequate levels of omega-3 fatty acids in the blood unless you feel lucky about the purity of the fish oil you are using since PCBs are known neurotoxins, carcinogens, and endocrine disruptors. Although there are no labeling requirements for PCB levels for an omega-3 fatty acid product, a few companies will actually post such data on their websites even though I pointed out this PCB problem in my 2001 book, *The OmegaRx Zone*.

Rancidity

The other marker of purity are the Totox levels in the final product. Totox is the universal marker of oil rancidity. In fact, this marker is the basis for worldwide trading of all edible oils. Because of the high concentrations of omega-3 fatty acids in these concentrates (50-85 percent omega-3 fatty acids), the likelihood of developing rancidity is quite high thus the importance of adequate antioxidant protection to prevent rancidity. Rancidity is the result of producing chemically reactive aldehydes and ketones (the breakdown products of fatty acids during oxidation) in an omega-3 fatty acid product during its stated shelf life. The lack of sophisticated antioxidant systems in typical fish oil products (including prescription omega-3 drugs) is why it is likely that most fish oil concentrates can quickly develop rancidity during shipping or while sitting on the store shelf. This is because the additional refining necessary to achieve higher EPA and DHA concentrations strips out the natural antioxidants in the fish oil that protect the omega-3 fatty acids from oxidation. Adding back relatively weak standard antioxidants will not be sufficient to protect the higher concentrations of EPA and DHA from oxidizing in the bottle.

The best way to overcome this oxidation problem is to develop far more sophisticated antioxidant systems for use in the omega-3 fatty acid concentrates to retard rancidity development. Over the years, I have developed such antioxidant systems that when coupled with low levels of PCBs in the finished product makes the long-term use of high-dose omega-3 fatty acid supplements to resolve residual cellular inflammation a reality.

Of course, the simplest way to test for rancidity may be simply to bite into the fish oil capsule and taste the oil. If it is bitter, it's rancid and will probably do more harm than good for you since you are tasting the aldehydes and ketones. Most omega-3 concentrates simply don't pass the taste test. Some health food grade products will try to bypass this problem by adding flavors (lemon being the most common) to mask the taste. These products will not taste bitter even though the resulting Totox values of such flavored products are often well above the standard that defines rancidity.

HISTORY OF OMEGA-3 FATTY ACID CONCENTRATES

The history of using fish concentrates started more than 2,000 years ago with the use of garum consisting of fermented fish intestines that were prized as a seasoning in ancient Roman times. Large garum factories were located throughout the Roman Empire as garum was considered far more valuable for health than olive oil. Unfortunately, with the fall of the Roman Empire, the recipe for garum was also lost.

The next major advance in fish oil supplementation occurred in the 1780s when the first cod livers from America were sent back to England where they were fermented (by rotting) in wooden vats. The oil released from the fermenting cod livers rose to the top of the vats and was considered a miracle treatment for rheumatoid arthritis. The fermented cod liver oil contained about 15 percent by weight of omega-3 fatty acids. In the 1850s, Norwegians started heating the cod livers in iron kettles rather than letting them rot in wooden barrels like the British. This greatly accelerated the extraction of the cod liver oil with a slightly better taste. This was the technique used for most fish oil production in the 20th century.

In the 1980s, the use of fish body oils began to replace cod liver oil for two reasons. One benefit was to nearly double the omega-3 fatty acid content to approximately 30 percent of the total fatty acids, and second, there was a dramatic reduction of vitamin A levels compared to cod liver oil, thus reducing the potential of vitamin A toxicity that could result in an increase of calcium levels in the blood.

In the late 1990s, manufacturing technology began using molecular distillation enabling the production of even higher concentrations of omega-3 fatty acids. This is the methodology used to make current prescription drugs containing omega-3 fatty acids. However, this older technology has been dramatically improved with the introduction of either super-critical fluid extraction or low-temperature thermal fractionation techniques to obtain even higher purity omega-3 fatty acid concentrates with far better taste and purity characteristics than thought possible using molecular distillation alone that I have described earlier. When you supplement with high-purity omega-3 fatty acid concentrates at therapeutic levels to resolve residual cellular inflammation, the results can be extraordinary.

TREATING "UNTREATABLE" CONDITIONS WITH HIGH-DOSE OMEGA-3 CONCENTRATES

The powerful benefits of high-dose omega-3 concentrates have been demonstrated in the treatment of conditions for which there is no known drug therapy. Such untreatable conditions fall into three major categories: severe brain trauma, age-related macular degeneration (AMD) and optical nerve damage, and the treatment of type 1 diabetes.

Raising the Dead: Treating Severe Brain Damage

In 2006, a major disaster occurred in West Virginia at the Sago mine. Thirteen miners were trapped in a carbon monoxide-rich atmosphere for more than 41 hours. No human being has ever survived such a prolonged period of carbon monoxide exposure. When the rescue team finally reached the trapped miners, twelve of the thirteen were dead. The one remaining survivor was as close to death as medically possible. He had heart failure, kidney failure, and liver failure. When they examined his brain by MRI, most of his myelin (i.e., white matter) was destroyed by inflammation induced by the carbon monoxide poisoning. That evening I received a phone call from the head physician of the Level 1 Trauma Center in West Virginia where the lone survivor (Randall McCoy) had been sent for treatment. That physician was Julian Bailes who is one of the top neurosurgeons in America. The reason Julian called me was to see if high-dose fish oil might keep Randall alive because he had read my book *The OmegaRx Zone* several years earlier. I agreed and suggested giving the miner 15 grams of EPA and DHA per day. After a long pause over the phone, Julian countered that his patient would probably bleed to death with such high levels. I assured him that wouldn't happen because there was a blood test to make sure that we could adjust the dose of omega-3 fatty acids, so the AA/EPA ratio would never drop below 1.5. Julian agreed, since he had no other options. That night I air-shipped several bottles of our omega-3 fatty acid concentrates to Julian, and the next day they started giving Randall 15 grams of omega-3 fatty acids per day through his feeding tube. Eight weeks later, Randall came out of his coma and was transferred to a rehab hospital where he continued the same daily dose of omega-3 fatty acids using a tablespoon to deliver the omega-3 concentrate for another eight weeks. Four months after the mine disaster, Randall went home. His heart was normal, his kidney was normal, his liver was normal, and he gave a press conference worthy of any politician. The press touted it as a miracle. Maybe it was, and perhaps Julian and I just got lucky. But I have consistently had similar results using the same aggressive use of ultra-refined high-dose omega-3 fatty acid concentrates in a number of patients with a wide variety of severe brain trauma subtypes over the years.

One recent case study involved a young adult who had a drug overdose and choked on his vomit causing hypoxia (lack of oxygen) to the brain requiring him to be placed onto a ventilator to survive. Two months later, the physician told the parents that they should pull the plug since it was unlikely their son would ever recover. That night I got a call from the parents. I told them that I wish they had contacted me earlier, but nonetheless I shipped out an even more highly purified omega-3 concentrate that I had recently developed and an appropriate blood test kit to test his AA/EPA ratio levels. He started to improve after a few weeks, and within a few months they took him completely off his ventilator. Some 14 months after he had started with the EPA and DHA supplementation, they sent me photographs of him canoeing with his father. Four months later, I received another picture of him at his sister's wedding. Not a bad outcome for a young man whose parents were told to pull the plug a year and half earlier. Every case is different, but supplementation with purified high-dose omega-3 fatty acid concentrates makes a lot more sense than the standard practice of putting the patient on a ventilator and hoping that time will resolve the neuroinflammation in the brain.

Curing the Blind: Restoring Sight in Macular Degeneration and Optic Nerve Damage

Ocular damage is really brain damage. One type of ocular damage is age-related macular degeneration (AMD), which is the primary cause of blindness after age 50. There are two types of AMD; dry and wet. There is no known treatment to improve dry AMD (which accounts for 90 percent of the cases) and usually most of the patients become legally blind within 10 years after developing the condition. The intervention for wet AMD (only 10 percent of AMD cases) is not to cure it, only to prevent it from getting worse with monthly injections of monoclonal antibodies directly into the eye.

Since the retina is rich in omega-3 fatty acids, it would make sense that supplementation with omega-3 fatty acids should be useful for either type of macular degeneration. Of course, that is true only if you are using therapeutic doses of EPA and DHA to reduce your AA/EPA ratio in the blood to the appropriate range. If you use placebo levels of omega-3 concentrates (like 0.8 grams of omega-3 fatty acids per day) to treat dry AMD not surprisingly you get placebo results. That's exactly what the large-scale clinical trials confirm.

I had the opportunity to work with an ophthalmologist in Cyprus to undertake pilot studies to see if higher doses (5 to 7.5 grams of omega-3 fatty acids per day) might provide a different clinical result. That's actually what we did for six months in his patients with dry AMD. All the patients improved. Furthermore, the clinical benefits were totally dose-dependent on the final AA/EPA ratio at six months. That is, the lower the final AA/EPA ratio after six months, the greater the vision improvement for this "untreatable" condition. In those patients that reached the lowest final AA/EPA ratio (1-1.6) after six months, their vision was improved by 100 percent.

The same holds true in our unpublished observations treating optical nerve damage. It is commonly assumed that once the optical nerve is damaged, it can never repair itself. But using high-dose omega-3 concentrates (10 grams of EPA and DHA per day), dramatic vision improvements were observed after six months, even though a significant period of time (like more than a year) had passed after the optical nerve damage first occurred. During the course of the treatment, it was possible to actually observe the optical nerve regenerating as measured by the growing response to light when shined on the retina. The underlying mechanism for the regeneration of the optic nerve probably starts with the reduction of neuroinflammation similar to the repair process seen in the patients with severe brain trauma.

Treating Type 1 Diabetes

Type 1 diabetes is an autoimmune disease like rheumatoid arthritis, lupus, and multiple sclerosis. This means the body's own immune system is attacking the target tissue. What cause autoimmune diseases remains unknown. But of these conditions, early onset type 1 diabetes in children may be the most terrifying, because if you are a parent of a child with type 1 diabetes the data strongly suggests that if they have developed type 1 diabetes before the age of 10, their lifespan will be shortened by 14-18 years. Furthermore, there is nothing in the current medical literature that can stop its development. Maybe that can change?

Two recently published case studies from Italy suggest that using high-dose omega-3 fatty acids may be able to stop the inevitable destruction of the beta cells in the pancreas. Furthermore, it appears that regeneration of the beta cells that produce insulin may be occurring as long as the AA/EPA ratio is maintained below 3 using high-dose omega-3 concentrates.

Based on these encouraging case studies, a large-scale FDA-allowed clinical trial has begun to determine if using ultra-refined high-dose omega-3 concentrates at 7.5-10 grams of omega-3 fatty acids per day can potentially increase the body's natural production of insulin in a wide variety of type 1 diabetes. If so, this may be the first real breakthrough for treating type 1 diabetics since the development of insulin injections nearly 100 years ago.

SUMMARY ▶

Without adequate levels of EPA and DHA in your blood, your ability to resolve cellular inflammation will be a constant struggle. Ideally, you should eat enough fatty fish to get adequate levels of both omega-3 fatty acids (as do the Japanese and especially the Okinawans). However, the contamination of fish with environmental toxins (such as mercury and PCBs) makes the use of ultra-refined omega-3 fatty acid supplements the preferred approach for significantly improving the resolution of cellular inflammation. This is one of the few times that refined is better than natural.

At moderate levels of EPA and DHA supplementation (about 5 grams of omega-3 fatty acids per day), the elevated levels of these two omega-3 fatty acids in the blood can begin to generate powerful resolvins. At still higher levels (greater than 7.5 grams of EPA and DHA per day), they become remarkable dietary complements to any drug intervention to better manage a wide variety of chronic diseases including those for which there currently is no known treatment. Regardless of the amount of EPA and DHA you are taking, make sure it is pure as well as sufficient in quantity for the resolution of residual cellular inflammation. That requires testing, not guessing.

11

Polyphenols

ACTIVATORS OF OUR GENES, GUARDIANS OF OUR GUT

ONCE YOU HAVE reduced diet-induced inflammation by the Zone Diet, and then sufficiently resolved residual cellular inflammation by producing adequate levels of resolvins using omega-3 fatty acids, the third and most complex stage of the Resolution Response is to repair the tissue damaged by increased exposure to cellular inflammation. Your primary dietary tool to achieve that goal is high-dose polyphenols.

The story of polyphenols is strongly intertwined with the activation of AMP kinase. AMP kinase is the master genetic switch that controls your metabolism (including the repair of damaged tissue). Thus, your ability to activate AMP kinase ultimately controls your healthspan. How activation of AMP kinase accomplishes this goal is complex, so I put the mechanisms in Appendices E and F.

Just as the Zone Diet reduces the activation of the genetic master switch of inflammation (NF-κB) that causes inflammatory damage, polyphenols activate the genetic master switch of metabolism (AMP kinase) that heals that inflammatory damage. This represents the final stage of the Resolution Response.

BACKGROUND

Polyphenols are the complex chemicals that give plants their color. The more colorful the plant, usually the higher the polyphenol content. This is why vegetables and fruits are the plants that have the highest concentrations of polyphenols. Although there are approximately 8,000 known polyphenols, and probably twice that number that have not been structurally analyzed, little was known about the biological activities of polyphenols before 1995. This was because we didn't have the technology to understand how they activate genes. It is now clear that the levels of polyphenols in the diet are critical for the final stage of the Resolution Response to be activated. The extent of the repair process depends on the remaining level of the inflammation caused by the initial injury that may have been further amplified by continuing diet-induced inflammation. Unfortunately, this often leads to fibrosis if the final step of the Resolution Response is not completed.

There is a great deal of epidemiological data that shows the increased dietary intake of foods rich in polyphenols (primarily vegetables and fruits) is associated with lower rates of chronic disease and mortality. We also know that increased levels of polyphenols in the urine (indicating their absorption into the blood) are also strongly associated with reduced mortality and frailty in elderly populations.

We are now beginning to understand how polyphenols work. They activate the master genetic switch of your metabolism. This is the function of the gene transcription factor of AMP kinase and represents the key to a longer healthspan. The story of AMP kinase and its vast array of actions is complex so I put it Appendix F. However, the repair process of the Resolution Response is governed by the ability of AMP kinase to maintain the quality control of your mitochondria that generate the energy needed for the repair of damaged tissue.

AMP KINASE AND POLYPHENOLS

Polyphenols are natural activators of AMP kinase, but through an indirect route. They work by activating another gene transcription factor called SIRT that in turns activates AMP kinase as described in Appendix E. This begins to explain why the consumption of high levels of vegetables and fruits are associated with greater health and longevity. That's also why you have to eat a lot of vegetables and fruits (about 10 servings per day) to consume enough polyphenols to start observing the benefits of activating AMP kinase. But there is another challenge with this dietary approach because the vast majority of polyphenols are not very water soluble, so only relatively small amounts of polyphenols get into the blood. This is actually good news for your gut since their concentrated presence in the gut will activate AMP kinase in the cells that line the gut wall thus improving gut health and reducing a potential source of inflammation. This means that for increasing your healthspan you will need a combination of both water-soluble polyphenols and water-insoluble polyphenols.

This importance of water-soluble polyphenols for human health is reinforced by studies in Italy studying elderly individuals following the traditional Mediterranean diet in remote regions of Tuscany. When the researchers initially looked at the amounts of polyphenols consumed by these individuals and their mortality, they found no relationship. However, when the researchers looked at the levels of polyphenols in their urine (which is a marker of the polyphenols that actually entered the blood), they found those individuals with the highest levels of polyphenols in their urine had a 30 percent reduction in mortality.

Therefore, the optimal activation of AMP kinase in your body requires finding appropriate polyphenols that not only activate AMP kinase, but also are water-soluble so they can enter into the blood. Now the number of potential polyphenol candidates for a longer healthspan drops dramatically. The primary candidates belong to a subclass of polyphenols known as delphinidins found in berries, and in particular blueberries. The secret is how to get as many delphinidins in your diet as possible.

POLYPHENOL EXTRACTS

The levels of polyphenols found in vegetables (about 0.1 percent by weight) and fruits (about 0.2 percent by weight) are low. Of course, the levels found in refined carbohydrates like white bread and white pasta are zero. Thus, you need to eat a lot of fruits and vegetables every day to maintain the adequate intake of polyphenols for improving gut health. Getting adequate levels of water-soluble polyphenols necessary to maximally activate AMP kinase in your body is an even greater challenge.

A potential solution is the processing of unique polyphenol sources to yield concentrated extracts. These extracts make it possible to consume adequate levels of polyphenols to generate consistent therapeutic benefits for your body's cells as well as in your gut. The two best dietary sources are the blueberry family for water-soluble polyphenols and cocoa beans for water-insoluble polyphenols.

The extraction methodology for most polyphenol extracts starts with making a slurry of the raw material source, followed by dehydration of the slurry generating a dry crude powder. This dehydration step usually doubles the polyphenol concentration. The dried powder can then be further extracted using alcohol to further increase the polyphenol content because polyphenols have a higher solubility in alcohol compared to other components in the dried crude polyphenol powder. This explains why drinking red wine has been the classical way to consume higher levels of polyphenols as opposed to eating massive amounts of grapes or other fruits (like blueberries). Finally, the alcoholic extracts can be further purified using chromatography to generate refined polyphenol extracts approaching 40 percent polyphenols by dry weight.

Unlike fruits, cocoa beans contain very little water, but a lot of fat. To produce cocoa powder, the cocoa nibs are first separated from the seeds, then milled to produce a slurry of cocoa powder and cocoa butter called a chocolate liquor. Now you can separate the cocoa butter from the cocoa powder to get an isolated cocoa powder that is relatively rich in cocoa polyphenols. That's why raw cocoa powder is so bitter when you taste it. The reason is that polyphenols interact with your bitter taste receptors in the tongue. Just as you can extract dried polyphenols powders with alcohol, you can also extract the cocoa powder with other organic solvents to get an even higher percentage of polyphenols also approaching 30 percent by weight.

Blueberry and cocoa polyphenol extracts have provided most of our clinical data on the benefits of polyphenols. Bottom line, blueberry polyphenol extracts are good for the blood, and cocoa polyphenol extracts are good for the gut. You need them both.

POLYPHENOL PURITY

Just like omega-3 fatty acids, the purity of polyphenols is critical for their use in high-dose applications. The best indication of polyphenol purity is whether or not the polyphenol extract has been purified by column chromatography. Try to look for those very limited number of polyphenol extracts that have undergone such refining. To date, only selected polyphenol extracts from the maqui berry (a member of the blueberry family) meet this criteria. Furthermore, such purified maqui extracts represent the highest levels of delphinidins available.

Although no cocoa polyphenol extracts are available that have been refined by column chromatography, a few products have been extracted by specialized organic solvents to remove much of the inherent cadmium. This is important as most crude cocoa polyphenols extracts (as well as cocoa powders and cocoa nibs) are naturally high in in the heavy metal cadmium. Using these specialized solvent-based refining techniques can dramatically lower cadmium levels. The only way to know if a cocoa polyphenol extract is low in cadmium is to check on the cadmium levels of the final product. If that information is not posted on the website of the product, then assume the cadmium levels are probably too high. As with omega-3 fatty acid concentrates, this is another example where refined is often better (and safer) than natural.

POLYPHENOL EXTRACT FACTS AND FANTASIES

Given the complexity of polyphenol science, it is quite easy for marketing hype to overwhelm scientific fact. Here is one statement that is constantly repeated as the truth: "Resveratrol is the primary polyphenol found in red wine." First, that is simply not true. There are some fifty different polyphenols in red wine, and resveratrol is a minor polyphenol among them. The highest concentration of polyphenols in red wine come from a specific class of polyphenols known as anthocyanins. Anthocyanins are the primary polyphenols found in berries and grapes. Second, pure resveratrol is a highly astringent off-white powder. It is highly unlikely that a white powder is going to give red wine its color. Third, resveratrol is not very water soluble, so very little of it will ever reach the blood to activate AMP kinase. Finally, virtually all commercial resveratrol comes from the Japanese knotweed, which as its name implies is a weed that is highly invasive to crops. That kind of takes all of the mystique away from resveratrol and red wine, as well as resveratrol supplements. This is why resveratrol supplements may not be a very good choice to increase AMP kinase activity in your body.

If resveratrol in red wine isn't the key to the health benefits, then what is? It certainly can't be the alcohol since no one talks about the health benefits of vodka. Maybe it's one of the other polyphenols found in red wine. The most likely candidate is a sub-class of anthocyanins known as delphindins. These unique polyphenols are everything resveratrol is not. First, delphindins are water soluble (remember that wine is primarily water), meaning they can enter into the bloodstream. Second, purified delphinidin extracts have extensive clinical benefits ranging from reducing blood glucose levels to decreasing oxidative stress, both important factors in managing diabetes. Third, they can be purified to high potency using column chromatography.

So, how do you get adequate levels of delphindins and begin to activate AMP kinase more effectively? You could drink a lot of red wine (about 56 glasses per day), but you can imagine there might be some health problems with that approach. Although red grapes contain some delphinidins, those levels are low compared to other fruits, in particular blueberries. Even with the blueberry family, there is a considerable variation in delphinidin content. American blueberries contain relatively low levels of delphinidins, bilberries (also known as Russian blueberries) contain higher levels, but the richest source of delphindins is the maqui berry (also known as the Patagonian blueberry). In fact, during the French wine crisis in the 1970s, tons of maqui berries were sent from Chile to France to blend with the weakened grapes to maintain the red color of the wine and thus save their red wine industry.

Research has shown that the delphinidins in purified maqui polyphenol extracts can easily enter the blood intact, thus they are more effective than other polyphenols to activate a wide number of gene transcription factors by increasing the activity of AMP kinase (see Appendix E for more details). Increased AMP kinase activity is the final key necessary to complete the Resolution Response.

On the other hand, cocoa polyphenols are primarily composed of polyphenol polymers which are not water-soluble but can be broken down to individual polyphenols by the bacteria in the gut. In this regard cocoa polyphenols are great for the gut.

WHAT ARE ADEQUATE INTAKE LEVELS FOR POLYPHENOLS?

The answer depends on which benefit generated by activation of AMP kinase you are trying to achieve. A general suggestion for water-soluble polyphenols (like maqui polyphenols) might be:

Benefit	Polyphenol intake required
Reduces oxidative stress	500 mg per day
Reduces inflammation	1,000 mg per day
Increase mitochondrial efficiency	1,500 mg per day

For water-insoluble polyphenols (like cocoa polyphenols), a general suggestion might be:

Benefit	Polyphenol intake required
Gut health	1,000 mg per day

SUMMARY ▶

Polyphenols have a remarkable range of physiological actions in both your cells to control your metabolism and in your gut to reduce the likelihood of a leaky gut and promote the growth of beneficial bacteria such as *Akkermansia*. Most importantly, polyphenols play a unique role in the final step of the Resolution Response by increasing the energy needed to repair damaged tissue. However, those repair benefits will be maximized only if you have first reduced diet-induced inflammation with the Zone Diet followed by the resolving of residual cellular inflammation with adequate levels of omega-3 fatty acids. Only after those two stages of the Resolution Response are completed can you begin to repair damaged tissue (and that includes the gut wall) caused by prior diet-induced inflammation. This is the final step of the healing process of the Resolution Response, which can be greatly accelerated with the use of polyphenol extracts that can increase AMP kinase activity. With that increase in AMP kinase activity comes a longer healthspan. This is why using purified polyphenol extracts can be considered gene therapy in the kitchen.

12

Personalizing
the Zone Pro-Resolution
Nutrition System

IN THE PREVIOUS chapters, I have outlined the key dietary components necessary for the Zone Pro-Resolution Nutrition system to work
most effectively plus the clinical markers that enable you to chart your
progress. Now it's time to put this all together in a personalized, lifelong
program based on your biochemistry, your dietary philosophy, and your
personal taste preferences to increase your healthspan. This is critical
since everyone is not the same genetically and we all have different dietary philosophies as well as diverse personal goals at each stage of life.
The power of the Zone Pro-Resolution Nutrition system is that it can
easily be adjusted to your genetics and dietary philosophy (neither which
is likely to change) as well as achieving your goals (which will change
during the course of your life).

Those changing goals (described in later chapters) may include childhood nutrition (especially in the first 1,000 days of life), achieving peak
physical performance, improved weight management, maintaining wellness, or improved managing of chronic diseases to enjoy a longer
healthspan. The more important these goals are to you, the more you
want to follow the Zone Pro-Resolution Nutrition system to reach them.

• • •

THE THREE R'S OF THE RESOLUTION RESPONSE

As I have mentioned earlier reaching the Zone requires an orchestrated three-pronged dietary approach that constitutes the Resolution Response. Those 3 R's needed for optimizing your internal Resolution Response can be summarized as:

- Reduce
- Resolve
- Repair

To *reduce* the intensity of diet-induced inflammation you must reduce the levels of eicosanoids in the blood as well as decrease the activation of the genetic master switch for inflammation (NF-κB). This is accomplished by the macronutrient balance of each meal plus consuming adequate levels of fermentable fiber to maintain a healthy gut. Both these tasks are the job of the Zone Diet.

Once you have reduced the levels of diet-induced inflammation by the Zone Diet, you then must *resolve* residual cellular inflammation by increasing the levels of the resolvins that control its ultimate resolution. This is the task of high-dose omega-3 fatty acids. Unless you are eating large amounts of fatty fish, to maintain adequate levels of omega-3 fatty acids in your blood as well as your organs you will probably require additional supplementation with ultra-refined omega-3 fatty acid concentrates as discussed earlier.

Finally, after residual cellular inflammation is resolved, the final step of the Resolution Response is to *repair* the tissue damage caused by previously unresolved cellular inflammation by maximizing the activation of AMP kinase to orchestrate your metabolism. This is the job of polyphenols, and most likely will require additional supplementation with a combination of refined water-soluble and water-insoluble polyphenols. It is only when all three steps of the Resolution Response are successfully completed, that healing takes place.

The exact levels of supplementation with omega-3 fatty acids and polyphenols are not only determined by your genetics, but also by how strictly you follow the Zone Diet to reduce diet-induced inflammation. Your success will be confirmed by the three clinical markers of the Zone as I described earlier.

Each dietary component of the Zone Pro-Resolution Nutrition system works synergistically and in a controlled sequence to optimize the Resolution Response. You first must reduce the ongoing diet-induced inflammation with the Zone Diet before you can adequately resolve residual cellular inflammation with high-dose omega-3 fatty acids. Likewise, you have to resolve residual cellular inflammation before you can optimally repair the damaged tissue with high-dose polyphenols. This sequential progression is no different than backing your car out of the garage. First, you get behind the wheel of the car. Next you turn on the ignition. Finally, you have to put the gear into reverse. Each step must be completed in the appropriate sequence, or it is unlikely the car is going to leave the garage. The Resolution Response is no different, except that all three components must be ready to go on-demand because random injuries can occur at any time. The only way to ensure that your internal Resolution Response is ready to immediately respond to the inflammation generated by such random injuries is by making certain you are in the Zone.

So, let's start with the first step necessary to get to the Zone: The Zone Diet.

MAKING THE ZONE DIET WORK FOR A LIFETIME

The Zone Diet is the foundation of Zone Pro-Resolution Nutrition system if you want to maintain an optimal Resolution Response. It is a personalized strategy based on three factors: (1) your unique protein requirements needed to maintain your muscle mass that depends on your exercise levels, (2) your current level of insulin resistance that determines the type of carbohydrates you can eat, and (3) your dietary philosophy ranging from vegan to Paleo.

Nonetheless, there are also several important dietary habits you want to develop that are fundamental to *reduce* the intensity of diet-induced inflammation that in turn will reduce insulin resistance:

- Maintain a consistent balance of the protein-to-carbohydrate ratio at each meal to stabilize your blood glucose levels, so you are never hungry or mentally fatigued between meals. This is usually about one-third more carbohydrates than protein.
- Ensure adequate intake of fermentable fiber and polyphenols

from your carbohydrate choices in the course of the day to maintain gut health.

- Try to consume low levels of total fat, but the fat you do consume should be rich in monounsaturated fat.
- Consume about 400 calories at each meal. This will be enough to maintain hormonal balance without feeling hungry or fatigued for the next four to five hours.

As pointed out in earlier chapters, getting adequate levels of polyphenols and omega-3 fatty acids to ensure an optimal Resolution Response may likely require additional supplementation with omega-3 fatty acid concentrates and purified polyphenol extracts.

GETTING STARTED

There are four unique factors that make the Zone Diet uniquely personalized to each individual. The first is your unique protein requirements to maintain your current muscle mass. Once you determine this, you spread that total protein requirement evenly throughout the day at each meal. The second factor is your current level of insulin resistance, which determines the type of carbohydrates you can eat to balance out your protein for optimal hormonal responses at each meal. The third factor is the type and amount of fat you consume at each meal. This means adding enough fat to increase satiety, but not too much to overload your calorie intake. The fourth and final factor is your personal dietary philosophy. Once you optimize each of those four factors, you have a dietary system to employ and enjoy for the rest of your life.

So, let's look at each factor in more detail.

PROTEIN REQUIREMENTS FOR THE ZONE DIET

The Zone Diet is based on your unique protein requirements, not how many calories you need. You most likely have plenty of excess calories stored in your fat cells for energy production, but your hormonal balance in the blood may prevent those fatty acids from being released and being metabolized primarily in the muscle cells to provide energy. Although calories do count, it's the hormonal response of those calories after each meal that counts far more. Furthermore, the Zone Diet is designed to balance your hormones, but without hunger or fatigue because you are also stabilizing blood glucose levels between meals.

This is why making any Zone meal starts with the amount of protein you need to maintain stable blood glucose levels in the blood as well as stimulate the flow of satiety hormones from the gut to the brain. The amount of protein you need at each meal depends on your current muscle mass as well as the type and intensity of exercise you actually do.

The calculation of your protein requirements has nothing to do with your weight, but everything to do with lean body mass. To know the amount of lean body mass you have, you first must know your percent body fat. There are a lot of ways to calculate your body fat percentage, but if you go to www.zonediet.com/resources-body-fat-calculator, you can use a simple calculator I have developed that will do all the work for you in a few seconds. All you need is a tape measure and your current weight and height.

Calculating your percent body fat instead of using body mass index (BMI) to determine your level of obesity can be an eye-opening experience. You will be surprised how many people (probably including yourself) who might be considered slightly overweight by their BMI measurements are actually considered obese by their percentage of body fat. Once that shock wears off, you now multiply your current body weight by that body fat percentage to get your total body fat. Then you subtract that number from your total weight to get your lean body mass as shown below:

Percent body fat times your weight in lbs. = Body fat in lbs.

Total weight in lbs. minus your body fat in lbs. = Lean body mass in lbs.

Finally, you must also determine how physically active you are. The more active you are, the more muscle mass is broken down during periods of physical activity and this means you need more dietary protein to replace it. Here are your daily protein requirements depending on your physical activity as shown below.

Activity level	Amount of protein required
Sedentary	0.5 grams of protein per lb. of lean body mass
Light activity (walking)	0.6 grams of protein per lb. of lean body mass
Moderate exercise (30 minutes per day, 3 times a week)	0.7 grams of protein per lb. of lean body mass

If you do more intense exercise, your protein requirements increase as I will explain in chapter 17 on peak performance. If you happen to be obese, then use 0.6 grams of protein per lb. of lean body mass to determine your protein requirements since you are essentially weight training every day because of the extra weight you carry on your body stored as body fat.

You are almost there. Now multiply your lean body mass by your activity factor and you can now determine how many grams of protein you need each day. That seems like a lot of work, but if you use my free body fat and protein requirement calculator at www.zonediet.com/resources-body-fat-calculator all of these mathematical calculations are done automatically for you allowing you to continually adjust your real protein requirements.

It turns out the amount of protein you need at each meal is probably not that great. Let's use the mythical 154 lb. male who is likely 5'9", sedentary, and with 28 percent body fat (the average percent body of American males between 1999 and 2004). If you make all those calculations (including the higher protein requirements because he is obese), his daily protein requirement would be about 66 grams per day or about 22 grams of protein at each meal. Regardless of your calculated protein requirements, divide your total protein intake and consume it evenly throughout the day to optimize blood sugar control as well as generate maximum satiety.

On average you are going to need approximately 25 grams of low-fat protein at every meal following the Zone Diet to maintain four to five hours satiety from meal to meal. This is the average of the amount of protein a typical female (3 oz. of low-fat protein or 21 grams of protein) or a typical male (4 oz. of low-fat protein or 28 grams of protein) would consume at a meal. So here are examples of the protein levels in 3.5 oz. (100 grams) of various protein sources according to the USDA nutrient database.

Sources	Grams of protein	Grams of carbohydrate
Veal	22	0
Beef	20	0
Lamb	21	0
Pork	21	0
Chicken	22	0
Turkey	24	0
Tuna	24	0
Salmon	21	0
Sardines	21	0
Egg whites	11	0
Cheese (semi-soft)	21	4
Cheese (hard)	36	3
Lactose-free milk (8 oz.)	8	13
Almonds	18	32
Tofu (extra firm)	5	1
Lentils (dry)	25	63
Black beans (dry)	21	62

You can see that animal protein is rich in protein and you don't need much at a meal to consume 25 grams of protein per meal. However, animal protein and fish are not sustainable sources of protein. On the other hand, eggs and dairy are sustainable sources consisting of high-quality protein. The only downside to eggs is their yolks; they are very rich in AA that will increase the production of pro-inflammatory eicosanoids. So, use the egg whites and toss the yolks. Egg whites are the highest quality protein source available except for human breast milk. Furthermore, egg white protein will have a much lower effect on insulin secretion. Although dairy products also have an excellent protein quality (almost equal to egg whites), this source of protein will have a higher impact on insulin secretion. Vegan protein-rich favorites like extra firm tofu are low in carbohydrates, but other vegetable protein sources like lentils and black beans are rich in carbohydrates and often contain undesirable anti-nutrients like phytates (that bind minerals), isoflavones (that interfere with thyroid action), and lectins (that require more extensive cooking to degrade them). So, for the vegan, this generally means eating a lot of extra firm tofu and plant-based imitation meat products that tend to be lower in these anti-nutrients due to the processing of the source (soy and pea are the most common) used to make plant-based imitation meat products.

Carbohydrates

The levels of protein at each meal determines the amounts of carbohydrates you can eat to prevent an oversecretion of the hormone insulin. You need some carbohydrates, but not too much. However, the types of carbohydrates you can use will be determined by your current levels of insulin resistance that I discussed in Chapter 6.

HOW MUCH INSULIN RESISTANCE DO YOU HAVE?

It's highly unlikely that you are going to take a blood test to determine your TG/HDL ratio more than once a year. Fortunately, there are subjective indicators that don't require a blood test that you can use to estimate your level of insulin resistance. One of those is a simple questionnaire that I have developed that provides a good estimate of the severity of insulin resistance at www.zonediet.com/insulin-resistance-quiz. The levels of insulin resistance from this quiz correlate well with your TG/HDL ratio, which is a more objective blood marker of insulin resistance. A more subjective indicator of insulin resistance is if you are constantly hungry and mentally fatigued. You can use these subjective markers as a guide to adjust the types of carbohydrates you are consuming to better control cellular inflammation, which is the underlying cause of insulin resistance.

WHAT CARBOHYDRATES CAN YOU EAT ON THE ZONE DIET?

The types of carbohydrates you consume following the Zone Diet is determined by your current level of insulin resistance. Don't worry because your current level of insulin resistance can rapidly change the more closely you follow the Zone Diet.

If you have high levels of insulin resistance, you must be more restrictive with your carbohydrate choices. As long as your level of insulin resistance is high, the primary carbohydrates that you should consume on the Zone Diet are non-starchy vegetables to optimize the levels of fermentable fiber and polyphenols with the least amount of carbohydrates to reduce insulin secretion. The best non-starchy vegetables (spinach, kale, mushrooms, asparagus, broccoli, cauliflower, and artichoke hearts) are surprisingly rich in protein compared to their carbohydrate content. Since insulin resistance can be rapidly reduced following the Zone Diet, you should soon be able to add a greater variety of other vegetables to your Zone meals.

If you have moderate levels of insulin resistance, then you can begin to introduce a greater variety of non-starchy vegetables as well as consuming more fruits, but still in moderation because of their higher glycemic load compared to non-starchy vegetables. Berries (especially blueberries) are the best choice because of their polyphenol content compared to other fruits.

If you have low insulin resistance, then you have even more carbohydrate flexibility as you can begin to include some whole-grain products such as brown rice and whole-wheat bread products in moderation with your Zone meals. Moderate means maybe a half a piece of whole grain bread or a very small serving of brown rice. Whole-grain products means they are richer in polyphenols and fermentable fiber than refined carbohydrates (but not as rich as non-starchy vegetables and fruits). Unfortunately, they will have the same impact on blood sugar levels as typical refined carbohydrates so use them in moderation regardless of your insulin resistance levels.

Finally, if you have very low levels of insulin resistance (as do many elite athletes because of the intensity of training), you have the greatest carbohydrate flexibility for increasing the levels of whole-grain carbohydrates as long as you don't overwhelm the amount of protein consumed at a meal.

Using my Insulin Resistance Quiz (www.zonediet.com/insulin-resistance-quiz), you can easily determine your level of insulin resistance on a weekly basis to make adjustments in the types of carbohydrates you can eat and still maintain the hormonal balance of the Zone Diet.

Fats

Finally, the easiest of the other macronutrients for a Zone meal is the fat. Just eat primarily monounsaturated fat (olive oil, nuts, or avocados), but how much? A dash. That means a small amount. A small amount is about half the amount of protein you consume at a meal. If you are consuming 25 grams of protein at a meal, then you want to consume about 12 grams of total fat in the same meal. Since even low-fat animal sources (like chicken breast) contain some fat, the amount of added fat is not going to be very much. That's about ½ tablespoon of olive oil, ⅓ oz. of almonds (about eight almonds), or a ¼ of an avocado. However, the more fat you consume, the less fat you will release from your own stored body fat and most Americans have plenty of stored body fat.

The fats you want to avoid are saturated fats (especially palmitic acid) and omega-6 fatty acids as both generate pro-inflammatory responses. The reason you need some fat in a meal is to stimulate the hormone cholecystokinin (CCK) from the gut to help stimulate additional satiety.

CONSTRUCTING ZONE MEALS

Once you know your protein requirements and your current level of insulin resistance that determines the types of carbohydrates you can eat, all you need to do is personalize a customized diet program so that each meal has about 40 percent low-glycemic carbohydrates, 30 percent low-fat protein, and 30 percent monounsaturated fat.

It is easier than you think to determine that balance using two methods I have developed over the years. The first is the hand-eye method to balance your plate (which is the easiest, but the least precise) that is fine for most individuals with low and very low levels of insulin resistance and the other is using Zone Food Blocks for individuals with moderate and high levels of insulin resistance (which is more precise because it allows you to fine-tune adjustments for your personal metabolism and genetics) described later in this chapter.

HAND-EYE METHOD

The easiest but least precise method for making Zone meals is the hand-eye method. Using this method, you simply divide your plate into three equal sections. The portion of low-fat protein should be the size and thickness of the palm of your hand; this should fill one-third of your plate. The size and thickness of the palm of your hand takes into account differences in sex and bone structure, but you will find the average Zone meal portion is about 25 grams of low-fat protein. Next, fill the other two-thirds of the plate with colorful carbohydrates (colorful because they are rich in polyphenols). Primarily these will be non-starchy vegetables with limited fruits (save those for dessert). Remember, the higher your initial insulin resistance levels, the more restrictive the carbohydrates choices. Finally add a dash of a monounsaturated fat source (olive oil, nuts, or avocado) to finish the meal.

If you do so, then your plate will visually look like this:

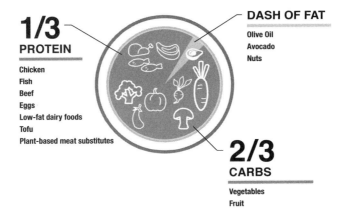

1/3
PROTEIN

Chicken
Fish
Beef
Eggs
Low-fat dairy foods
Tofu
Plant-based meat substitutes

DASH OF FAT

Olive Oil
Avocado
Nuts

2/3
CARBS

Vegetables
Fruit

If you aren't hungry or fatigued during the next four to five hours after consuming a Zone meal, then the hand-eye method worked just fine for you. Just remember this method is less precise than the other method in both protein and carbohydrate balance and calorie content and so there may be some trial and error before you get the balance right. But have some fun and experiment with the hand-eye method knowing that when you aren't hungry for the next four to five hours after a meal you have it mastered.

BRINGING PEACE TO DIETARY WARS

While the hand-eye method is not the most accurate for planning Zone meals, it illustrates the fourth factor for personalizing the Zone Diet; your personal dietary philosophy. This is because virtually every possible dietary philosophy, ranging from Paleo to vegan as well as lacto-ovo vegetarians and omnivores, can easily be accommodated using the general Zone Diet guidelines.

Regardless of your dietary philosophy, two-thirds of the plate will always be virtually the same: It will be filled with colorful carbohydrates (primarily non-starchy vegetables with limited amounts of fruit). It is only the last third of the plate containing your protein source that depends on your dietary philosophies as shown below:

Vegan: No animal protein, no dairy, and no eggs

Lacto-ovo vegetarian: No animal protein

Paleo: No legumes, no dairy, no soy meat substitutes, and no grains

Omnivore: No protein restrictions whatsoever

The only requirement for each of the different dietary philosophies is that the protein content of the meal should contain approximately 25 grams of protein. Other than the types of protein on that third of your plate, the Zone Diet blueprint is totally compatible with virtually every dietary philosophy, except ketogenic diets (i.e., Atkins) and very low-fat, low-protein, and high-carbohydrate diets (i.e., Ornish). I guess you can't please everyone. Other than those two exceptions, it is difficult to fail on the Zone Diet since you are following your personal dietary philosophy using foods tailored for your personal tastes and based on your unique protein requirements and current levels of insulin resistance.

THE ZONE FOOD BLOCK METHOD

As I stated earlier, if you have moderate to high levels of insulin resistance, then you may initially need a more detailed plan than simply using the hand-eye method to balance your plate. That's why I developed the Zone Food Block method many years ago. It also allows you to fine-tune the Zone Diet based on your unique biochemistry, genetics, and current level of insulin resistance.

Although protein is fairly consistent in nutrient density, carbohydrates are not. The density of carbohydrate can vary widely from very low density as found in non-starchy vegetables to very high density as found in grains and starches. I developed the Zone Food Block method many years ago to make it easier to better match carbohydrate density to the protein intake at a meal. The end result is more precise hormonal control. This method allows you to add Zone Blocks for protein, carbohydrate, and fat in defined proportions to create the necessary hormonal balance for improved appetite control.

The most important goal for any Zone meal is to maintain hormonal balance to maximize the stabilization of blood sugar levels for the next four to five hours. This means the total calorie content of any Zone meal is usually the same; with approximately 400 calories, at least 25 grams of protein, and less than 12 grams of fat per meal with most of the carbohydrates coming from non-starchy vegetables. That means for every *one* gram of fat in a Zone meal, you want *two* grams of protein, and *three* grams of low-glycemic carbohydrates to achieve the appropriate hormonal balance. Consider this the 1-2-3 method. Frankly, very few individuals are going to do the math (this is why the hand-eye method is so useful). On the other hand, using Zone Food Blocks you simply balance the blocks of protein, carbohydrate, and fat for every meal necessary to the reach the same final hormonal balance.

A typical male will consume four Zone Blocks of protein, carbohydrate, and fat for a Zone meal, whereas a typical female would consume three Zone Blocks of protein, carbohydrate, and fat for a Zone meal. A complete listing of Zone Food Blocks and a wide of variety of other helpful tools can be found at www.zonediet.com/resources/food-blocks). Using this information will help you make an infinite variety of Zone meals compatible for virtually every dietary philosophy.

ADJUSTING YOUR HORMONAL CARBURETOR

Your hormonal "carburetor" is the balance of protein to the glycemic load of carbohydrates at each meal. Just like a carburetor in the car that can be adjusted to provide maximum mileage from the gas in your car's fuel tank, your hormonal carburetor can be adjusted to provide the maximal hormonal control from a meal. The real benefit of using the Zone Food Block method is that you can adjust your hormonal carburetor to take into account potential differences in biochemistry, genetics, and current levels of insulin resistance to provide better control of blood sugar levels. As a result, you are not hungry or mentally fatigued for four to five hours after a meal.

Your hormonal carburetor is really the balance of glucagon and insulin generated by a meal that determines how stable your blood sugar levels will be after a meal. That hormonal balance is a consequence of adjusting the protein-to-glycemic load in a meal.

How to adjust that hormonal carburetor is actually quite easy. Simply consume a Zone meal using an equal number of Zone Food Blocks and then look at your watch four to five hours later. If you have no hunger or mental fatigue at the four-to-five hour time point, then that Zone meal is ideally suited for both your metabolism and your genetics meaning you can make that same meal over and over and produce the same hormonal response.

If you are hungry within four to five hours after a making a meal using the Zone Food Block method, you'll need to make some adjustments for your personal biochemistry and genetics. If you were hungry and mentally fatigued after a meal, this indicates that the previous meal had too high of a glycemic load. The slight excess of carbohydrate in that meal was enough to increase blood insulin levels that drove blood sugar too low during the next five hours inducing a slight hypoglycemic effect. Simply remake that same meal in the future and subtract one Zone carbohydrate block from the recipe. If this modified Zone meal keeps you satiated and mentally alert for four to five hours after eating, then it is ideal for your personal biochemistry.

On the other hand, if you are hungry but mentally alert within four-to-five hours after a making a Zone meal, then you consumed too few carbohydrates because not enough insulin was making its way to the hypothalamus to reduce hunger (insulin acts as a satiety hormone in the brain). Remake that same meal in the future and add one extra Zone carbohydrate block to the recipe. After making that meal, you should enjoy four-to-five hours of satiety without mental fatigue. This is how you can modify any Zone meal to ideally suit your biochemistry.

In reality, we actually don't eat a highly varied diet. For most, our diet at home consists of two different breakfasts, three different lunches, and five different dinners. Likewise, when you go to eat, you might frequent five to ten different restaurants and eat essentially the same meals. Once you have developed ten Zone meals you enjoy at home and another ten meals you like at the restaurants you frequent that work for you, you are pretty well set for life.

Finally, keep in mind you never "cure" chronic problems caused by diet-induced inflammation. To achieve better weight management, improved athletic performance, maintenance of wellness, or healthy aging, you are using the Zone Diet like a "drug" managing those problems more successfully. Once you stop following the Zone Diet, the more likely those chronic problems will begin to reappear.

MEAL TIMING

The best stabilization of blood sugar levels will only last about five hours. This means you want to constantly maintain stable blood sugar levels to be successful, so you are never hungry or mentally fatigued. So, plan your day accordingly.

Try to eat a Zone breakfast within an hour after waking. Your body has been in an overnight fast and is essentially running on empty. For most people that will be about 7 a.m. in morning. Then plan to eat lunch no later than noon to maintain stable blood sugar levels. However, most people eat dinner around 7 pm in evening. Therefore, eat a small Zone snack at around 5 pm. Finally, before you go to bed, you might want to consider another small Zone snack because even though you are going to bed, your brain is not. That's why you will wake more refreshed the next morning. You can find hundreds of Zone meals and snacks at www.zoneliving.com in the Tools and Resource section.

MAKING MISTAKES ON THE ZONE DIET

We don't live in a perfect world, and more importantly we are not perfectly disciplined in our eating habits. There will always be times when it will be impossible to have a Zone meal. Birthday parties, holidays, vacations, sporting events, etc. are good examples. Although you will try to make good choices using the hand-eye method, reality often dictates otherwise. The end result is you are likely going to consume meals that will most likely be hormonal disasters on these special occasions.

Fortunately, the hormones generated by your diet can change rapidly once you return to the Zone Diet. Of course, the longer you have been following the Zone Diet in the first place, the greater the resilience you will have to bounce right back into hormonal balance after consuming any hormonal disaster of a meal.

EATING OUT

The most convenient way to consume Zone meals at restaurants is to use the hand-eye method to balance your plate. Pass on the bread, ask for non-starchy vegetables to replace the grains and starches in the meal, and then have fresh fruit for dessert. This is always a lot easier to do if you have had a Zone snack before going to the restaurant.

BECOMING TOO THIN ON THE ZONE DIET

Can you become too thin following the Zone Diet? Of course you can because the Zone Diet is a calorie-restricted diet designed to enable your body to use its own stored body fat for energy. How do you know if you are getting too thin? The answer is when you can clearly see all of your abdominal muscles (the proverbial "six-pack" you see in fitness magazines). This means you are about 5 percent body fat for a male and 11 percent body fat for females. These are unrealistic levels of body fat for elite athletes as well as the general population The reason you can't see your abdominal muscles is because they are covered by a layer of excess fat. By that criteria, very few Americans are too thin. You have plenty of calories stored as excess body fat to call upon to make up for any calorie deficiency assuming you can more effectively access your stored body fat by reducing insulin resistance. So, how do you alter the Zone Diet if by some chance you get too lean? You simply add more nuts (almonds or walnuts are good choices) that are rich in monounsaturated fat, until you can just barely see your abdominal muscles. (This would a be "two-pack" as opposed to a "six-pack.") Keep in mind most Olympic swimmers have a "two-pack" (10 percent body fat for males and 15 percent body fat for females). Also keep in mind that it is very easy to overconsume nuts. Even healthy fat consumed in excess will be stored in your fat cells to the extent that your abdominal muscles completely disappear again. This is why the only difference between the Zone Diet for the overweight diabetic and the elite athlete is that the elite athlete may have to add some extra fat to their diet over and above their increased need of protein and carbohydrate that I will discuss in more detail in Chapter 17.

WHAT ABOUT PERSONALIZING RESOLUTION AND REPAIR?

The Zone Diet is the ideal dietary intervention to reduce the intensity of diet-induced inflammation, but it will have a limited effect on increasing the resolution of existing cellular inflammation as well as the repair of damaged tissue necessary to complete the Resolution Response. However, it is very difficult to build new tissue, unless you resolve the residual cellular inflammation causing the damage in the first place.

This is why the optimization of the Zone Pro-Resolution Nutrition system will usually require the use of additional omega-3 concentrates and polyphenol extracts as supplements to optimize your Resolution Response. How much? It depends on how closely you follow the Zone Diet. The more closely you follow the Zone Diet, the fewer Pro-Resolution supplements you should need to stay in the Zone. On the other hand, the less closely you follow the Zone Diet, the more Pro-Resolution supplementation using highly purified omega-3 fatty acid concentrates and refined polyphenol extracts rich in delphindins you need to get to the Zone. In either case, your blood will tell exactly how much of omega-3 fatty acids and polyphenol supplements you need by using the Zone markers I described earlier in Chapter 7.

Frankly the reason everyone needs Pro-Resolution supplements is because it is very difficult to get enough EPA and DHA to resolve inflammation or enough water-soluble polyphenols to activate AMP kinase from the foods we eat following any diet.

HOW MUCH OMEGA-3 FATTY ACIDS AND POLYPHENOLS DO YOU NEED?

A good starting dose for omega-3 fatty acids would be 2.5 grams of EPA and DHA per day whereas a good starting dose for polyphenol extracts would be 500 mg. per day. These are minimum suggested levels. The optimal level for optimal resolution of residual cellular inflammation can be determined by a simple blood test requiring only a drop of blood that was discussed in Chapter 7. In particular, the AA/EPA ratio will determine the ideal amount of omega-3 fatty acids required for resolving residual cellular inflammation.

For determining the levels of polyphenol extracts that you need, use the level of glycosylated hemoglobin (HbA$_{1c}$). Reaching the appropriate range for this marker will determine the ideal levels of polyphenol extracts required for activating AMP kinase to enhance tissue repair.

LIFETIMES OF THE DIETARY COMPONENTS OF THE ZONE PRO-RESOLUTION NUTRITION SYSTEM

The concept of the Zone is based on classical drug pharmacology, which describes a therapeutic zone for a drug. Too little of the drug in the blood will have placebo effects, too much drug in the blood will be toxic. Furthermore, every drug has a unique lifetime in the blood, and that lifetime determines how often you have to administer the drug to maintain the blood levels needed for a therapeutic effect. Some drugs require you to take them every few hours, some once a day, and still other drugs only require a weekly injection.

The physiological responses to your diet are no different. Some effects take place rapidly (within minutes as is the case with hormones generated by a meal), within days relative to gene expression, or weeks depending on the rate that a particular dietary component (especially omega-3 fatty acids) is accumulated in the target organ.

The lifetime of the hormonal changes generated by a Zone meal is four to five hours which means to maintain the benefits of the Zone Diet you should be as consistent as possible with balancing the protein-to-glycemic load of each meal. After five hours, your hormone levels have returned to their starting levels and it's time to eat again.

The lifetime of polyphenols in the blood is even shorter (2-3 hours), meaning they should be consumed at every Zone meal either by a large serving size of non-starchy vegetables or by using polyphenol supplements. On the other hand, fermentable fiber is slowly metabolized in the large intestine. The primary benefits of fermentable fiber are the production of short-chain fatty acids that play a major role in gut health, but only for the time period that the fermentable fiber is in the colon before finally being eliminated in the stool. Since that time period is about 30 hours after consumption of a meal, theoretically you could consume all your required fermentable fiber once a day. However, since you want to consume about 8-10 servings of vegetables per day, it makes better sense to consume that amount over the course of several meals. The fermentable fiber content (or lack of it) of your diet can quickly begin to alter the microbial composition of the gut for better or worse within five days. Furthermore, entire colonies of friendly bacteria in the gut may become extinct without a constant supply of fermentable fiber as shown in animal models.

Finally, the half-life (the time during which the levels in the blood decrease by one half) of omega-3 fatty acids in the body is about two days in the blood. This also means you can take all of your required omega-3 fatty acid supplements only once a day to maintain constant levels in your blood.

You want to be as consistent as possible with the Zone Pro-Resolution Nutrition system to ensure that all the dietary components needed for optimizing the Resolution Response are at or near their peak levels throughout the day. This is no different than taking medications at the right dose and the right time to maintain adequate drug levels to manage the symptoms of a chronic disease.

SUMMARY ▶

The ideal Zone Pro-Resolution Nutrition system is unique to you and no one else because of your biochemistry and genetics. In addition, your diet must be personalized for the foods you like to eat as well as your diet philosophy. The Zone Pro-Resolution Nutrition system represents the future of personalized nutrition because it is based on four elements unique to you:

1. The daily amount of total protein you require to maintain your current muscle mass. The amount of protein at a meal also determines the amount of carbohydrates and fats you should also consume at the same time.
2. Your current level of insulin resistance that determines the type of carbohydrates you can eat to maintain stable blood sugar levels.
3. Your diet philosophy.
4. The levels of Pro-Resolution supplements you require to resolve residual cellular inflammation and then to repair tissue damage to complete the Resolution Response. The amounts of supplementation are determined by the blood tests that are the markers of the Zone.

The Zone Pro-Resolution Nutrition system is a dietary technology that allows you to optimize your Resolution Response. Like any technology, you need to follow a system like the Zone Pro-Resolution Nutrition system for it to work. The Zone Pro-Resolution Nutrition system is also a highly personalized dietary program compatible with virtually every dietary philosophy. Most importantly, your Zone blood markers allow you to determine how well you are maintaining an optimal Resolution Response, which is the key to extending your healthspan.

13

Dietary Facts and Fallacies

NUTRITION IS CONFUSING because it is complex. Because it is so complex, there are also many fallacies about specific dietary ingredients that lead to constant confusion as to what we should be eating and why. This is why it is best to view nutrition as a systems-based approach to better understand how the foods we eat affect a wide variety of outcomes that we term metabolism.

UNDERSTANDING METABOLISM

Metabolism is defined as the chemical processes that occur within a living organism necessary to maintain life and this includes the healing of injuries. Metabolism may be best understood as a mysterious biological black box that controls your life. Within this black box inflammation is generated in response to an injury as well the Resolution Response being generated in response to inflammation. If inflammation and Resolution Response remain balanced, you remain well. However, the Resolution Response is generated "on demand" so you must ensure the "fuel tanks" necessary for each stage of the Resolution Response to work most effectively are always full. The best way you can ensure that outcome is to be in the Zone. If for some reason these separate mechanisms of inflammation and the Resolution Response are not continually balanced, their mismatch generates cellular inflammation that can be amplified to a higher level by diet-induced inflammation. As the levels of unresolved cellular inflammation increases, this only accelerates your progression toward developing a chronic disease and a shorter healthspan. It's often not the initial injury that causes the chronic disease, but the relentless increase of unresolved cellular inflammation that is the real underlying cause of development of any eventual chronic disease.

One of the primary jobs of metabolism is to convert incoming dietary calories into energy (primarily the chemical adenosine triphosphate or ATP), to repair and build tissue, to maintain your immune system to fight off infections and heal physical injuries, keep your body warm, etc. However, most of the excess incoming dietary calories beyond those needed for your immediate metabolic needs will be stored as fat.

In my book, *Toxic Fat*, I discuss how excess body fat could be considered a potential staging area for the spread of cellular inflammation to other organs that can eventually result in chronic disease. This is why diet-induced inflammation makes us sick and age at a faster rate, because it amplifies existing levels of cellular inflammation. Therefore, the Zone Pro-Resolution Nutrition system depends on reducing diet-induced cellular inflammation as the obligatory first step in activating the Resolution Response. This requires you to consume the least number of calories you need to maintain your metabolism without compromising nutrition. What ultimately controls your metabolism is not the diet per se, but the hormonal and genetic changes induced by the diet.

HOW DIETARY CALORIES GET CONVERTED TO ENERGY

About 90 percent of the body's ATP is generated in your mitochondria found in every living cell. Mitochondria are essentially your metabolic factories that maintain life. However, the constant generation of ATP to keep us alive creates a lot more heat than the body can handle so there is a constant need to dissipate that excess heat by evaporation through the skin. This is why you feel so miserable on a hot and humid day since it becomes very difficult to get rid of the excess heat generated by your mitochondria. The generation of ATP also produces excess free radicals in the process. Scientifically, this is called oxidative stress. Unless you have adequate levels of antioxidant enzymes in the body, those excess free radicals will start damaging tissue by increasing inflammation and making it far more difficult to repair damaged tissue. The more calories you consume at a meal, the more oxidative stress you generate.

When it comes to generating ATP, you have two types of fuels: high octane and low octane. Consider the fatty acids found in the diet and stored as body fat as your high-octane fuel because you can generate a lot more ATP per gram of fat (i.e., high-octane fuel) than you can per gram of glucose (i.e., low-octane fuel). However, if you consume either potential fuel source (fat or glucose) in excess, whatever is not immediately used will ultimately be stored as excess body fat.

The absolute number of calories needed to make adequate levels of ATP depends on whether or not the body is using fat or glucose for fuel. One of the secrets of the Zone Pro-Resolution Nutrition system is that it allows you to consume the least number of calories, yet produce adequate ATP that maintains your metabolism. This is the result of reducing insulin resistance in your fat cells, thereby allowing you to release more stored body fat as high-octane fuel burned by your mitochondria to produce ATP in other organs.

ESSENTIAL NUTRIENTS

Maintaining adequate ATP production with the least number of dietary calories is only the first step in the Zone Pro-Resolution Nutrition system. You also have to ensure those calories contain the essential nutrients that the body cannot make. The first three are the classical essential nutrients including (1) essential amino acids, (2) essential fatty acids, and (3) vitamins. The other two classes of essential nutrients have only recently been investigated and can be considered as essential for gut health. These include polyphenols and fermentable fiber, which are both necessary for maintaining the health of a complex ecosystem composed of trillions of bacteria in the gut as well as the human cells that line the gut wall.

Protein

Although dietary protein is a poor source to generate ATP, it is required to constantly synthesize enzymes, structural proteins (like hair, skin, and muscle), and proteins for the immune system. This enables you to maintain your muscle mass and immune system. Only nine of the twenty dietary amino acids are considered essential, meaning they cannot be made by the body and therefore must be supplied by the diet. High-quality protein is defined as protein sources that supply adequate levels of those nine essential amino acids. The highest quality protein source is egg whites, followed by dairy protein, because both are rich in essential amino acids. However, egg white protein has a much lower effect on insulin secretion than does dairy protein making it the best overall protein source. Without adequate levels of those essential amino acids, it is impossible to have efficient protein synthesis to maintain, let alone build, muscle mass, support adequate immune responses, or repair damage caused by cellular inflammation. Furthermore, adequate dietary protein at every meal is also required to release certain satiety hormones (PYY and GLP-1) from the gut that travel directly to the hypothalamus via the vagus nerve to reduce hunger so that you don't overconsume calories.

Fat

There are two classes of fatty acids that constitute dietary fat. One class consists of essential omega-6 and omega-3 fatty acids that the body cannot synthesize and thus must be supplied by your diet because they are required to turn on and turn off inflammation. The other class consists of non-essential fatty acids (saturated and monounsaturated) that the body can synthesize.

You not only need both omega-6 and omega-3 fatty acids in your diet, but they must be in the correct balance to maintain a proper inflammatory response. Dietary intake of total essential fatty acids should have an approximate 2:1 ratio of omega-6 and omega-3 fatty acids. Today that ratio in Americans is about 20:1 of omega-6 fatty acids to omega-3 fatty acids. This mismatch generates an overproduction of pro-inflammatory eicosanoids.

Even though essential fatty acids are critical for life, the majority of your dietary fat intake consists of non-essential fatty acids, consisting of either saturated or monounsaturated fatty acids. These fats provide the materials for maintaining membrane structure and provide much of the fuel for ATP production. However, saturated fatty acids (especially palmitic acid) also stimulate inflammation, whereas monounsaturated fatty acids are non-inflammatory. This is why you want most of your incoming dietary fat to consist of monounsaturated fat. Olive oil, nuts, and avocados are great sources of monounsaturated fatty acids.

Vitamins

Vitamins are co-factors for a wide number of enzymes. Without adequate vitamin levels in the diet, enzymatic activity throughout the body will begin to slow, decreasing the efficiency of your metabolism.

The need for vitamins was only discovered with the advent of food processing in the late 19th century that removed them from natural foods (such as removing the outer bran of brown rice to make more shelf-stable white rice). Only when vitamin deficiencies began to develop from the increased use of refined carbohydrates was it realized that something in natural foods (i.e., vitamins) were essential to human health. In fact, one of the sure pathways to winning a Nobel Prize in the early part of the 20th century was to discover a new vitamin. The richest source of vitamins with the least number of calories are non-starchy vegetables. These are also excellent sources of minerals, so if you are getting enough fermentable fiber, you are probably getting adequate levels of minerals.

Polyphenols

In my opinion, polyphenols should also be considered essential nutrients since we now know they function as activators of various gene transcription factors critical for managing inflammation, metabolism, tissue repair, and the rate of aging as well as maintaining gut health. These essential nutrients are found primarily in non-starchy vegetables, fruits, legumes, and nuts. However, their naturally occurring concentration in these foods is low ranging from 0.1 to 0.2 percent of the total weight. Since your daily intake should be between 500 mg and 1,500 mg of polyphenols, this requires the consumption of large amounts of these foods. Since improved blood glucose control is another major goal for the Zone Pro-Resolution Nutrition system, the primary sources of polyphenols should come from low glycemic-load carbohydrates (such as non-starchy vegetables, fruits, and nuts). This means consuming primarily non-starchy vegetables with limited amount of fruits or nuts. Although whole grains also contain polyphenols, they are considered high-glycemic load carbohydrates, since the entry rate of glucose from whole grain products into the blood is virtually the same as the same products made with re-fined carbohydrates. Thus, both refined and whole-grain carbohydrates generate an excessive insulin response that can rapidly drive down blood glucose levels leading to hunger and fatigue within a few hours after their consumption.

Fermentable fiber

Fiber is also not currently considered an essential nutrient but it does contain a subclass of total fiber known as fermentable fiber. Fermentable fiber is an absolute requirement for maintaining a healthy gut. This is because the fermentation by-products of fermentable fiber (short-chain fatty acids or SCFA) are critical for maintaining gut health as I described earlier. The percentage of fermentable fiber in total fiber is highly vari-able ranging from zero in refined carbohydrates to nearly 50 percent in raw asparagus. I and most health authorities feel that you have to con-sume at least 30 grams of total fiber per day to provide adequate levels of fermentable fiber for the bacteria in your gut.

Carbohydrates

Theoretically there are no essential carbohydrates. However, the brain is the primary user of the body's glucose intake as it consumes nearly 20 percent of the body's total daily energy production even though it ac-counts for only 2 percent of your body's weight. Unlike other organs that can use both fatty acids and glucose to produce ATP for energy, the brain can only use glucose. To produce that amount of energy the brain con-sumes much of the circulating blood glucose. Therefore, maintaining an adequate intake of dietary carbohydrates to maintain stable blood glucose levels is essential for optimal brain function. The brain requires about 130 grams of glucose per day. If you consume too few carbohydrates to main-tain brain function, then the brain increases the secretion of the hormone cortisol that starts breaking down protein in your muscles to make glu-cose for the brain. This process is called neo-glucogenesis. On the other hand, if your carbohydrate intake is too high, then your pancreas secretes excessive levels of the hormone insulin that can accelerate cellular in-flammation (especially in the presence of excess omega-6 fatty acids) as well as promoting the storage of excess carbohydrates as body fat (primarily as palmitic acid). If you want to maintain an optimal metabolism, you also need to maintain a zone of carbohydrate intake.

Furthermore, there are also carbohydrate-containing glycoproteins and glycolipids that are critical for cellular signaling. These glycoproteins and glycolipids often contain unique carbohydrates (such as fucose, mannose, sialic acid, etc.) that theoretically can be synthesized by the body from glucose. However, if there is a defect in their synthesis, then eating mushrooms or sea vegetables (primarily seaweeds) that are rich in those unique carbohydrates can help ensure that adequate levels of these specialized carbohydrates are maintained in the body.

The key factor of the Zone Diet is to obtain adequate levels of these essential nutrients with the least number of calories. At the same time, you need to eat enough calories to produce ATP, maintain stable blood glucose levels, manage inflammation, and maintain the ongoing renewal process for the tissue in every organ. Beyond those levels, any excess incoming calories will be stored as body fat that can become a reservoir for the potential development of future diet-induced inflammation leading to the early development of chronic disease and accelerate the rate of aging.

Although it seems that balancing all of these nutrients with the least number of calories may seem difficult, following the Zone Diet makes it easy to adapt this as a lifelong habit leading to a longer healthspan. This is why the first step to optimizing the Resolution Response starts with the Zone Diet.

DIET FALLACIES

The complexity of metabolism makes it a fertile ground for many misconceptions. I have advocated for more than thirty years that diet-induced inflammation makes you fat and keeps you fat as well as increasing the likelihood of developing chronic disease and accelerating the rate of aging. Unfortunately, this is a difficult concept to convey to the general public. What people want to hear is that there is some dietary villain that only needs to be banished from the diet that will magically reverse our growing epidemics of obesity and diabetes yet doesn't require much thinking or commitment on their part, especially relative to any thought of calorie restriction. They are looking for some magic formula that allows them to eat as much food as possible and never gain weight. So, let me outline some of the usual suspects of this flawed thinking.

IF IT IS TOO GOOD TO BE TRUE, THEN IT PROBABLY IS

In an effort to maintain wellness (usually defined by most people as not yet having enough organ damage to require chronic medication to manage its symptoms), we often jump from one popular dietary panacea to another to better manage our weight, try to stay well, or at least better manage an existing chronic disease. We love to hear things in the media that give us a license to indulge and ignore the scientific research that we know is probably true but is not to our liking. Here are some of the likely myths you will find.

Fat is bad

Since obesity is really defined by the accumulation of excess body fat, then simply following a dietary program based on the concept that "if no fat touches your lips, no fat will reach your hips" would make perfect sense. However, not all fats are bad. Some are pro-inflammatory, others non-inflammatory, and still others are pro-resolution fats. Excess omega-6 fatty acids and palmitic acid are the real culprits because of their inflammatory consequences. Monounsaturated fats are non-inflammatory and omega-3 fatty acids are pro-resolution fats. Therefore, taking much of the omega-6 and saturated fatty acids out of the diet and replacing them with monounsaturated fat and omega-3 fatty acids makes good sense.

Unfortunately, this "fat is bad" thinking has usually been interpreted as a scorched earth policy that also removes monounsaturated fats such as oleic acid that are non-inflammatory and the omega-3 fatty acids that are necessary to generate the hormones needed for the resolution of cellular inflammation. Furthermore, since proteins contain fat, they are also usually restricted on a typical low-fat diet. As a result, you'll feel less satiated because the hormones PYY and GLP-1 are not released in high enough amounts by the gut as the protein content of the meal decreases. These low-fat, low-protein, and high-carbohydrate diets remain consumer-friendly (who doesn't like bread, rice, and pasta), but often result in hormonal disasters especially if the carbohydrates are rich in high-glycemic load grains and starches. The industrialized food giants were able to seize upon this "fat is bad" trend to churn a wide number of fat-free foods in the early 1980s that contributed greatly to the beginnings of our current obesity and diabetes epidemics because they had a high-glycemic response that contributed to constant hunger as well as being deficient in fermentable fiber and polyphenols. The result was not only excess calorie consumption caused by increased hunger, but also a corresponding decrease in gut health which is one of the causes of gut-induced inflammation that leads to obesity and early development of chronic disease.

Carbohydrates are bad

The carbohydrate-insulin theory states that carbohydrates make you fat because they increase insulin levels, whereas fat, especially saturated fat, doesn't. This has led to the vigorous advocacy of ketogenic diets that supposedly give you a "metabolic advantage" so you can eat more calories and lose weight. It is true that radically reducing carbohydrates in the diet will rapidly deplete the glycogen stores in your liver needed to help maintain blood glucose levels. However, it takes a lot of bound water to hydrate that stored liver glycogen. So, as liver glycogen levels rapidly decrease, this bound water is also released. As a result, on a ketogenic diet you rapidly lose retained water via urination and see a rapid weight loss on the scale. However, losing stored water is different than losing stored body fat. When researchers compared a high-fat ketogenic diet to a high-carbohydrate diet containing an equal number of calories, there was no difference in the fat loss between the two diets.

It is also stated that ketogenic diets provide a "metabolic advantage", so you can theoretically eat more calories and lose weight. Yet carefully controlled experiments published in 2006 compared the Zone Diet to a high-fat ketogenic diet demonstrated there was no "metabolic advantage" of ketogenic diet compared to the Zone Diet. However, the high-fat ketogenic diet dramatically increases cellular inflammation compared to the Zone Diet in only six weeks. Other publications using the same subjects also demonstrated that a high-fat ketogenic diet also induces greater fatigue upon mild exercise and causes accelerated loss of calcium potentially leading to bone loss. Both of these adverse metabolic consequence were observed as early as two weeks after starting a high-fat ketogenic diet.

If your intake of carbohydrates is too low, then brain function becomes compromised. Even under conditions of complete starvation, blood sugar levels in humans never drop below 65 mg/dL (90 mg/dL is considered a normal glucose level). This is because glucose is the primary fuel used by the mitochondria in the brain to generate the tremendous amount of ATP needed to maintain cognitive function. Therefore, to maintain minimal glucose levels in the blood, the body increases cortisol production to breakdown muscle mass into glucose (i.e., neo-glucogenesis). Unfortunately, the increased cortisol secreted in this process also depresses the immune system and increases fat storage by promoting insulin resistance. It is insulin resistance, not insulin per se, that makes you fat and keeps you fat.

Finally, advocates of high-fat ketogenic diets tend to forget that carbohydrates don't cause constantly elevated levels of insulin because insulin levels rapidly rise and fall with blood glucose levels unless you have insulin resistance. What actually causes insulin levels to remain elevated in the blood all the time is insulin resistance, and that is ultimately caused by cellular inflammation.

Fructose is bad

This theory came from the observation that the rise in obesity coincided with an increase in fructose content due to the introduction of high-fructose corn syrup as a sweetener in the American diet. It is true that fructose is more reactive than glucose, thus at unnaturally high (i.e., supra-physiological) levels, fructose can cause increased oxidative stress leading to increased fat formation in the liver. What hurts this hypothesis is that the use of high-fructose corn syrup in the United States peaked in 1999 and has been declining ever since, whereas obesity has not. Furthermore, recent animal and human studies show that when equivalent levels of fructose and glucose are provided, there is no difference between the two carbohydrates on any metabolic functions, let alone fat accumulation in the liver. Recent research also indicates that at normal levels of fructose consumption, the microbes in the small intestine will metabolize most of the fructose before it ever enters the body and possibly reach the liver. Also overlooked is the role of polyphenols in preventing oxidative stress. This is why an apple (rich in both fructose and polyphenols) is good for you, and excess amounts of high-fructose corn syrup (as well as table sugar) is not. Finally, humans don't absorb fructose from the small intestine efficiently unless it is in the presence of glucose that co-transports fructose into the blood via a glucose transporter located on the walls of the small intestine. It doesn't matter if it is high-fructose corn syrup (55 percent fructose/45 percent glucose) or table sugar or sucrose (50 percent fructose/50 percent glucose), these usual suspects will provide the necessary glucose to aid the entry of fructose into the blood. So, simply stated only use either table sugar or high-fructose corn syrup with great moderation.

One reason we are consuming less fructose since 1999 is because we are consuming more artificial sweeteners. Unfortunately, recent research indicates that the most commonly used artificial sweeteners disturb the bacterial composition in the gut resulting in a condition called metabolic endotoxemia, which increases inflammation. This helps explains why artificially sweetened soda consumption appears to increase hunger and weight gain. And if you eat more calories, you will gain weight even if your fructose consumption is decreased.

It should also be noted that fructose (especially in the form of fructose polymers) is one of the best fermentable sources of energy for the gut microbes to increase the production of short-chain fatty acids critical for gut health.

Gluten is bad

This theory states that gluten (the protein found in wheat products like bread, pizza and pasta, and certain grains such as rye and barley) causes inflammation that produces obesity as well as virtually every other chronic condition because of its negative impact on the gut. There are certain genetic markers that are necessary for an inflammatory response to gluten. Nearly 40 percent of the American population has those genetic markers, but less than 1 percent of the population has a true gluten intolerance that leads to celiac disease. So why don't the vast majority of those genetically susceptible people have celiac disease? The reason is that it depends on how healthy their gut is, and in particular the integrity of the mucus barrier that prevents any large protein fragment (defined as containing more than three amino acids) from getting close to the gut wall where it can cause an inflammatory response. This is why approximately 1 percent of any population will have an intolerance to any large protein fragments coming from products such as egg, casein, nuts, fish, etc. Large protein fragments that can cause allergenic responses can't reach the gut wall if there is a healthy mucus barrier. In addition, the permeability of the gut barrier itself is controlled by the balance of two proteins, occludin and zonulin. As discussed earlier, occludin is the protein in the gut wall that maintains a tight gut barrier whereas zonulin is a protein that causes a leaky gut by increasing the permeability of the gut wall. The synthesis of occludin can be stimulated by the presence of short-chain fatty acid by-products of the metabolism of fermentable fiber in the gut and its assembly into the gut wall is activated by AMP kinase stimulated by dietary polyphenols. While it is true that gluten increases zonulin synthesis, it does so only if gluten gets past the mucus barrier, which is the first line of protection for the gut wall. It also has to penetrate the barrier of the gut wall, which is your second line of protection, before interacting with the immune cells behind the gut wall. One of the key benefits of the Zone Pro-Resolution Nutrition system is to rebuild the mucus barrier and maintain a healthy gut wall by supplying adequate levels of fermentable fiber to activate mucus production by the goblet cells in the gut wall as well as activating AMP kinase to maintain a tight junction in the gut wall making it difficult for gluten or any other large protein fragments from reaching the immune cells in the gut.

Another unexpected cause of a leaky gut are high levels of eicosanoids, in particular, leukotrienes. That gives rise to not only a leaky gut, but also leaky blood vessels as well as a leaky brain. Over the past forty years, celiac disease and food allergies to proteins have significantly increased. At the same time, the intake of fermentable fiber has significantly decreased due largely to the increasing consumption of refined carbohydrates. This combination could very well lead to both a weakened mucus barrier as well as a more permeable gut wall (i.e., a leaky gut). Add to this a growing increase in the generation of eicosanoids such as leukotrienes, coming from the excess intake of omega-6 fatty acids and you have gut trouble. Gluten was simply caught in the crossfire of these two dietary trends.

Furthermore, individuals who have "gluten-sensitivity" are more likely to have sensitivity to FODMAPs (Fermentable Oligo-, Di-, Monosaccharides, and Alcohol Products) also found in bread products. Carefully controlled studies have indicated that when "gluten-sensitive" individuals are put on a low FODMAP diet and then challenged with gluten, there are no adverse effects. It appears that FODMAPs may be the cause of "gluten sensitivity," not gluten per se. It should be noted that lactose is one of the FODMAPs, meaning if you have lactose-intolerance (as does 65 percent of the world's population), then it is likely you will also have a FODMAP intolerance.

I agree that increased inflammation will definitely make you fat, but making gluten the cause of that inflammation is unsupported although it has created a multi-billion dollar "gluten-free" processed food industry similar to the rapid rise of the "fat-free" processed food industry in the 1980s.

Finally, the gluten-free products developed by the food industry for "gluten-sensitive" individuals are very low in fermentable fiber. Lack of fermentable fiber is a primary dietary reason for developing a leaky gut. In addition, these gluten-free products having a higher glycemic response than the wheat products they are replacing thus making you hungrier the more of them you eat. This is great news for the food manufacturers whose sagging sales of fat-free products are now being replaced by the growing sales of gluten-free products without missing a beat.

Dairy is bad

Another food group that has gotten a bad reputation is dairy, and many popular diets restrict "evil" dairy products altogether.

It is true that about 65 percent of the world's population is lactose-intolerant, but human breast milk is very rich in lactose, and is considered nature's most perfect food. What gives? Human breast milk is recommended as the infant's sole source of nutrition during the first four to six months of life. This makes sense since it's rich in high-quality protein, omega-3 fatty acids (and resolvins), and unique sugar polymers needed to establish and maintain the ideal microbial composition in the gut for an infant. The down side is you'll be hard pressed to find human breast milk in your local supermarket aisle, whereas you will find a massive selection of cow's milk that also contains lactose. So, why is human breast milk good, but dairy milk is bad? The answer is epigenetics.

All newborn children have the enzyme (lactase) in their gut that allows them to breakdown the disaccharide lactose found in human breast milk into two simple sugars (galactose and glucose) that can easily be absorbed. This is important because if the lactose makes its way to the colon, then it is often the cause of gastric disturbances (i.e., lactose intolerance).

Children and other mammals nourished by maternal milk are genetically programmed to lose the lactase enzyme activity with time. This is part of your epigenetic programming where certain genes are turned off with development. In children who become lactose intolerant, the lactase activity is usually gone by age seven, whereas other mammals lose this enzyme activity in a much shorter period of time. The most likely reason is that it becomes very difficult for the maternal milk supply alone to provide the increased calorie needs for a growing infant or calf and therefore shutting down lactase production is a good way to force the growing child or calf to start using other food sources.

That all changed with the advent of dairy farming. For that very small number of humans (probably less than 1 percent) that continued to keep generating the lactase enzyme, they now had a survival advantage over those who didn't because dairy milk could be used as a source of high-quality protein in times of famine and was also a relatively uncontaminated source of liquid.

Today about 35 percent of the world's population is lactose persistent. For them, dairy products are an excellent source of high-quality protein. On the other hand, the other 65 percent of the world's population will have a difficult time consuming any dairy at all. Considering 10,000 years ago virtually no one maintained the continued expression of the gene for lactase persistence, this is a dramatic increase of a particular gene pool. The development of lactose-tolerant individuals has become the best example of natural genetic selection in humans caused by a cultural change. In other words, dairy milk gave this otherwise small segment of the human population a significant survival advantage over everyone else.

One of the first applications of biotechnology some 6,000 years ago was to reduce the lactose levels in dairy products. This provided new protein sources for those individuals that were still genetically lactose intolerant. Two of these early biotechnology products were yogurt and cheese. Yogurt was only a partial solution since the lactose concentration was still relatively high, being reduced from about 5 percent lactose in whole milk to about 3-4 percent lactose in traditional yogurt. However, for many, that reduction was enough for them to tolerate the remaining lactose. Yogurt production uses live bacteria (i.e., probiotics) to partially reduce the lactose levels in yogurt by converting lactose into lactic acid thereby giving yogurt its bitter taste. On the other hand, cheese production was much more efficient in lactose removal from dairy milk. First, you remove much of the lactose by acidifying the milk. This precipitates out the casein fraction (i.e., curds) of milk protein from much of the whey protein and lactose remaining in solution. Then you treat the curds with rennet (a complex of enzymes isolated from the stomachs of ruminants like cows, sheep, and goats) to better digest the lactose completely to galactose and glucose instead of using probiotics as in the production of yogurt. Then you age the cheese to ferment it even further to remove still more lactose. This is why some hard cheeses are nearly lactose-free depending on the production method and extent of aging.

The production of yogurt and cheese that gave many humans (in particular those who did not maintain lactase production) a vastly improved survival advantage using a sustainable source of protein as a growing reliance was now being placed on farming instead of hunting for protein requirements. These individuals had a greater chance for survival because they had a more consistent and plentiful source of high-quality protein. The newest technology that can take this a step further is the development of lactose-free milk. Using a similar enzyme technology compared to cheese making, it is possible to reduce the lactose level in dairy milk to zero. Most importantly, you don't need to a have an epigenetic mutation (only 35 percent of humans have such a mutation) to enjoy these nutritional benefits of high-quality sustainable protein as long as you are consuming lactose-free dairy milk. The same is true of food products such as shakes and bars made with lactose-free dairy protein.

Then there is another argument that dairy products cause cancer. A little common sense goes a long way to address that statement. People in northern Europe have little lactose intolerance and consume considerable amounts of dairy products with no decimation of their populations by cancer.

The cancer-promoting theory is based on the association of insulin-like growth factor 1 (IGF-1) with cancer. Dairy products do increase IGF-1, but so does intense exercise. IGF-1 is a hormone released from the liver in response to growth hormone secreted by the pituitary gland after intense exercise as discussed in my book, *The Anti-Aging Zone*. IGF-1 is structurally similar to insulin and is partially responsible for muscle growth. Furthermore, when you perform calorie-restriction studies in humans, their general health increases, but there is no change in their IGF-1 levels. So, something doesn't make sense here. If there is a shred of potential for the idea that dairy has a connection to cancer, it's because dairy protein, egg whites, and human breast milk are rich in the essential amino acid leucine. This is why they are termed high-quality proteins. Leucine is the only amino acid that can stimulate another gene transcription factor known as mTOR that is essential for muscle building. mTOR is more strongly related to cancer than is IGF-1, but without stimulation of mTOR you lose muscle mass creating sarcopenia (i.e., loss of muscle) as you age. Obviously neither cancer nor frailty are desirable outcomes as both can lead to an earlier death.

This is where the Zone Pro-Resolution Nutrition system comes to the rescue. The gene transcription factor AMP kinase is stimulated by following the Zone Pro-Resolution Nutrition system (especially supplementation with adequate levels of polyphenol extracts) and will reduce the levels of mTOR by activating AMP kinase. As a result, by following the Zone Pro-Resolution Nutrition system program you can maintain the correct intake of leucine needed to maintain muscle mass to prevent frailty as well as preventing any increase in mTOR. As usual in nutrition, it is a matter of balance.

Lectins are Bad

Lectins are proteins used by plants to defend themselves against microbial invaders. Think of them as a sort of a stripped-down human immune system. The lectins bind to glycoprotein or glycolipid surface components of the potential microbial invaders and makes it difficult to penetrate into the interior of the plant cell. Commercially, isolated lectins are used to distinguish blood group types, so you don't get the wrong red blood cell group type during a transfusion that could kill you. But there is a big difference between testing isolated blood for transfusions and eating plants that contain high levels of lectins. The primary plants that contain lectins are legumes, wheat (keeping in mind that gluten is not a lectin), and members of the nightshade family (peppers, tomatoes, eggplant, potato, and Goji berries). The contention that lectins create inflammation is only likely if the lectin reaches the gut wall and actually enters into the blood via a leaky gut to cause trouble. For most individuals, this means gaining weight and developing diabetes. Frankly, following the Zone Pro-Resolution Nutrition system will have a far greater effect on preventing weight gain and developing diabetes than trying to remove lectins from the diet. Lectins, like gluten and other proteins, are relatively harmless if you have a healthy gut. Furthermore, lectins are easily denatured by heat especially using a pressure cooker. If you are concerned about lectins causing inflammation, then I would first rebuild the gut with a combination of omega-3 fatty acids, polyphenols, and fermentable fiber described earlier, before you consider avoiding the consumption of food products containing lectins which are the hallmarks of the Mediterranean diet.

Just as we are constantly reminded about the "evil" food ingredients that should be eliminated, there is a corresponding list of "good" ingredients coming from social media that we are constantly told should be included our diet.

Alcohol is good

We are told that alcohol is good for the heart and therefore good for our health. This is great news for the alcoholic beverage industry, but not so true for the rest of us. Alcohol is a toxic substance. Furthermore, about one in seven who drink alcohol will ultimately develop a dependency on alcohol because it has the potential to hijack your dopamine reward system. The only benefit to drinking red wine is that it contains polyphenols. Keep in mind that the key polyphenols in red wine are most likely delphinidins and this means drinking a lot of red wine to consume enough delphinidins to see any significant health benefits.

Red wine is actually a poor man's polyphenol delivery system just as alcoholic herbal tinctures were the primary drugs of the 19th century. Of course, a lot of people don't like the strong taste of red wine and find white wine more pleasing. That is because white wine contains 10 times fewer polyphenols than red wine, but with the same amount of alcohol. Beer is even lower on the polyphenol delivery chart, and finally vodka brings up the rear, containing absolutely no polyphenols whatsoever.

But what about all the research that supports drinking? Most of that comes from epidemiological studies, which means the conclusions are highly dependent on how the trial was organized. Furthermore, if it is a purely observational study, then it only suggests a possible intervention trial should be undertaken to see if the hypothesis has any true validity.

A recent analysis of all the epidemiology trials suggesting that alcohol may be beneficial for heart disease may be suspect since most of the studies included former drinkers who had stopped drinking in the "abstainer" group. If you drank alcohol in excess in the past, you are going to have a lot of residual collateral damage. Since true alcohol abstainers are also included in that overall group, this dilutes the actual benefits of never consuming alcohol. If you are comparing everything to that "currently abstaining" group, then moderate drinking groups might look good in comparison. This is reinforced by a recent British study over a 30-year period strongly suggesting that any drinking at all will cause a shrinkage of the hippocampus in the brain. This makes sense since it is estimated that every alcoholic drink causes the death of about 10,000 nerve cells in the brain. Over thirty years, that can add up. Finally, a recent large-scale global study has indicated the optimal alcohol intake for decreasing all-cause mortality should be zero.

SUMMARY ▶

The food ingredients in your diet and how they affect your metabolism are incredibly complex. Once you know the facts about dietary ingredients, then you can begin to understand how various unsupported food fallacies have emerged. How these facts and fallacies shape our current nutritional debates about diets is discussed in the next chapter.

14

Diet Wars

COMPARISON OF THE ZONE DIET TO OTHER DIETS

IN THE PREVIOUS chapter, I discussed some of the facts and fallacies of various dietary nutrients. In this chapter I want to discuss how many of those dietary fallacies have been turned into diet philosophies that have left most Americans totally confused as to what to eat and why.

There are three things in life that are based on belief: politics, religion, and diets. Once you are convinced of a belief, you will defend that belief to the death. At least with diets, you can measure them objectively in controlled clinical trials and let the facts speak for themselves.

THE ZONE DIET VERSUS POPULAR DIETS

Zone Diet versus the Mediterranean diet

As I pointed out in my book, *The Mediterranean Zone*, there is no real definition of a Mediterranean diet. There are some 16 different countries that line the Mediterranean Sea and the cuisine is very different in each country. (For example, only in Italy do people eat a lot of pasta.) However, all the diets of this region put an emphasis on fruits and vegetables, just like the Zone Diet. Also, fish and chicken are the primary sources of lean protein which is similar to the Zone Diet and at consumption levels similar to the Zone Diet. Finally, olive oil and nuts are the primary sources of fat just like the Zone Diet.

The major difference between the Zone Diet and the Mediterranean diet is the reduced intake of grains (breads and pasta) and starches (potatoes and rice) with a corresponding increase in non-starchy vegetables and fruits. That one seemingly small dietary difference has significant hormonal implications. By replacing the grains and starches found in the Mediterranean diet with even more vegetables and fruits, the Zone Diet represents the evolution of the Mediterranean diet with fewer calories, more fermentable fiber, and more polyphenols and with far better blood glucose control. While the Mediterranean diet is a good (even if totally undefined) diet, the Zone Diet represents a hormonally superior choice with a high degree of dietary definition that results in the reduction of insulin resistance and cellular inflammation.

What about the studies that "prove" the Mediterranean diet is the best diet? The most quoted study (Prevention with the Mediterranean Diet or PREDIMED) was designed to show that changing the diet of individuals (primarily located in the Spain) to a more Mediterranean diet could be useful in preventing cardiovascular disease. Initially all the subjects were eating a relatively high-fat diet. The subjects were then divided into three groups. One group was given free nuts and regular intensive counseling on how to incorporate the principles of the Mediterranean diet (more fruits and vegetables) into their daily diet. The second group was given free olive oil and intensive regular counseling on how to incorporate the principles of the Mediterranean diet (more fruit and vegetables) into their daily diet. The third group (the control group) was given nothing outside the advice to consume less fat.

You are probably thinking to yourself, that's not a very good study. You are right, yet the PREDIMED study was published in the *New England Journal of Medicine* in 2013 and was considered the most import dietary trial in the last decade. Of course, you would never realize this design flaw by simply reading the article. You must go to the supplemental material embedded only in the electronic files of the *New England Journal of Medicine*. Here is what it stated:

"The initial dietary protocol for the Control group started with the delivery of a leaflet summarizing the recommendations to follow a low-fat diet and scheduled one yearly visit. In October 2006, three years into the trial, we realized that such a low-grade intervention might potentially be a weakness of the trial and amended the protocol to include quarterly individual and group sessions with delivery of food descriptions, shopping lists, meal plans, and recipes (adapted to the low-fat diet) in such a way that the intensity of the intervention was similar to that of the Mediterranean diet groups, except for the provision of supplemental food for free."

In essence, the PREDIMED study was not very well designed. The reason why is the control group never changed their diet to a low-fat diet. Yet this terribly designed and executed study has generated more than 200 additional papers on the "superiority" of the Mediterranean diet. In fact, this trial demonstrated two things. First, if you give people free food, they will eat it and second, it is hard for people to change their diet without giving them free food. The original study was retracted in 2018 and republished with amended results acknowledging that they should have done a more controlled study even though the data were relatively similar to the first trial.

I personally spend a lot of time in Italy and Spain and I always have the same meal for lunch and dinner: grilled vegetables as my appetizer, grilled fish with more grilled vegetables as my entrée, and fresh fruit for dessert. It works every time. Of course, I add olive oil to my meals. I guess you would call my diet in Italy and Spain the Zone Diet Mediterranean style.

Zone Diet versus ketogenic diets

What about ketogenic diets? A ketogenic diet is a high-fat, very low-carbohydrate diet designed to generate ketosis. Ketosis is a condition in which the liver becomes deficient in stored carbohydrates and therefore can't completely convert fat into carbon dioxide and water to produce ATP. This deficiency of stored carbohydrates in the liver produced by following a ketogenic diet also means that there is no way to stabilize blood sugar levels between meals. Furthermore, instead of a normal clean oxidation of the fatty acids to carbon dioxide and water for the generation of ATP, you now get metabolic by-products termed ketone bodies circulating in the blood that the body tries to reduce by increased urination. The Zone Diet, on the other hand, is a protein-adequate, carbohydrate-moderate, low-fat diet that prevents ketosis.

Ketogenic diets were first made popular by Robert Atkins in the 1970s, and they rise and fall in popularity with each new generation. With the resurgence of ketogenic diets in the early part of this century, I published a carefully controlled head-to-head clinical comparison of the Zone Diet and a ketogenic diet in 2006. Using overweight and obese subjects, each group ate meals prepared for them and consumed the same number of calories (about 1,500 calories per day) and the same levels of protein at each meal. The only variable was the fat-to-carbohydrate ratio at each meal. The results? The subjects following the Zone Diet lost more weight and body fat than the subjects following the ketogenic diet meaning there was "no metabolic advantage" to the ketogenic diet. In fact, those who followed the ketogenic diet saw their levels of cellular inflammation (as measured by the AA/EPA ratio) double in six weeks. Additional analysis demonstrated that those following the ketogenic diet had higher levels of fatigue when performing mild exercise and they lost calcium most likely from their bones. These are not strong selling points for a ketogenic diet.

Compared to all other high-carbohydrate diets under less controlled clinical conditions, the ketogenic diets do show more initial weight loss, but after one year there are no differences in terms of weight loss between the two types of diets. Furthermore, a very recent study under metabolic ward conditions in which all food consumed is tightly controlled demonstrated that a ketogenic diet actually generates less fat loss than a high-carbohydrate diet. More ominously, in animal studies conducted at Yale Medical School in 2010 it was demonstrated that while a ketogenic diet did reduce total body weight and serum insulin levels, there was a significant increase of insulin resistance in the liver. This is usually the first step toward developing type 2 diabetes.

Zone Diet versus longevity diets

We also hear a lot of talk about areas in the world that people seem to have greater longevity and a longer healthspan. Unfortunately, most of these regions also have poorly documented birth and medical records meaning the stated ages of those being interviewed may be somewhat suspect. The only region of reported longevity that does have legitimate birth and medical records is the island of Okinawa. So, how does the Zone Diet stack up against the Okinawan diet?

There are several similarities between the two diets. First both diets tend to be calorie-restricted with the typical Okinawan diet providing about 1,800 calories per day. The Okinawans also eat significant amounts of fish, eat little rice (it's hard to grow rice on a volcanic island), and consume more pork and tofu than other Asian populations. The carbohydrate content of the Okinawan diet comes primarily from a purple potato unique to Okinawa, which is exceptionally rich in polyphenols (that's why it is purple). While the Okinawan diet contains fewer non-starchy vegetables than the Zone Diet, it is a calorie-restricted diet rich in omega-3 fatty acids and polyphenols making it similar to the Zone Pro-Resolution Nutrition system. Okinawa also has the highest percentage of centenarians per capita in the world as well as having the longest healthspan on the planet. This might suggest that following the Zone Diet would potentially generate the same results.

Zone Diet versus intermittent fasting

It's clear that calorie-restriction can have significant health benefits. Can those benefits be enhanced or easier to obtain by adding the concept of intermittent fasting? Intermittent fasting is based on the idea that continuous calorie restriction is too hard to follow on a long-term basis. So maybe you can just do it for a couple of days with mini-fasts, knowing you can overeat the next day. In one version of intermittent fasting, you eat normally (of course this is what probably caused the weight gain in the first place) for five days and then do a limited fast of about 500 calories per day for two days. This is known as either the 5:2 diet or the Fast diet. Another version has you alternating partial-fasting days (25 percent of your normal calorie diet) with mini-feast (125 percent of your normal calorie intake) days as reward days resulting in an overall diet consisting of 75 percent of your normal calorie intake instead of following a constantly calorie-restricted diet providing 75 percent of your normal calorie intake every day. Regardless of the approach, recently published long-term studies have demonstrated no benefits of intermittent fasting compared to consuming the same number of restricted calories day in and day out. Furthermore, there is no difference in weight loss. However, the subjects were less compliant on the intermittent fasting diet—probably because they were hungrier on their mini-fasting days. The same lack of differences between consistent calorie restriction (like the Zone Diet) and intermittent fasting is also found in a recent long-term study with type 2 diabetics.

On the other hand, on the Zone Diet you are never hungry or mentally fatigued because of consistent hormonal control you can easily follow for a lifetime.

Zone Diet versus Paleolithic diets

As I stated in my first book, *The Zone*, the Zone Diet was developed based on a short article describing the potential composition of Paleolithic diets published in the *New England Journal of Medicine* in 1985. I am very big on the idea of attribution. That's why I included an entire chapter in *The Zone* (it's Chapter 9: Evolution and The Zone) outlining the origin of what eventually became the Zone Diet.

In 2010, various academic scientists including Boyd Eaton, one of the authors of the 1985 *New England Journal of Medicine* article published the most up-to-date data on the best analysis of the macronutrient composition of the Paleolithic diet some 15,000 years ago. Their estimates were that it consisted of 39–40 percent low-glycemic load carbohydrates (i.e., vegetables and fruits), 25–29 percent low-fat protein, and 31–39 percent fat. That's close enough for me to the average macronutrient composition of the Zone Diet (40 percent low-glycemic load carbohydrates, 30 percent low-fat protein, and 30 percent fat). Moreover, it is clear that based on those macronutrient percentages that neither the Zone Diet or a real Paleolithic diet are ketogenic diets.

There are two primary differences between a Paleo diet and the Zone Diet. The first difference is that the Zone Diet starts with your calculated protein requirements that are unique to you. Since the absolute levels of protein consumption is left unstated in Paleo diets, this potentially could lead to the potential overconsumption of protein as well as consumption of excess calories. The second difference is that wheat, legumes, dairy, and alcohol are not to be consumed on the Paleo diet because they didn't exist 15,000 years ago. As I described in the previous chapter, the absolute elimination of wheat, legumes (as well as lectins), and dairy protein may not stand up to closer examination. Relative to alcohol, I always caution moderation to the extreme because of alcohol's effects on developing a leaky gut as well as a leaky brain. However, I personally agree with the recent study in *Lancet* that the ideal consumption of alcohol is probably zero. Other than those differences, the Paleo diet and the Zone Diet are like two peas in a pod (even though peas are legumes).

ZONE DIET VERSUS MEDICAL DIETS

The Zone Diet was not developed as a weight-loss program, but a lifelong dietary program to better manage diet-induced inflammation which I believe is a major factor in the development of most chronic diseases. Medical diets are designed to manage a chronic disease condition meaning that they should be followed for a lifetime to better manage that specific condition. Many medical diets like the American Heart Association diet and the American Diabetes Association diet have pretty much been failures in managing heart disease and diabetes. However, others have had more success. Three of those are the DASH diet, MIND diet, and Joslin Diabetes diet.

DASH diet (1997)

This diet started as a research study put together by Harvard and Johns Hopkins researchers to lower blood pressure. The study was initially called Dietary Approaches to Stop Hypertension. That's a mouthful, so it was shortened to the DASH diet.

The major breakthrough for the DASH diet was recommending more vegetables and fruits (they are rich in potassium) and more protein (like low-fat dairy) than the recommendations of the American Heart Association diet. Somewhat like a poor man's Zone Diet.

Somehow in the subsequent years, the annual ratings of the *U.S. News and World Report* has ranked the DASH diet as the best diet in America for everything ranging from weight loss to diabetes as well as treating hypertension. But let's see how this diet stacks up against the Zone Diet in both percent macronutrients and total calories.

For comparison, I have taken the caloric average for males (1,500 calories/day) and females (1,200 calories/day) on the Zone Diet to get an average of 1,350 calories/day to compare to the 2,000 calorie daily recommendation for the DASH diet.

	Zone Diet	DASH diet
Calories/day	1,350	2,000
% Carbs	40	55
% Protein	30	18
% Fat	30	27
Servings of fruit/day	2	4-5
Serving of vegetables/day	8	4-5
Servings of grains/day	0-1	7-8

Notice that you would be eating a lot more vegetables, a little less fruit, and a lot fewer grains on the Zone Diet compared to the DASH diet. That's means the glycemic load on the Zone Diet is far lower than the DASH diet.

To underscore this point, I did the math to see how these recommendations would translate into grams per day.

	Zone Diet	DASH diet
Carbs per day	135 grams	275 grams
Protein per day	101 grams	90 grams
Fat per day	45 grams	60 grams

Following the Zone Diet, you would be consuming less fat, about the same amount of protein, and far fewer carbohydrates (and with a much lower glycemic load) than the DASH diet and have a protein-to-glycemic load ratio that would provide better hormonal responses. So, based on the actual amount of protein, carbohydrates, and fat grams consumed, the Zone Diet seems to make more medical sense.

I also made similar calculations on sodium, potassium, and fiber based on the two diets.

	Zone Diet	DASH diet
Sodium	1,600 mg	2,300 mg
Potassium	5,200 mg	4,700 mg
Fiber	40 g	30 g

The Zone Diet supplies more fiber and potassium than the DASH diet because it contains more vegetables. In addition, vegetables are the richest source of nitrates of any food group known. This is important for the treatment of hypertension since nitrates can potentially be converted (especially in the presence of polyphenols) into nitric oxide (NO) that is the most powerful agent known to reduce blood pressure. Finally, the Zone Diet contains significantly less sodium than the DASH diet. Isn't reducing sodium one of the ways to treat hypertension? I guess this makes the Zone Diet the equivalent of the "super-DASH" diet.

MIND diet (2015)

MIND stands for Mediterranean-DASH Intervention for Neurodegenerative Delay diet. This is a strange mixture of both the DASH diet and the Mediterranean diet to potentially slow the course of Alzheimer's disease. I say potentially, since only observational studies have been conducted on such a dietary approach.

There are ten "good" things to eat on the MIND diet and five "bad" things not to eat. Here is the list.

HEALTHY BRAIN FOODS

Green leafy vegetables: Six servings per week
Non-starchy vegetables: One serving per day
Nuts: Five servings per week
Berries: Two servings per week
Whole grains: Three servings per day
Fish: Eat fatty fish once a week
Beans: Eat four times per week
Chicken: Eat twice a week
Olive oil: Use as your main cooking oil
Wine: One glass per day

UNHEALTHY BRAIN FOODS

Red meats: No more than 3 servings per week
Butter and margarine: Eat less than 1 tablespoon per day
Cheese: No more than once per week
Pastries and sweets: No more than four times a week
Fried and fast foods: No more than one meal per week

I was expecting a little more detail on the MIND diet, but you take what you can get. Nonetheless, a published observational study indicated that the risk of Alzheimer's disease was 53 percent lower in people who closely followed the guidelines of the MIND diet and 35 percent lower in those who followed its guidelines only moderately well. Another purely observational study using the MIND diet suggested that better dietary adherence to its guidelines resulted in a slower decline in brain function. Interesting observations, but that's the type of current nutritional science that makes the PREDIMED study actually look good. Since the daily consumption of healthy brain foods are much greater following the Zone Diet, it would it seem to me that the Zone Diet would appear to be the more appropriate diet to follow for lowering the risk of Alzheimer's and decline in cognitive function.

Joslin Diabetes Center diet (2006)

When the Joslin Diabetes Center announced their new dietary guidelines for managing diabetes in 2006, they struck me as exceedingly similar to the ones spelled out in *The Zone*, published more than a decade earlier. Their guidelines were a calorie-restricted (1,200 to 1,500 calories per day) diet containing 40 percent low-glycemic carbohydrates, 30 percent low-fat protein, and 30 percent fat.

The Joslin Diabetes Center published a five-year study in 2017 on the effects of their diet on type 2 diabetics—one of the longest controlled diet studies of type 2 diabetics who have not undergone gastric bypass surgery. In this study, obese type 2 diabetics who had had lost 7 percent of their body weight by the end of the first year were able to keep much of the initial weight loss from returning over the next four years. And at the end of the five years, they were successful with keeping the weight off as well as having a lower HbA_{1c} (one of the clinical markers that defines the Zone) indicating better long-term control of blood sugar levels.

Of course, once you add high-dose omega-3 fatty acids and polyphenols to the Zone Diet to optimize the Resolution Response you now have the potential to regenerate beta cells in the pancreas and perhaps begin to reverse diabetes?

All of these comparisons to existing medical diets would strongly suggest that following the Zone Diet would be an appropriate dietary treatment for the improved management of hypertension, Alzheimer's, and diabetes. Adding supplemental high-dose ultra-refined omega-3 fatty acids and purified polyphenols to the Zone Diet will only further enhance the optimization of the Resolution Response.

SUMMARY ▶

People will always have strong opinions about diets. That's why you must analyze them in the crucible of controlled clinical trials where the diet is highly controlled. More than 30 clinical trials have been published demonstrating that the Zone Diet is superior in terms of appetite control, fat loss, reduction of blood sugar, blood lipids, and most importantly, the reduction of cellular inflammation compared to all other diets.

The Zone Diet is an anti-inflammatory diet because it represents a combination of both hormonal and gene therapy. It reduces the formation of pro-inflammatory eicosanoids and reduces the activation of NF-κB (the master genetic switch for inflammation) by reducing both diet-induced and gut-induced inflammation. That's why the Zone Diet is the necessary first step for improving the Resolution Response. But to optimize the Resolution Response, you will also need supplemental omega-3 fatty acids and polyphenols. That is the description of the Zone Pro-Resolution Nutrition system. With such a comprehensive nutritional system, you have all the dietary components needed for your journey back toward wellness.

15

Zone Protein

MAKING THE ZONE DIET
EVEN EASIER TO FOLLOW

AS **SHOWN IN** the previous chapter, if you want to follow a dietary program to reduce inflammation in order to better manage a chronic disease, then the Zone Diet seems like the obvious choice. Unfortunately, dietary reality can be summarized in this quote from Margaret Mead, the great American anthropologist, when she said: "It is easier to change a man's religion than to change his diet."

One of the major hormonal benefits of the Zone Diet is achieved by simply giving up many foods (the 3 Ps; pizza, pasta, and pastries) because of their adverse effects on hormonal responses. Unfortunately, those are exactly the foods most people love to eat. Another potential challenge for the Zone Diet is that you must constantly think about balancing protein, carbohydrates, and fat at each meal to achieve the hormonal equilibrium essential for reducing the intensity of diet-induced inflammation.

In 2004 my late wife and I wrote the definitive "how to" book about making Zone meals. The book was entitled *Zone Meals in Seconds*. There wasn't much else I could say about making it as easy as possible to follow the classic Zone Diet. However, once the molecular mechanisms behind the success of gastric bypass surgery for treating obesity and diabetes were understood, I realized I could potentially replicate those same mechanisms with an innovative new food technology that could be used to make great tasting replacements for pizza, pasta, pastries, or virtually anything else (like tortillas) that one could make using traditional wheat or corn flour. I termed this new form of protein as Zone Protein. To realize why Zone Protein is so revolutionary, you have to understand how gastric bypass surgery actually works.

THE SECRETS OF GASTRIC BYPASS SURGERY

The best long-term clinical approach to treat obesity and diabetes is gastric bypass surgery. This is the first time in medical history that cutting out normal healthy tissue is considered "evidence-based medicine." Actually, it is a barbaric and desperate intervention, but it works. In particular, diabetes is characterized by severe insulin resistance. As discussed earlier, insulin resistance occurs when the metabolic signals carried by insulin are no longer getting through to the target tissues such as your adipose tissue, liver, muscles, or to the hypothalamus in the brain that controls appetite. Insulin resistance causes insulin levels in the blood to rise and these increased insulin levels, especially if you consume excess levels of omega-6 fatty acids, make you fat, sick, and age faster by increasing cellular inflammation as I explained earlier.

The truly unexpected benefit of gastric bypass surgery is the incredibly rapid reduction of insulin resistance and almost miraculous reversal of diabetes prior to any weight loss. Obviously, part of this was due to calorie restriction as a result of rerouting the intestine to bypass much of the middle portion of the gut. But there was another critical change being the location in the gut of where protein is absorbed. Instead of being absorbed in the middle of the intestine (the jejunum), now most of the ingested protein is absorbed in the lower part of the intestine (the ileum). Why would that be important? The lower part of the intestine contains the vast majority of cells (L-cells) that secrete hormones that respond to the protein content in a meal. If these cells are stimulated by protein, they secrete unique satiety hormones (PYY and GLP-1 in particular) that go directly to the brain to signal you to stop eating. That's exactly what happens to patients undergoing gastric bypass surgery. Beginning with their first meal after surgery patients experience freedom from hunger due to the increased production of these satiety hormones. This lack of hunger is followed by a rapid reduction in insulin resistance. If you reduce insulin resistance, you reduce elevated blood sugar levels. And because the surgery is permanent, your diabetes is managed far better than with diet or drugs.

Gastric bypass surgery is a pretty drastic way to lose weight or manage diabetes, besides being an indictment of modern medicine's failure to treat both conditions. But what if you could reduce insulin resistance eating pasta and rice replacements as well having the ability to make a new generation of bread, pizza, and pastry replacements to achieve the same goal? Now you are talking.

Once the biochemical reasons for the rapid reduction of insulin resistance after gastric bypass surgery was understood, it appeared to me that a potential solution was to develop a food technology that could replicate the appetite suppression of gastric bypass surgery and yet supply the same hedonic pleasure as eating pizza, pasta, and pastries. In other words, if you couldn't bring Mohammed to the mountain, then bring the mountain to Mohammed.

To achieve that goal, I needed to microencapsulate a small core of carbohydrate with an outer layer of protein to alter the location in the gut for protein absorption to replicate as much as possible what was observed with gastric bypass surgery. This was not all that different than my early cancer drug delivery technologies I had developed 40 years earlier. In addition, I had to make sure this new technology could be used to produce diverse foods such as pizza, pasta, tortillas, breakfast cereals, and even pastries.

The key to Zone Protein was developing a unique patented flour that when heated would be exposed to relatively high temperature (that occurs during baking) which would cause the protein in the flour to form a protein-rich outer layer held together by sulfur bonds in the protein itself so that both the inner core of carbohydrate and the outer layer of protein would not easily be absorbed until it reached the lower part of the small intestine.

My first attempts to make food products using Zone Protein generated excellent appetite suppression, but not the greatest taste. After all, I am a scientist, not a chef. This was never a problem in cancer drug delivery since the cancer drugs are injected intravenously. But food is different as taste is always paramount. I figured the people who knew best how to solve this problem would be located in Italy and in particular working with Daniela Morandi who is my co-author of several Zone cookbooks that have been published in Italy. After a lot of continued development working with highly trained chefs in Italy, I finally had a second-generation Zone Protein technology that generated appetite suppression, but now coupled with excellent taste.

Now it was time to start testing the products to see if they delivered the Holy Grail of lowering insulin resistance in a clinical trial. Our first published trial was relatively clever. First, we recruited obese individuals who had significant insulin resistance. Then we split these insulin resistant obese subjects into two groups and told all the subjects we were going to supply them with freshly prepared pasta meals and provide pre-packaged breakfast cereals that would supply half their calories for the next six weeks. The only thing both groups would have to do was follow the exact same meal plans for six weeks for the other half of their calories. The overall diet was designed to reduce their total calorie intake by about 500 calories per day so there would be the same amount of weight loss in both groups. What they weren't told was that those in the active group would be getting pasta and cereal made using Zone Protein and the other half would be getting gluten-free pasta and gluten-free cereal as the controls. Since the subjects were not only getting half their food for free, but also getting to eat the foods they like to eat (pasta and breakfast cereals), the compliance in both groups was excellent as confirmed by their food diaries. Furthermore, they couldn't tell the difference between the Zone Protein pasta and cereals and the corresponding gluten-free varieties. This marked the first time in a diet study that you had a truly controlled study using real foods.

So, what were the results? Since calorie restriction was the same in both groups, the weight loss was exactly the same. No surprise there. However, weight loss can be a highly misleading number. When the body composition of the two groups was analyzed, very different results emerged. Those consuming the pasta and cereal made with Zone Protein lost more body fat and actually gained muscle compared to the control group. On the other hand, the group consuming the gluten-free products lost muscle mass as well as losing less body fat than those consuming the Zone Protein. That's why there was no difference in weight between the two groups. Losing fat and gaining muscle while restricting calories is the Holy Grail of weight loss and it was being delivered by the Zone Protein.

More important, those consuming the products made with Zone Protein had a much greater effect on the reduction of insulin resistance. In fact, the level of insulin resistance in those who consumed the Zone Protein products was decreased by 250 percent compared to those who consumed the gluten-free products even though the calorie intake and total weight loss was identical.

Keep in mind, only half the total calories were replaced by prepared meals using Zone Protein. If I were a betting person, I would suspect if all the protein was coming from products made with Zone Protein, then this dietary technology might give gastric bypass surgery a good run for its money without surgically removing normal tissue in the gut.

This new technology of making Zone Protein makes it even easier to follow the Zone Diet because now you only have to add non-starchy vegetables and a dash of monounsaturated fats to your Zone Protein pasta or rice replacements (as well as in the future potentially making your own bread, tortillas, pizza crusts, and pastries using the appropriate Zone Protein flour) to make a complete Zone meal. Furthermore, the Zone Protein pasta or rice replacements become "vegetable helpers" because somehow when you add vegetables to a bowl of pasta or rice, they are more readily consumed. In fact, just eating the Zone Protein pasta or rice replacements with some olive oil is also a complete Zone meal that greatly reduces insulin resistance while increasing satiety. It doesn't get much easier than that.

SIMPLE WAYS TO USE ZONE PROTEIN TO MAKE ZONE MEALS

The simplicity of using Zone Protein pasta and rice replacements coupled with its superior hormonal effects now makes following the Zone Diet incredibly easy to follow. Here are some of the ways that I use it.

Eating at home

It is a good idea to make three or four servings of the pasta or rice replacements made with Zone Protein and store them in the refrigerator for whenever you make your meals.

If you want a quick hot meal with vegetables, microwave some frozen non-starchy vegetables (creamed spinach or mashed cauliflower are good choices because the protein-to-carbohydrate ratio in each is almost identical to the Zone Protein) and then add a serving of the pre-cooked Zone Protein pasta or rice replacement and re-heat for 30-60 seconds in a microwave. Likewise, a cold pasta salad can be made with the Zone Protein pasta or rice replacement and then adding Italian vegetables like sun-dried tomatoes, artichoke hearts, olives, capers, and roasted peppers and finishing it off with some olive oil. Likewise adding some of the Zone Protein rice replacement to slow-cooked oatmeal is a quick Zone breakfast. However, the ultimate quick Zone breakfast may be adding some lactose-free milk to Zone cereal made with Zone Protein.

Eating out

If you are eating out, simply bring the pre-cooked Zone Protein pasta or rice replacement with you to your favorite local restaurant. If it is an Italian restaurant, ask them to replace their pasta with your own pre-cooked Zone Protein pasta replacement, but have them warm it up in the kitchen and use their sauces to top it off. The same would be true for going to a Mexican or Indian restaurant. Just ask them to replace their rice with your pre-cooked Zone Protein rice replacement and steam it in their kitchen and use with their sauces and side vegetable dishes. Likewise, going out to lunch is just as simple. Just take some of the pre-cooked Zone Protein pasta or rice replacement products with you and add them to any salad.

Now you can enjoy all of the social benefits of going out to eat knowing you are controlling hormonal response to your meal at the same time. Currently, products made with Zone Protein are only available at our website (www.zoneliving.com).

16

Your First 1,000 Days
and Beyond

I AM OFTEN ASKED the appropriate ages to begin following the Zone Pro-Resolution Nutrition system? My answer is from birth to 102. That's not a flip answer. Although the goals at each stage of your life may change, the dietary reason that prevents you from reaching your health or performance goals is usually unresolved cellular inflammation. In other words, not being in the Zone. In this chapter and those that follow, I will discuss some of those problems that can be addressed by the Zone Pro-Resolution Nutrition system during different stages of life.

STARTING OFF LIFE

The term childhood nutrition is often misunderstood. It encompasses the period of time in the womb until early adulthood. However, the child's most critical time in life may occur during the first 1,000 days. This period of time includes the nine months in the womb as well as the next two years as a newborn child. This is the same time frame when neural circuits are established not only within the brain, but also between the gut and brain that will last a lifetime. In other words, the greatest impact on your child's future wellness may often occur during those first 1,000 critical days.

In the womb

Obviously, the nutrition of the fetus is determined by the mother's diet. If there is ever a time a woman should be in the Zone, it is during the period of her life when she is considering becoming pregnant and after she has become pregnant. In fact, there is a growing body of knowledge that indicates the ability to conceive is strongly influenced by the levels of inflammation and its effect on the hormonal patterns of every potential mother. Once the fetus begins to grow, the stakes grow much higher.

In the past, maternal malnutrition was the major problem for the fetus. This could include the lack of adequate protein and/or lack of calories leading to stunted fetal growth. Today the problem is generally reversed as existing maternal obesity is now increasing the likelihood of even further insulin resistance during pregnancy and increased risk of gestational diabetes. Obesity is not a major barrier to becoming pregnant, but it will have a significant negative effect on fetal development. In particular, it increases the likelihood of setting epigenetic marks in the DNA of the fetus that will affect its future metabolism as a child and adult. However, the biggest immediate nutritional problem of the American maternal diet may be the lack of omega-3 fatty acids.

During the final trimester in the womb, the fetal brain grows at an extraordinarily rapid rate with 250,000 new brain cells generated every minute. Without adequate levels of omega-3 fatty acids in the maternal diet, the neural development of the brain will be compromised. Recent research has shown that American women are woefully deficient in their intake of omega-3 fatty acids during pregnancy. Animal models are all too conclusive as to how an omega-3 fatty acid deficiency during fetal development affects the newborn. These offspring are not as cognitively adept as those whose mothers were getting adequate levels of omega-3 fatty acids in their diet. They are also more anxious and less socially active after birth. Those defects could be corrected with a very early dietary intervention using high-dose omega-3 fatty acids, but only for a short period of time after birth. However, after that short window closes, those cognitive and social defects induced by a deficiency of omega-3 fatty acids in the womb appear to be permanent and can't be corrected by future supplementation with omega-3 fatty acids. This observation in animal models potentially suggests that our growing epidemics of childhood depression and attention deficit disorders may be the consequence of decreased omega-3 fatty acid intake. This is further supported by the very low levels of omega-3 fatty acids in the breast milk of American mothers compared to other populations in the world.

Furthermore, the setting of genetic marks on the fetal DNA can also be determined by the mother's diet. This is known as epigenetics and the impact of the epigenetic marks on the fetal DNA can last a lifetime. This is true for both under-nutrition (starvation) or over-nutrition (obesity) of the mother as well as the stress experienced by the mother during the fetal period. This is called fetal programing. Bottom line, the closer the mother is to being in the Zone during pregnancy, the more likely the correct epigenetic marks will be set on the DNA of the fetus to reduce the likelihood of developing obesity, diabetes, and heart disease in the child's future.

Epigenetic marks set in the womb prepare the fetus for the type of world they will likely encounter when they are born, especially in terms of food supply. This was demonstrated in the analysis of children born during the Dutch famine in the winter of 1944. As the Nazi armies were retreating from the Allied invasion, they took most of the food in Holland with them. It was estimated that the remaining Dutch population survived on an intake of about 600 calories per day. Fetuses exposed to this severe calorie restriction in the last trimester of pregnancy were malnourished. Epigenetic marks were set in the womb to expect similar calorie shortages after their birth. However, after their birth, food supplies and calorie intake were quickly restored in Holland and there was an epigenetic mismatch of the fetal expectation for continued calorie restriction and what the newborn child was actually exposed to. Fifty years later, it was found that the adults born in this time period had higher levels of obesity, diabetes, and heart disease than Dutch children born either before or after the Dutch famine. Epigenetic marks established during the Dutch famine in 1944 set in motion metabolic changes leading to hyperinsulinemia as adults. However, similar famine-like conditions were experienced by Russian mothers during the siege of Stalingrad. Unlike the Dutch, the epigenetic marks set on their fetuses were perfectly matched for the continued calorie restriction that their unborn children would be exposed to in the future. Those Russian children born in that period did not demonstrate any increase in obesity, diabetes, or heart disease compared to those born before or after that famine period.

Today our problem is not calorie restriction during pregnancy, but obesity and the accompanying hyperinsulinemia that comes with it. Epigenetic marks set on fetal DNA reflect the hyperinsulinemia of the mother and will be expressed as metabolic problems later in life. This may help explain the rapid increase of childhood obesity in America.

Another example of epigenetics induced by diet is the transgenerational effects of a high omega-6 fatty acid diet. This is seen in the effects of the continued feeding of excess omega-6 fatty acids to mice for three generations. The third-generation offspring demonstrate significant abnormalities in excess obesity and fat deposits in the liver and the heart tissue. Additional studies have indicated that a prenatal diet rich in omega-6 fatty acids will produce substantial obesity in the first-generation offspring. Even supplementation with omega-3 fatty acids could not completely reverse the negative metabolic consequences of an excessive intake of omega-6 fatty acids by the mother during pregnancy.

Post-natal nutrition

After birth, there are two areas of the body that grow rapidly for the next two years; (a) the brain and (b) the composition of the bacteria colony in the gut (i.e., microbiota) that comprise the microbiota-gut-brain axis. One of the reasons that breastfeeding is so highly recommended is that it supplies the necessary omega-3 fatty acids (assuming the mother has adequate levels in her own diet) for the brain and the short sugar polymers (oligosaccharides) containing very unique sugars to support the building of an optimal gut microbiota. If omega-3 fatty acid levels in the child are insufficient, normal brain development can be delayed. Upon birth, the initial colonization of the newborn child's gut comes from microbes passing though the mother's birth canal. Unfortunately, a growing number of children are being delivered by Caesarian section. This means the first microbes that get the chance to establish themselves in the sterile colon of the newborn infant are those on the skin, and not the more beneficial microbes found in the birth canal. However, the child's nutrition in the first two years after birth will significantly alter the initial bacterial composition established at birth. After that time, the bacterial composition of the gut in the child is pretty well set for the rest of their lives for better or worse.

Which bacteria get the best start in establishing their colonies depends on the types of fermentable fiber as well as the oligosaccharides the newborn child is exposed to. The oligosaccharides in human breast milk are very different than those found in infant formulas. As a result, it is likely that the newly adjusting bacterial competition for gut colonization will also be different for breast milk compared to using standard infant formulas. This is important because the fermentation products produced from the digestion and metabolism of fermentable fiber by the microbes in the gut can have a significant impact on the critical gut-brain connections that are being developed. Research indicates that potential imbalances in these fermentation metabolites may be linked to the likelihood of developing autistic spectrum disorders that begin to occur later in early childhood. I have already discussed that one of those fermentation metabolites coming from the child's fiber intake are short-chain fatty acids (SCFA). In particular, the three main SCFA's are acetate, propionate, and butyrate. The SCFA ratio is determined by the microbial composition of the gut. If the ratio of propionate is off compared to the other two short-chain fatty acids, then it is likely the child may have a greater likelihood of developing autistic spectrum disorders. In animal experiments, injections of propionate directly into the brain can induce autistic-like symptoms within minutes. The same can potentially occur in a young child through the passage of propionate from the gut directly to the brain via the vagus nerve. For the parents this means they want to try to get their newborn child exposed to a wide variety of fermentable fibers coming from vegetables and fruits to promote the maximal amount of microbial diversity in the gut during the post-natal period for the next two years after birth.

EARLY BEHAVIORAL PROBLEMS

After the first 1,000 days the child becomes more aware of controlling their behavior as well as their diet. As a child becomes more selective in making their own food choices, usually the first things to go are vegetables because they have a more bitter taste than other carbohydrates, especially compared to refined carbohydrates such as those found in bread and breakfast cereals (like Cheerios). Unfortunately, vegetables are the primary food items rich in fermentable fiber necessary to maintain a healthy gut. This can lead to a leaky gut as well as a reorganization in the microbial composition of the gut allowing for the potential colonization of pathogenic microbes.

In addition, deficits in omega-3 fatty acid intake also become very likely. Several generations ago, many parents routinely gave their children a daily tablespoon of cod liver oil (providing 2.5 grams of EPA and DHA). The stated reason for taking the cod liver oil was to prevent the development of rickets (a disease caused by the lack of Vitamin D). However, cod liver oil is rich in omega-3 fatty acids and relatively low in vitamin D. Wrong reason, but right outcome.

The combination of these dietary factors (lack of fermentable fiber and omega-3 fatty acids) can set the foundation for the potential future development of a wide number of neurological problems such as attention deficit disorders, autistic spectrum disorders, depression, and even schizophrenia. If there was ever a time for dietary "tough love" with the child, it would be during this pre-adolescent phase of childhood given the potential for the development of behavioral conditions related to increased neuroinflammation in the brain.

In addition, the bacteria in the gut can produce many neurotransmitters that allow them to sense similar bacteria by "quorum sensing," which enables them to communicate with other members of their species. Among these neurotransmitters are serotonin, dopamine, and gamma butyric acid (GABA) that are also used by our brain for neural communication. The neurotransmitters produced by the bacteria in the gut can travel directly to the brain via the vagus nerve to affect the child's brain function. If the gut bacteria are not producing adequate levels of these neurotransmitters, it could lead to deficiencies in any one of those neurotransmitters. Lack of serotonin is associated with depression, lack of dopamine is associated with ADHD, and lack of GABA is associated with anxiety. Perhaps the best way to help reduce the development of these behavioral conditions in early childhood may start with providing the bacteria in the gut with adequate levels of fermentable fiber such as pureed vegetables with a dash of purified fish oil as soon as the child begins to eat solid food as opposed to going to the pharmacy later in childhood for prescription drugs to manage neurological conditions.

EARLY CHILDHOOD OBESITY

The fastest growing segment of the obese population since the 1970s is represented by children according to the Centers for Disease Control. Animal studies mentioned earlier indicate that this may be due to a combination of hyperinsulinemia and increased omega-6 fatty acid consumption leading to the development of insulin resistance. Just as neuroinflammation can be a major contributing cause for behavioral disorders, it will also disrupt the energy balance system in the hypothalamus making it difficult to maintain satiety between meals. As I discussed earlier, a very well-designed experiment in 1999 at Harvard Medical School demonstrated that changing the protein-to-glycemic load composition of a single meal results in dramatic hormonal changes in obese children. The meal that had the most profound beneficial effects on hormonal changes was a Zone meal consisting of 40 percent low-glycemic carbohydrates (slow-cooked oatmeal), 30 percent protein (an egg white omelet), and 30 percent fat (low-fat cheese). Furthermore, when the obese children had the same Zone meal for breakfast and lunch, they reduced their calorie consumption after the second Zone meal by 46 percent compared to meals they consumed with the same number of calories, but with a lower protein-to-glycemic load. If you aren't hungry, then you simply eat fewer calories. If you eat fewer calories, you lose excess body fat. If you lose excess body fat, you reverse obesity.

The Zone Diet for kids is pretty simple. Never consume anymore protein at a meal than they can fit on the palm of their hand (that's 15 grams of protein or about 2 oz. of low-fat protein) and let them eat as many vegetables as they want. When you are using Zone Protein in the form of pasta or rice replacements, it's pretty easy.

PUBERTY

Puberty marks a time of tremendous hormonal changes with corresponding mood changes. The hormonal changes that drive physical growth result in a corresponding increase in appetite to sustain that growth. In the past much of that growth in adolescents has been vertical. Today we are seeing increased horizontal growth (i.e., obesity). The solution is to provide enough protein for vertical growth while restricting excess carbohydrates and calories that promote horizontal growth. In other words, following the Zone Diet.

Likewise, residual cellular inflammation in the brain can increase mood disorders in teenagers, particularly anxiety and depression. There are two likely dietary contributors to this increase. The first is an increase in gut-induced inflammation caused by a leaky gut allowing the increased transport of microbial fragments into the blood to promote systemic cellular inflammation. The second is the decrease of omega-3 fatty acids in the child's diet that would otherwise resolve neuroinflammation in the brain. This is why high-dose omega-3 fatty acids have been clinically effective in treating childhood depression. It also reduces inflammation in the brain that distorts the information signaling mediated by neurotransmitters making it very useful in managing attention deficit hyperactivity disorder (ADHD).

Since puberty is a time of accelerated growth, teenagers should be considered as adults when it comes to constructing Zone meals and their omega-3 fatty and polyphenol needs.

COMPLETION OF THE FINAL WIRING OF THE BRAIN

Teenagers tend to undertake risky behavior because the final establishment of the connections between the limbic system (i.e., just do it) and the pre-frontal cortex (i.e., think about the consequences) are not completed until around age 22. Without adequate omega-3 fatty acids in the diet, it is unlikely that those connections will ever be fully functional.

SUMMARY ▷

The first stage of life when the Zone Pro-Resolution Nutrition system can potentially have its greatest effect is during the first 1,000 days. This is not only because critical neural connections are established in the brain as well as between the brain and the gut, but also because epigenetic marks are established on the DNA that control gene expression (especially relating to metabolism) for the rest of the child's life. Furthermore, another critical event during the last part of that first 1,000 days is the establishment of the bacterial composition of the gut that will affect metabolism for the child's future. Likewise, there is a constant need for omega-3 fatty acids for optimal brain development that continues up to age 22. To maintain those connections, you will need to maintain (or even increase) the dietary level of omega-3 fatty acid intake for the rest of the child's life.

By following the Zone Pro-Resolution Nutrition system, your child will have every advantage they will need for entering adulthood. It is always much easier to do it correctly at the start of life, rather than going back at a later date in an effort to correct the initial dietary mistakes (assuming they can ever be totally corrected) that occurred early in life.

17

Reaching Peak Performance

AS YOU MOVE into early adulthood, peak performance (both physi-cal and mental) becomes your growing focus. This is the second stage of life when you want to be in the Zone. Both physical and mental performance require energy. In particular, you need chemical energy in the form of adenosine triphosphate (ATP) to fuel the brain and our mus-cles (as well as every other organ in the body).

You might be asking how a calorie-restricted diet like the Zone Diet can improve athletic performance. The answers are complex, as I will explain in this chapter. But here's a start. First, any type of performance is based on your ability to generate ATP. For that you need highly efficient mitochondria in your muscle cells as well as in your brain. It's not the size of the muscle that counts, but the amount of ATP it can generate that is important. By restricting calories, you are activating the gene transcrip-tion factor AMP kinase in every organ to produce more efficient mito-chondria especially in your muscles. This provides the power you need for improved athletic performance. Second, the Zone Diet is based on the level of daily protein intake required to maintain your lean muscle mass. This is a major problem in professional sports because muscles are con-sistently damaged during training and competition. The amount of pro-tein an athlete requires to maintain their muscle mass is unique to them and must be consumed evenly throughout the day like the intravenous drip of a drug in order to constantly activate another gene transcription factor (mTOR) that supports muscle protein synthesis. Likewise, the calorie content of the Zone Diet should also be evenly spread throughout the day to maintain AMP kinase activity which is critical for the efficient removal of damaged mitochondria and replacing them with new, more efficient ones to generate more ATP using fewer calories. Consuming too many calories (especially carbohydrates) at any one meal will inhibit AMP kinase activity, thus stopping the biogenesis of new mitochondria. This means the athlete should be consuming additional Zone meals throughout the day, but with fewer calories per meal. (Later in this chapter, I will give you an example of the Zone Diet requirements for a typical Olympic male swimmer.) Third, the Zone Diet is a low-fat diet that allows the athlete to access their own stored body fat for high-octane fuel throughout the day which is necessary to generate the increased levels of ATP required not only for performance, but also to repair damaged tissue that dictates their recovery time. The Zone Diet is a carbohydrate-moderate diet designed to maintain adequate blood sugar levels for optimal brain function without causing the excess secretion of insulin as well as decreasing AMP kinase activity. All of these hormonal and genetic responses are the foundation that help explain why the Zone Pro-Resolution Nutrition system has improved the athletic performance of a wide range of elite athletes including the winners of 25 Olympic Gold medals to teams that have won world championships ranging from the NBA, NFL, MLB, the World Cup, and the Tour de France.

However, maximum performance in elite athletes also requires significant pro-resolution supplementation to enhance the Resolution Response. In particular, higher intakes of omega-3 fatty acids are needed to generate the levels of resolvins to reduce exercise-induced inflammation. Likewise, higher levels of polyphenol extracts will be needed to maximize AMP kinase activity to repair tissue damaged by the same high-intensity exercise.

MITOCHONDRIA AND ATHLETIC PERFORMANCE

The real key to enhanced performance is based on the levels of ATP in a cell. The only trouble is you can't store ATP because it is made on demand in every body cell. The biological factories that make ATP are the mitochondria. These factories are the microbial ancestors that made multi-cellular life possible over 600 million years ago, and we still depend on them to sustain us today. So, if you want peak mental or physical performance you have to start with understanding why healthy functioning mitochondria are essential and you have to keep them in tip-top condition for as long as possible. When your mitochondria become dysfunctional, they start producing more free radicals and less ATP. Excess free radicals accelerate cellular inflammation and this inhibits the body's ability to repair the damage caused by that exercise-induced inflammation. As result, performance begins to decrease and recovery times begin to increase.

WHY DO WE EAT?

The obvious answer whether you are an athlete or not is to live. The less obvious answer is because we need a constant supply of fats and carbohydrates (protein is a very poor fuel source for ATP production) that can be converted into ATP that fuels the metabolism needed for the survival of every cell in every organ. The heart only uses fatty acids for fuel, the brain uses only glucose for fuel, and other organs (especially the muscles) can use both. The ability to use either fatty acids or glucose for making ATP is called metabolic flexibility. You also have to consider ATP as the "currency of life." The more you have, the better you live. You think faster, your muscles work better, and your overall metabolism becomes far more efficient. The end result is that you perform better.

As stated earlier, mitochondria are incredibly small organelles (think of them as very tiny organs inside the cell) that consume 85–90 percent of the incoming oxygen you breathe to convert either dietary fats or carbohydrates into ATP. They do this by a process called oxidative phosphorylation—a term that only a biochemist would love. Your mitochondria almost magically combine the oxygen in the air you breathe with the carbohydrates and fats you eat to make the ATP essential to keep you alive. That's the good news. The bad news is they also generate free radicals (X-rays and atomic bomb blasts do the same thing) in the process. These free radicals not only damage the mitochondria, making ATP production less efficient, but also damage both the mitochondrial and nuclear DNA giving rise to mutations as well as increasing the oxidation of protein, lipids, and carbohydrates. These oxidized products interact with structures inside the cell known as inflammasomes that are designed to sense the presence of damaged cell components thereby mistakenly activating the gene transcription factor NF-κB that creates increased cellular inflammation. All of this oxidative damage decreases your daily mental and physical performance.

Your typical cell in the body usually has a lifetime of about 10 years. However, because of this constant exposure to free radical radiation, the lifetime of the mitochondria in your cells is measured in days and in mice with even higher metabolic rates, the lifetime of their mitochondria is measured in minutes. This means the mitochondria must constantly be replaced if you are going to maintain peak performance by generating enough ATP. This need for constant replacement is another big problem since the cell can store just enough ATP to give you about 10 seconds worth of chemical energy. Furthermore, active cells like those in the muscles (remember the heart is also a muscle working 24/7) might have upwards of 2,000 mitochondria per cell. The liver is the central hub for your metabolism and is also rich in mitochondria. However, the ultimate ATP user is your brain. The brain uses 20 percent of the body's total ATP production at rest for its own internal needs even though this organ only accounts for 2 percent of your total weight. Bottom line, every organ in your body requires your mitochondria to function at peak efficiency for peak performance (both physical and mental).

If one mitochondrion (and there might be thousands in a cell) becomes damaged, how do you pick it out of the crowd of other mitochondria, get rid of it, and then replace it with a new one without missing a beat in ATP production? The constant demand for ATP production means replacing a damaged mitochondrion is the responsibility of AMP kinase acting as your master metabolic switch, and in particular it is the commander-in-chief of mitochondrial replacement. If you can activate AMP kinase, you will maintain your ATP generating capacity at maximum efficiency by continually replacing damaged mitochondria with new healthy and more efficient mitochondria allowing you to think faster and perform better.

So how do you activate AMP kinase? You have three useful lifestyle strategies:

■ Calorie restriction
■ Consumption of polyphenols
■ Intense exercise

Calorie restriction activates AMP kinase because it increases the body's efficiency for generating ATP with fewer calories. The body does this by making sure all the mitochondria in every cell are running at peak levels. Consider calorie restriction like taking your car for its annual tune-up, but now on a daily basis. Of course, the secret to successful calorie restriction is to never be hungry or fatigued in the process. The only way that is going happen is to follow the Zone Diet.

On the other hand, if you are not controlling satiety, you are always going to be hungry and will constantly consume more calories than you really need and that will decrease AMP kinase activity. The two particular groups who usually fall into this category of having constant hunger: diabetics and elite athletes. As I will discuss later in this chapter, the protein needs of elite athletes is obviously greater than the average individual so that their overall calorie needs are increased, but the composition of those calories for both groups is pretty much the same. The consumption of excess calories (usually more than 400 calories per meal) is one of the best ways to inhibit AMP kinase activity and therefore decrease the production of new, more efficient mitochrondria.

Dietary polyphenols can also activate AMP kinase as well as a wide number of other gene transcription factors, but only if they get into the blood. You consume polyphenols by eating colorful carbohydrates like vegetables and fruits as well as adding a wide variety of spices to every meal since they are all rich in polyphenols. But if you really want peak performance, then it is likely that you will need additional supplementation with refined polyphenol extracts, especially those that are rich in water-soluble polyphenols (such as delphinidins) that can easily enter the bloodstream intact to maximize AMP kinase activity.

Finally, intense exercise lowers the levels of ATP in the muscles used thus activating the AMP kinase in those muscle cells to rapidly replace damaged mitochondria with new healthy ones. That's fine for the muscles, but if the athlete consumes too many calories in a meal then those excess calories will decrease AMP kinase activity in muscles as well as other organs, like the brain. Of course, it's very difficult to exercise at high intensity for more than 30 seconds. This is why high-intensity interval training (HIIT) is so effective in activating AMP kinase, but unfortunately it can only be maintained for a short period of time (like 30-second intervals). This is why most high-intensity workouts have eight separate 30-second bursts of high-level intensity activity followed by 90-second recovery periods. Low-intensity exercise like walking will rarely activate AMP kinase activity.

HIGH-OCTANE VERSUS LOW-OCTANE FUEL

Even if you have a fully functioning array of mitochondria (and that's a big if), to maximize ATP production requires knowledge of the type of fuel you are using and the amount of oxygen you have available.

Let's start with your potential fuel choices. If you have adequate levels of oxygen available, you have three choices: fats, glucose, or ketone bodies. The amount of ATP that can be formed in the presence of adequate levels of oxygen is totally dependent on the number of carbon atoms in the molecule. Not surprisingly, each of these potential metabolic fuel sources are not equal in their ability to generate ATP. The best fuel source is long-chain fatty acids. For each long-chain fatty acid molecule (usually about 18 carbons in length), you can theoretically generate 130 molecules of ATP if adequate oxygen is available.

Glucose contains only six carbon atoms per molecule, making it a poor second place finisher compared to fatty acids because for each glucose molecule you can theoretically generate 38 molecules of ATP in the presence of oxygen.

Bringing up the rear for ATP production are ketone bodies that are even less efficient than glucose in generating energy because they contain fewer carbon atoms per molecule. But like fatty acids, ketone bodies can only make ATP in the presence of adequate oxygen, so using ketone bodies for exercise as your primary fuel may not be your wisest decision. In fact, I demonstrated in a 2006 article that the increased level of fatigue induced by even mild exercise was directly correlated with increased ketone levels in the blood. Recent studies have confirmed this also to be true in trained athletes.

All bets are off when you are operating under anaerobic conditions. Now the lack of adequate oxygen forces the mitochondria to use only glucose and with lack of adequate oxygen you don't make much ATP. Under anaerobic conditions the efficiency of ATP production from glucose drops down to about two molecules for each glucose molecule as opposed to the 38 molecules of ATP under aerobic conditions.

The muscle cells can only store enough ATP to work maximally for about 10 seconds. Running a 100-yard dash at your maximum speed will quickly eliminate those internal ATP stores. An elite sprinter can finish such a race. Most of us have to stop well before that 100-yard mark as we have run out of ATP and have to stop to rebuild its levels. This is why you have to reduce your rate of exercise intensity to increase your ability to use oxygen to generate more ATP or to have a significant recovery to re-build your ATP levels (this is called your oxygen debt). This is why you can't run a marathon at the same rate that you might run a 100-yard dash.

Fortunately, more than 99.9 percent of our lives is spent at a level of physical intensity that provides adequate oxygen. This is why the pre-ferred fuel for making the necessary ATP that fuels our body is always long-chain fatty acids, except for one organ. That organ is the brain.

Total fuel capacity

The theoretical ATP production doesn't matter much if you aren't carry-ing a lot of high-octane fuel as fuel reserves in the first place. Fortunately, you always have a massive storage capacity in your body fat even in elite athletes. Here are some fuel storage facts: Using the mythical 70 kg (154 lb.) male (he may actually exist), at any given time he might have 400 grams of glucose stored in his muscle cells, 100 grams of glucose stored in the liver, 15 grams of glucose circulating in the blood, and only about 2 grams of glucose in the brain. As I stated earlier, the brain uses 20 per-cent of the body's energy production at rest even though it accounts for only 2 percent of total bodyweight. The brain is able to maintain this high level of ATP production because it can continually pull glucose from the blood, which in turn can be replenished from the stored glucose in the liver if you have adequate liver glycogen. When following a ketogenic diet, you don't have such reserves. At the same time, this male would have about 10,000 g (10 kg) of stored fat if he has about 15 percent body fat (considered to be ideal for the average male). That is enough stored en-ergy in adipose tissue to potentially run more than 30 consecutive mara-thons if converted into ATP. A 154-pound elite male athlete will have less stored body fat (about 10 percent), so he could only run potentially 20 consecutive marathons.

The secret for performance is getting stored fatty acids out of your fat cells and into the blood so they can reach the muscles and be converted into ATP. That process is inhibited in the presence of high levels of insulin. This can occur if you are drinking a lot of sports "energy" drinks rich in carbohydrates or have insulin resistance caused by diet-induced inflammation. In either case the high insulin levels in the blood inhibits the hormone-sensitive lipase in your fat cells that in turn inhibits the potential release of this amazing amount of energy contained in your stored body fat for potential ATP production.

Translating to physical performance

By this time, you are thinking bacon fat might be the ideal performance food for athletes. Think again. Peak athletic performance starts in the brain. Analysis, focus, and the transmission of neural impulses to the muscles all start in the brain. The brain can't use fat for ATP production, otherwise it would digest itself. That's why its primary fuel source is glucose. Since the brain can't store glucose, it can only get it from the blood. As stated earlier, the brain is the major energy user in the body based on its weight compared to other organs. So, unless you are able to maintain constant blood glucose levels, ATP production in the brain slows. This is a consequence of low blood glucose or hypoglycemia. Not only does hypoglycemia make you hungry, but it also slows down thinking and causes lack of focus.

What about ketones as a fuel source for ATP production in the brain? First, they are not very effective in generating ATP compared to glucose. Remember the brain can't use fatty acids to produce ATP otherwise it would digest itself. Glucose remains a better fuel source for ATP production than ketone bodies. Even during extended periods of total starvation, the body continues to convert existing muscle mass into glucose to maintain brain function. This is why the levels of blood glucose do not drop below 65 mg/dL (keeping in mind that 90 mg/dL represents normal blood glucose levels) even under medically supervised periods (35 days) of complete starvation. That level of blood glucose is maintained by constant conversion of muscle into glucose. Should a total fast continue for 50 days, the subject usually dies from heart failure as the heart is the last source of muscle to be consumed in order to try to maintain blood glucose levels for the brain.

The other critical factor needed for ATP production is oxygen. Without adequate oxygen getting to the brain and the muscles, the efficiency of ATP production will be dramatically reduced whatever the fuel source.

Athletes are always concerned about the build-up of lactic acid in the muscle that causes pain. The reason lactic acid builds up is because there is insufficient oxygen reaching the muscle cells and ATP production grinds to a slow drip since lactic acid cannot be further converted into ATP very effectively without adequate oxygen. Eventually the muscle that is being actively exercised simply runs out of energy. The solution to the problem is not excessive carb-loading, but a combination of omega-3 fatty acids and polyphenols.

Getting more oxygen to the muscle cells (as well as the brain for peak mental performance) requires both greater blood flow and increased red blood cell flexibility because the red blood cell is the carrier of oxygen in the blood. The transfer of oxygen takes place within the capillary bed where the diameter of the capillary is actually smaller than the diameter of the red blood cell. This forces the red blood cell to slow its velocity to squeeze itself through the capillary bed so that oxygen can move more readily from the red blood cell into the adjoining tissue. Therefore, any dietary change that will either make the red blood cell more flexible or increase the size of the capillary bed will increase oxygen transfer and increase the efficiency of ATP production.

Increased amounts of the omega-3 fatty acids EPA and DHA in the red blood cell membrane increases the flexibility of the red blood cell traveling through the capillary bed making it more efficient in transferring oxygen to the adjoining tissue. The polyphenols work by a different mechanism to increase the size of the capillary diameter thus improving the rate of red blood cell transient times through the capillary bed.

Just exactly how polyphenols improve oxygen transfer is a little more complicated, but if you want better performance (physical or mental), it is worth the effort to understand why. Improving blood flow comes from the production of a gas known as nitric oxide or NO, which is a powerful vasodilator. Medically, the drug nitroglycerin is used to treat angina by increasing NO production. The only problem is that it can potentially be fatal as blood pressure may drop too low. Is there a more controlled way to increase NO production that can be used to improve performance? The answer is yes—with nitrates. Nitrates are primarily found in vegetables and they are particularly rich in arugula, spinach, and beets. Nitrates, however, must be converted into nitrites on their way to NO production. This conversion of nitrates into nitrites takes place by bacteria in the mouth (many of which are destroyed by mouthwashes). However, there is still a long way to go to increase NO production. The polyphenols play a key role in the metabolic conversion of the nitrites into NO, but only if you have adequate levels of polyphenols in the blood. The Zone Diet benefits athletic performance because it is rich in vegetables providing nitrates as well as polyphenols since most of your carbohydrate sources are derived from non-starchy vegetables with limited fruits, both of which are rich in polyphenols. Of course, you can also further increase NO generation with supplemental water-soluble polyphenols such as delphinidins.

There are additional neurological benefits for omega-3 supplements in trained athletes. For example, it was demonstrated more than a decade ago that supplementing with 2.5 grams of EPA and DHA per day in trained athletes significantly improved their reaction times, their mood, and changed their brain wave patterns to a more focused and relaxed mental state within 35 days after starting their omega-3 fatty acid supplementation.

Hormonal changes during exercise

When you exercise, your hormone levels can change dramatically depending on the intensity of your exercise. The more intense your exercise, the greater the hormonal changes. The better you manage those hormonal changes, the better your performance will be at every level of competition. The Zone Diet was designed to modulate these hormonal changes to achieve that goal.

Some of these hormonal changes are shown graphically below:

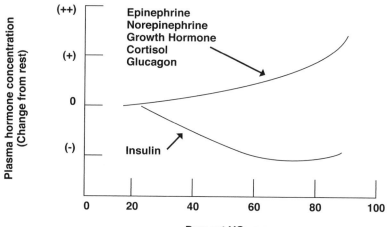

Hormonal Responses to Graded Exercise Intensity

Notice that the primary hormone that decreases during exercise is insulin. This is because as you increase the intensity of exercise, you need to release more stored high-octane fuel (i.e., fat) from your fat cells to enter the blood to meet the increasing need for ATP production required for muscle contraction. As insulin levels drop, its inhibition of the hormone-sensitive lipase in the fat cells is reduced, and free fatty acids can now flow more easily from your stored fat into the blood for transport to the muscle cells to make more ATP.

On the other hand, a lot of other hormones increase as you step up your exercise intensity. The metabolic effect of these other hormones helps stabilize blood glucose levels to maintain energy production for the brain.

Dietary training for peak athletic performance

How can the Zone Pro-Resolution Nutrition system enhance these metabolic events to give you a better physical performance? It starts with a hormonal warm-up. Just as you wouldn't start a workout or begin any type of athletic competition without first warming up your muscles, you should also be warming up your hormones to prepare for the dramatic changes that will take place during increased exercise. Furthermore, you can use the principles of the Zone Diet to orchestrate the other hormonal changes that take place after exercise that can lead to a more rapid recovery. These phases can be broken down into four distinct periods:

- Hormonal warm-up
- Immediate post-exercise recovery
- Intermediate glycogen recovery
- Long-term repair of damaged tissue

Hormonal warm-up (30 to 45 minutes prior to exercise)

Since blood sugar levels will drop during exercise, this is the time to stabilize it by increasing the secretion of the hormone glucagon (increased by protein) that will cause the release of stored carbohydrate from the liver (stored carbohydrates in the muscle can't be released into the blood) as well as adding some extra glucose to the blood. So about 30–45 minutes prior to exercise consume a small hormone-stabilizing snack. The snack should contain no more than 100 calories with slightly more low-glycemic carbs than protein. To further slow the entry of the glucose in the bloodstream, add a little fat. A good starting point for such a hormonal snack would a 3-2-1 balance of carbohydrates (9 grams), protein (6 grams), and fat (3 grams) on a gram basis or one Zone block of carbohydrate, protein, and fat. If you wanted to convert that balance to a per calorie basis that would be about 40 percent low glycemic carbohydrates, 30 percent protein, and 30 percent fat. Sound familiar? This was the composition of the hormonal warm-up snack the Olympic athletes I have worked with over the years ate prior to training and competition. Since these athletes have collectively won 25 Olympic Gold Medals, it seems to have made a difference.

Typically, you shouldn't eat while exercising as it might divert blood flow toward the gut for aiding digestion and away from your muscles when you need its oxygen and nutrients to make ATP. The only exception to this might be during an Ironman triathlon or during a four-hour ride when competing in the Tour de France in which it is easier to consume nutrients during the biking segments. Even under those conditions you still want to maintain the 3-2-1 balance of carbohydrates, protein, and fat.

Immediate post-exercise recovery (0 to 15 minutes post exercise)

Exercising intensely causes significant muscle damage. But the moment you stop exercising, growth hormone is secreted to begin repairing that damage. This is the best time to stabilize insulin levels because the otherwise rapid rise of insulin after exercise will inhibit growth hormone release. Insulin stabilization can be accomplished with the same small 100-calorie snack with the same 3-2-1 carbohydrate-protein-fat balance (in grams or more simply a Zone snack) that you consumed prior to exercise. So, have a snack at the ready to be eaten right after you finish exercising, when you are walking off the field before you ever get to the locker room.

Intermediate post-exercise recovery (15 to 120 minutes post exercise)

This two-hour window is the best time to replenish muscle glycogen levels that have been depleted by exercise. It has been shown that a balance of protein-to-carbohydrate will replenish muscle glycogen levels at a faster rate and to a greater extent than higher levels of carbohydrate alone. The best time to maximize muscle glycogen levels is within 30 minutes after stopping exercising and your ability to do so wanes completely after two hours post exercise. This is why this two-hour period right after exercise is an ideal time to consume a Zone meal.

Long-term repair of damaged tissue (2 to 24 hours post exercise)

This time period is often ignored in sports nutrition, but it's by far the most important because this is when damaged muscle is repaired and new muscle mass is synthesized. This requires massive amounts of energy in the form of ATP and the primary fuel source for the repair process will come from your stored body fat to make ATP, not stored glycogen. At the molecular level, the extra energy you need at rest to repair muscle damage will come from activation of AMP kinase. That is best done with supplementation with polyphenol extracts rich in delphinidins.

Furthermore, building muscle mass is a lot more complex than consuming tubs of protein powder. First, the human body can only utilize about 40 grams of protein at any one meal. Any more than that amount of protein will be converted into fat for future fuel use. There is only one key amino acid (leucine) that activates another gene transcription factor called mTOR that is key to the stimulation of muscle growth. However, the stimulation of muscle synthesis peaks at about 3 grams of leucine per meal and will only last for about three hours. The richest sources of leucine are egg whites and dairy protein. However, any more leucine consumption beyond that limited level will have no further stimulus on mTOR. The secret is to spread the leucine intake throughout the day like a drug to constantly stimulate muscle formation even while watching TV. For most of us, that would be three Zone meals and one Zone snack. For performance athletes, that would be four to five Zone meals with two Zone snacks.

It's a lot of work, but it is well worth the effort depending on what level of performance you wish to achieve. This is why the life of professional athletes usually consists of training, eating, and resting and then repeating the same routine day after day during the season.

HOW MUCH PROTEIN DOES AN ATHLETE REALLY NEED?

It depends on your existing muscle mass, your training intensity, and what type of training you do. As discussed in Chapter 7, your protein requirement has nothing to do with your weight, but everything to do with lean body mass. So, let's see how those calculations would apply to the elite athlete and their protein needs.

Active exercise (1 hour per day, 5 times a week)	0.8 grams of protein per lb. of lean body mass
Very active exercise (2 hours per day, 5 times per week)	0.9 grams of protein per lb. of lean body mass
Heavy weight training or twice a day training (5 days per week)	1.0 grams of protein per lb. of lean body mass

It turns out that not that much additional protein is needed to maintain your existing muscle mass, especially if you consume it evenly throughout the day. Once you know your protein requirements, then the levels of low-glycemic carbohydrates and monounsaturated fat you need at each meal is automatically set by the amount of protein you are consuming to end up with a calorie consumption that is about 40 percent low glycemic carbohydrates, 30 percent low-fat protein, and 30 percent monounsaturated fat. The calories may seem low, but that macronutrient balance is the hormonal key to allow access to your stored body fat for the high-energy fuel needed to repair damaged tissue at the maximum possible rate.

How does this translate to elite athletes? Let's take a look at Olympic swimmers. A typical Olympic male swimmer might weigh 80 kg (176 pounds), have about 10 percent body fat, and work out twice a day. This hypothetical male Olympic swimmer would need about 143 grams of protein spread evenly throughout the day. Since the body can't effectively use more than 40 grams of protein at one meal, this means he would have to eat about four to five Zone meals per day as well as two Zone snacks each containing about seven grams of protein. And his total calorie intake? If he follows the Zone Diet, he would consume about 2,000 calories per day keeping in mind that any extra needed energy for ATP production to repair damaged tissue is coming from stored body fat. I have already discussed in Chapter 7 that it is exceptionally difficult to consume 1,500 calories per day for the average male following the Zone Diet. It becomes even more difficult for an elite athlete following the Zone Diet to consume the higher levels of calorie intake they require.

But can't an elite athlete become too thin following the Zone Diet? Of course they can. How do you know? The answer is when you can clearly see your abdominal muscles. This means you are about 5 percent body fat for a male and 11 percent body fat for females. By that criteria, very few elite athletes are too thin. Remember stored body fat is your reservoir for the high-octane fuel necessary for the increased ATP production needed to repair damaged muscles caused by intense exercise. So, when you can clearly see your abdominal muscles, you probably don't have enough high-octane fuel on your body to rebuild damaged muscles to reduce recovery times. To rectify this "fat deficiency" you simply add more monounsaturated fat to your diet until you can barely see your abdominal muscles (that will be about 10 percent body fat for a male and 15 percent body fat for a female). Not surprisingly these are the typical body fat percentages for Olympic swimmers. The easiest way to get this extra fat is by eating more nuts like almonds or by adding more olive oil or avocados to your meals. But until that time that you can clearly see your abdominal muscles, realize that calories do count, and you don't have a blast furnace for a stomach simply because you work out. This is especially true as you age since you are losing mitochondrial capacity that converts stored fat into ATP. Also keep in mind, the fewer calories you consume, the more you activate AMP kinase to make more efficient mitochondria to increase the production of ATP for repair of muscle damage. This will further improve performance in any sport.

What if you want to build additional muscle? First, it is difficult. If you are already a highly trained athlete, it is difficult enough just to maintain your lean body mass during active training and competition. So, let's say the elite athlete wants to add six pounds of extra muscle mass per year to their existing muscle mass. Muscle is about 75 percent water, so the actual protein required for building the six additional pounds of added muscle would be about 1.5 pounds (700 g) of amino acids. Divide that by 360 days and you get a theoretical need for two extra grams of dietary protein per day. To give yourself some leeway, plan to add seven grams of protein every day over and above your daily protein requirement to maintain your existing muscle mass. For the male Olympic swimmer in this example, his daily protein requirements would increase from 143 grams of protein to 150 grams of protein per day. That isn't much. This is also why the gold-medal-winning Olympic swimmers I have worked with over the years have never consumed more than 2,500 calories per day. Less calories means more AMP kinase activity to replace damaged mitochondria and replace them with more efficient mitochondria. This means more ATP production to more rapidly repair damaged tissue and that means better performance.

Resolution of exercise-induced inflammation

Elite athletes live in a world of inflammation by choice. Intense exercise creates significant inflammation because of constant muscle damage caused by high-intensity exercise. The rate of recovery from exercise-induced inflammation determines your success in reaching whatever performance goal you have set for yourself. This is why the successful resolution of exercise-induced inflammation is absolutely essential to achieve peak physical performance. This will simply not happen unless you have optimized your Resolution Response.

The key to the optimal resolution of inflammation is the production of adequate levels of resolvins derived from the omega-3 fatty acids EPA and DHA. But how much? As usual, it depends. For the non-elite athlete, that level might range between 2.5 and 5 grams of EPA and DHA per day. For the elite athlete, an appropriate level would be 5 to 7.5 grams of EPA and DHA per day. Of course, if you want to dial in the exact amount you require for peak physical performance then try to maintain your AA/EPA ratio in the blood between 1.5 and 3.

Another problem with unresolved inflammation is delayed onset muscle soreness. This is a consequence of significant micro-tears in the muscle that are simply not healing, and until the damaged muscle heals there will be significant ongoing pain. This is a case of "lingering pain creates negative gain" because you will rapidly lose much of your conditioning the more extended the time you require for healing damaged muscle tissue. It has been demonstrated that muscle damage, and hence recovery times, can be reduced significantly with adequate supplementation with omega-3 fatty acids.

Overtraining

If training is good, then more training should be better? The answer is a resounding no. The harder you train, the more inflammation builds up in the muscles and the longer it takes to resolve it. If you are not taking enough omega-3 fatty acids to make resolvins, then overtraining forces the athlete into a far less desirable hormonal pathway to reduce inflammation via the increased secretion of the hormone cortisol. We think of cortisol as a stress hormone, but in reality, cortisol is actually an anti-inflammatory hormone associated with a significant amount of collateral damage. There is no such thing as an eicosanoid gland in the body since every cell is capable of making eicosanoids. Therefore, if exercise-induced inflammation is not effectively resolved due to a lack of adequate levels of omega-3 fatty acids in the diet, then increased cortisol secretion becomes a far less desirable alternative to stop the further production of eicosanoids. Cortisol works by inhibiting the release of free fatty acids for future eicosanoid synthesis from their primary storage depots (as phospholipids in the membrane of the cell), and this shuts down any further eicosanoid formation until the existing inflammation is hopefully reduced over time. The collateral damage is the result of excessive levels of cortisol in the blood that causes an increase in insulin resistance (making you fat), disturbs neurological action (making you more depressed and mentally fatigued), and disrupts immunological function (making you less likely to fight off microbial invasions). Performance-wise, excess cortisol leads to a downward spiral of decreasing performance. The common name is "over-training syndrome."

The number one prescription for reducing exercise-induced inflammation is lots of rest coupled with taking adequate levels of omega-3 fatty acids to generate the necessary levels of resolvins so the body is not forced to secrete excess cortisol. When the increased omega-3 fatty acids are part of the Zone Pro-Resolution Nutrition system, the speed of recovery from intense exercise is accelerated.

Rebuilding your mitochondria

Understanding the role of maintaining mitochondrial function is a central component of both mental and physical peak performance. These tiny factories found in every cell are the keys to performance since they control ATP production. Keeping them working at peak efficiency is the ultimate pathway to peak performance.

Earlier, I discussed the need for continued synthesis (i.e., biogenesis) of new functional mitochondria coupled with the simultaneous removal (i.e., mitophagy) of damaged mitochondria. This is an intricate dance that is controlled by the gene transcription factor AMP kinase. This means the future of sports nutrition is not about constantly consuming sports drinks enriched in excess carbohydrates, purchasing tubs of protein powder, or tablets containing some magical compound that you buy in a health food store, but instead it requires constant activation of gene transcription factors, and in particular AMP kinase. In other words, the future of sports nutrition will be based in gene therapy that can be orchestrated by the Zone Pro-Resolution Nutrition system.

One way to induce AMP kinase activity is by calorie restriction, but without hunger or fatigue. That is the goal of the Zone Diet. However, the activation of AMP kinase by the Zone Diet alone will not be sufficient alone to increase mitochondria efficiency. Maximum activation of AMP kinase will require both restricting calories and supplementation with polyphenol extracts to optimally activate AMP kinase.

POLYPHENOLS AND PERFORMANCE

Not all polyphenols will increase AMP kinase activity. First, they have to be water soluble, so they can more easily enter into the blood to reach their target cells. Unfortunately, the vast majority of polyphenols are not water soluble. The one class of polyphenols that are the most water soluble are called delphinidins, and very few plants are rich in these unique polyphenols. They are found in low concentrations in blueberries, higher concentrations in bilberries, but their highest concentration is the wild maqui berry found in Chile. However, to have a significant impact, these maqui berry polyphenols must be extracted, purified, and concentrated to achieve the necessary potency you need for optimal AMP kinase activation as I described earlier.

Even if an elite athlete consumes large amounts of vegetables and fruits per day, they will still need an additional 500 to 1,000 mg of purified polyphenol extracts to optimize AMP kinase production. That's a lot more budget friendly than purchasing a $10,000 bicycle or a $500 pair of running shoes in an attempt to improve your performance.

Concussion Injuries

There is a growing awareness (if not fear) of concussion injuries in sports. This is another benefit of having adequate levels of omega-3 fatty acids in the blood to be able to generate the production of resolvins to reduce the neuroinflammation caused by a concussion injury. I demonstrated this in 2011 working with Julian Bailes, who is one of the leading neurosurgeons in the United States, who I discussed in Chapter 10 on our research using high-dose omega-3 fatty acids to treat severe brain trauma. Julian also had served as the team neurosurgeon for the Pittsburgh Steelers for a number of years and was very aware of concussion injuries, which are a milder form of brain trauma. So, we decided to see if omega-3 fatty acids could also reduce neurological damage caused by concussions. Our experiment was simple. We would attach a tiny steel helmet to the head of a rat and then drop a weight onto the head of the rat replicating the same type of injury an NFL player might receive to cause a concussion. This type of experiment was sufficient to induce a mild concussion, but no apparent physical injury. To half the rats we immediately started feeding them high levels of omega-3 fatty acids for the next 30 days. The other half of the rats received no supplementation. After 30 days, we examined the brains of each group for damage. Those rats that received no omega-3 supplementation had significant neurological damage including the appearance of proteins associated with development of Alzheimer's. On the other hand, the damage in the rats supplemented by the omega-3 fatty acids was reduced by 98 percent.

Concussion injuries in sports (football, soccer, field hockey, etc.) are random. However, activation of the Resolution Response is programmed and must be ready on demand. If you want the ultimate brain insurance policy to reduce the neurological damage from such potential sports injuries then you want to make sure you have high enough levels of omega-3 fatty acids in the blood before the injury actually occurs. The best way to ensure that is to maintain your AA/EPA ratio between 1.5 and 3.

SUMMARY ▷

Peak performance comes from optimal generation of ATP coupled with the simultaneous resolution of exercise-induced inflammation. Using the Zone Pro-Resolution Nutrition system as a performance "drug" provides you with a powerful advantage for the greatest success in whatever area of performance (both mental and physical) that you want to achieve.

18

Why Do We Get Fat?

ALTHOUGH MAINTAINING WELLNESS using the Zone Pro-Resolution Nutrition system should be your number one health goal, for most Americans their primary dietary focus is usually weight loss. Actually, it should be fat loss.

For most of us, we wake up one day and see excess body fat beginning to appear in all the wrong places. Unfortunately, this is happening at a younger and younger age, as I discussed earlier. The underlying cause of the accumulation of excess body fat is increased cellular inflammation and your growing inability to resolve it. The central player in fat gain is increased insulin resistance. It is not insulin per se, but insulin resistance that makes you fat and keeps you fat. The reason you have insulin resistance is because of a blocked Resolution Response.

THE DIFFERENCE BETWEEN FAT LOSS AND WEIGHT LOSS

Successful weight management must start with an understanding of what you are really talking about. Your body weight is primarily composed of three distinct components: water, lean body mass (muscle and bone), and fat. If you want to lose water, go to a sauna. If you want to lose muscle, dramatically cut back on your protein intake. The only health benefits that come with weight loss are a consequence of fat loss.

Regardless of what you read, the only way to lose excess fat is to consume fewer calories than are being expended (keeping in mind that most calories are used just to keep your body warm). This must be accomplished without hunger or fatigue throughout the day if you have any hope to maintain any fat loss for the long term. This is critical because fat loss is a slow process controlled by a wide variety of hormonal systems. In addition, there are a variety of hormonal defenders of fat loss that often conspire to ensure that much of the initial loss of excess body fat will eventually return if you don't have a lifelong dietary strategy to follow.

We also are lot fatter than we think. Body mass index (BMI) is the easy way to determine obesity, but it is not a very precise method as many top male professional athletes would be considered obese based on their BMI. The best measurement for determining obesity is dual-energy X-ray absorptiometry (DEXA) measurements. This is the gold standard for determining your percent body fat. Using DEXA measurements, you can run, but you can't hide from the results. According to the American Council of Exercise an ideal body fat percentage for a typical male should be about 15 percent and for the typical female it should be 22 percent. From a functional standpoint, a male at 15 percent body fat would not have any love handles and a female at 22 percent body fat would not have any cellulite. Anything above 25 percent body fat for males and 32 percent body fat for females is considered obese. So how does obesity in Americans rank based on percent body fat using DEXA measurements? The results were published in 2009 in the *American Journal of Clinical Nutrition* on some 13,000 representative American males and females measured between 1999 and 2004. The average male had 28 percent body fat and the average female 40 percent body fat suggesting that nearly 20 years ago the average American was already obese. If you look closer at the data, more than 67 percent of the males had more than 25 percent body fat, and 75 percent of the females had more than 32 percent body fat. This study suggested that at the beginning of the 21st century about 70 percent of Americans were actually obese. Meanwhile, using BMI measurements, the estimated levels of obesity in Americans in the same time period was only 31 percent. It appears the real obesity rates in America determined by DEXA measurements was more than double those rates estimated from BMI measurements. The levels of obesity have only continued to increase since that time.

WHY DO WE GAIN EXCESS BODY FAT?

The simple answer is that we consume more calories than we expend. Regardless of what anyone tells you about losing excess body fat and keeping it off, it is difficult. To understand why you gain excess body fat and how to achieve long-term weight management requires understanding the complex interplay of your diet on the levels of cellular inflammation in the blood, brain, and the gut.

Surprisingly, the accumulation of excess body fat does not begin in your fat cells, but in your brain and in particular, your hypothalamus. The hypothalamus controls your decisions about when to eat and how much to eat. The information it relies upon comes from hormonal inputs throughout the body, especially the levels of hormones in the blood as well as those coming from the gut that are sent directly to the brain via the vagus nerve in response to the macronutrient composition of a meal.

Hormonal signals that are continually produced in other parts of your body are integrated in the brain that determine hunger or satiety. The levels of insulin that reach the hypothalamus in the brain acts as its carbohydrate sensor. The levels of the hormone leptin coming from your stored body fat that also reach the hypothalamus is used as the brain's fat sensor. And finally, the levels of the hormones PYY and GLP-1 sent from the gut to the hypothalamus are the protein sensors for the brain. If the input of any of these hormonal inputs received by the brain is low, the brain tells you to eat. This assumes the hormonal sensors in the brain are properly receiving and interpreting these hormonal inputs. As an example, the increased intake of palmitic acid (the most abundant saturated fatty acid) can go directly to the hypothalamus to increase inflammation thus disrupting the information coming from those various hormones acting as fuel sensors. Once the hypothalamus becomes inflamed, it develops both insulin and leptin resistance so that the actual levels of insulin and leptin in the blood are perceived by the hypothalamus as artificially low thereby increasing hunger. In animal models, it only takes 24 hours to develop inflammation in the hypothalamus after starting a high-fat diet rich in palmitic acid.

The hormonal inputs from the blood and gut also converge at the hypothalamus to make the final decision determining whether you should eat or not. This is known as the energy-balance system, and it is remarkably fine-tuned. Since the average American consumes at least 750,000 calories each year (if not more), it doesn't take much cellular inflammation to distort the precision of the brain's energy-balance system. For example, only a slight decrease in hormonal signaling efficiency that increases your calorie intake by 1 percent would generate an extra two pounds of accumulated fat over the course of one year. That is what the average American gains on a yearly basis. In fact, the increase in calorie consumption since 1970 is more than adequate to explain today's obesity crisis.

To understand how this calorie mismatch occurs, consider your stored body fat as an "energy" bank. The ultimate "currency" used by every living cell in the body is chemical energy in the form of ATP made primarily by the mitochondria. Stored body fat is your ultimate energy bank filled with high-octane fuel. When you consume more calories in a meal than is immediately needed, the excess carbohydrates that can't easily be stored as glycogen in either your liver or your muscles are converted to fat that can be stored safely in your fat cells. The same is also true of any excess protein in a meal. However, the conversion of protein into fat takes more energy than converting excess carbohydrates into fat thereby generating a thermogenic effect as your protein intake increases. This is why isocaloric diets containing higher levels of protein compared to carbohydrate produce more initial weight loss because it takes more metabolic energy to convert any excess protein into stored body fat compared to converting excess carbohydrates into stored body fat. Of course, any excess dietary fat intake in a meal requires the least amount of metabolic energy to be converted into stored body fat.

Your goal is to reduce the level of excess stored body fat by using it for fuel in the muscles to make ATP. The first step is the reduction of insulin resistance by reducing diet-induced inflammation. The only way that is going to happen is to consume fewer calories without hunger or fatigue by improved hormonal control.

In an ideal world, your levels of insulin fall after a meal thus making it possible for your stored body fat to be released providing "high-octane" fuel for the mitochondria in other organs to produce energy in the form of ATP. I use the term "high-octane" since you can make far more ATP per gram of stored fat than per gram of stored carbohydrate. The release of stored body fat when insulin levels are decreased is like taking a withdrawal from the energy bank.

The wild card that can decrease this orderly withdrawal of energy is your level of insulin resistance. Insulin resistance as discussed earlier maintains elevated blood levels of insulin that blocks the release of stored body fat from the adipose tissue by inhibiting the gate-keeper (the hormone-sensitive lipase) that controls this withdrawal process in your fat cells. If you have high levels of insulin resistance, you are generally constantly hungry and fatigued. And what do you do if you are hungry or fatigued? You eat more calories.

Another factor that plays a role in this "banking" process is the energy-balance system located in the hypothalamus. If the hypothalamus determines the levels of insulin and leptin are adequate, you get signals not to eat. Of course, this assumes your hypothalamus is not inflamed. If it is, then all bets are off. This is because cellular inflammation also causes hormonal resistance (for both insulin and leptin) in the hypothalamus. The result is that hormonal signals of insulin and leptin levels in the blood are not received correctly, and the hypothalamus perceives their levels in the blood are actually lower than they really are. Increased insulin and leptin resistance caused by cellular inflammation in the hypothalamus has fooled the brain into thinking there is less energy coming into the body than there actually is. As a result, it activates hunger neurons to increase food intake. This results in a mismatch between calorie intake and calorie expenditure, so that you consume more calories than you actually need. This is particularly true of leptin, your fat fuel sensor. To compound the effects of insulin and/or leptin resistance, the lack of adequate protein at the meal will reduce the levels of satiety hormones (like PYY and GLP-1) released from the gut that go directly to the brain to tell your hypothalamus to stop eating. The combined result of insulin/leptin resistance and lack of adequate satiety hormones is that you are constantly hungry and you will consume more calories than you require. Thus, the key to long-term weight control is not to be hungry between meals. To achieve that goal, you need a diet that is balanced in protein, carbohydrates, and fat at every meal with the least number of calories to prevent hunger and fatigue. This is the foundation of the Zone Diet.

Another unexpected source of increased inflammation in both the hypothalamus and the blood is caused by a leaky gut that allows bacterial fragments to enter the blood that will also cause an inflammatory response that can eventually lead to disruption of the energy-balance system. This is called metabolic endotoxemia. The higher the saturated fat in your diet, the more likely these microbial fragments will enter into the blood that can piggyback with these saturated fats to enter the bloodstream more easily.

Even if the energy balance system in the hypothalamus is perfectly balanced, it can be overridden by the hedonic reward system. This system in the brain is activated by neural inputs from your taste receptors in the tongue. In particular, these taste receptors are activated by salt, sugar, and fat. These are also the primary food ingredients used by the processed food industry to make their products so irresistible since the 1970s. That was also the start of our current obesity epidemic in America.

MAINTAINING INITIAL WEIGHT LOSS IS HARD

Finally, there is the cognitive aspect to weight loss. Keeping lost body fat from returning requires a lifetime of constant decision making. The National Weight Control Registry is a program for individuals who have lost more than 30 pounds and kept the lost weight off for at least one year. Although it was established in 1995, currently there are only 10,000 registered members. This only demonstrates that keeping lost weight from returning is very difficult. However, this registry also provides a unique opportunity to see what dietary strategies have been useful for long-term weight management. The first dietary strategy is not to consume more than 1,500 calories per day and the other dietary insight is always eating breakfast. What this means is *the only way you are going to lose excess body fat and keep it from returning is to consume fewer calories and spread the consumption of those calories evenly throughout the day.* There is nothing magical about this. However, this means a long-term commitment to calorie restriction. As a consequence, restricting calories without hunger or fatigue and eating pleasing meals with the least amount of thinking is the real challenge. The Zone Diet makes this "impossible dream" a potential reality.

WHY WE REGAIN LOST BODY FAT

Losing excess body fat is relatively easy. Keeping it from returning is the hard part. Here are the five common reasons why fat regain is so common:

- Constant hunger and fatigue
- Restricting your favorite foods
- Too much thinking involved
- Too much preparation time involved
- Activation of powerful hormonal defenders that increase the likelihood of regaining all the initially lost body fat

So, let's look at each one of these factors in more detail.

Constant hunger and fatigue. Following a diet that simply restricts calories without regard to hormonal responses will always make you constantly hungry and tired. You are hungry because you are not consuming enough protein to stimulate satiety hormones generated in the gut (such as PYY and GLP-1) and fatigued since you usually are also cutting back on carbohydrates. Both nutrients are needed at every meal to stabilize blood sugar levels on a constant basis for optimal brain function. This hunger and fatigue might be fine for a few weeks, but not for a lifetime. The only way to overcome this problem is to restrict calories without hunger and fatigue. The best dietary pathway to achieve lack of hunger and fatigue is following the Zone Diet.

Restricting your favorite foods. You are also restricting your favorite foods (the ones that probably got you into trouble in the first place), thus causing the hedonic reward system constant distress. Once you have found the ten meals that work at home and ten meals that work for the restaurants you eat at as described in Chapter 12, you are always eating your favorite meals as you are losing excess body fat. Furthermore, you continue those same meals to keep the lost body fat from returning.

Too much thinking involved. Diets that restrict one or more food groups become very tiresome after time. This is especially true since cognitive thought requires a stable supply of glucose for the brain to function optimally. Once you have your top-ten Zone meals you can easily make at home and a similar number of Zone meals to order when dining out, you simply don't have to think anymore.

Too much preparation time involved. Time compression is greater than ever. The most obvious casualty is time to prepare food. That is why fast food restaurants exist. They are fast, cheap, and they meet your hunger needs. Once you have your ten proven Zone meals at home and dining out developed, the amount of time in buying and preparing those Zone meals at home is dramatically reduced and you don't have to think about what to eat off the menu when dining out.

Defenders of lost body fat. Diets ultimately fail because there are many powerful hormonal defenders that are activated with loss of excess body fat. The most important of these is the return of insulin resistance. This can occur in insulin-sensitive tissues like fat, muscle, and the liver, but the most insidious target of insulin resistance may be the hypothalamus because it is the command center for these defenders of body fat. Unless you reduce cellular inflammation in each of these locations you will continue to have powerful hormonal urges to eat excess calories. In addition, the cellular inflammation that causes insulin resistance, is also responsible for generating leptin resistance. The combination of both insulin and leptin resistance in the hypothalamus virtually guarantees the return of excess body fat. Furthermore, there is a corresponding increase in hunger hormones (such as ghrelin) coming from the gut after any diet-induced weight loss that also increases hunger. The end result is that hunger significantly increases after your initial weight loss. Finally, with the loss of body fat comes loss of muscle mass. Usually about 25 percent of your total weight loss consists of lost muscle mass. Loss of muscle decreases your metabolic rate. This is why you don't see any reunion specials for prior contestants of *The Biggest Loser* television series. Invariably almost everyone will regain their lost weight, it's just a matter of how fast the lost body fat will return. This is also why the chances of going from being obese to normal weight and staying at a normal weight is less than 1 percent. This is why you need to follow a defined, personalized dietary program on a continual basis not only to lose excess body fat, but also keep it from returning.

Unless you address each of these five major points, you can easily expect that much of any initial fat loss will return and all of the health benefits of losing that excess body fat will be lost too.

WHAT ABOUT LIPOSUCTION?

Why not just suck out the excess body fat? The interesting thing about liposuction is that within one year after removing the excess fat by lipo-suction, it reappears in other parts of the body, so the net loss of body fat is zero. The only trouble is that before the liposuction the excess fat was safely stored in your fat cells. After liposuction, the reappearance of the new excess body fat occurs in other tissues that are not designed to safely store fat. This type of fat is called ectopic fat and leads to lipotoxicity that disrupts hormonal signaling as discussed in my book, *Toxic Fat.*

WHAT ABOUT DRUGS?

If liposuction simply moves fat around, wouldn't it just be simpler to take a drug to reduce hunger and thus reduce calorie intake? Of course, it would, but such drugs have failed to provide a safe solution. It's not that they haven't tried.

One of the first weight-loss drugs developed was dinitrophenol (DNP) in the early 1930s. It worked by poisoning your mitochondria leading to a rapid decrease in ATP production and thereby increasing heat produc-tion produced from excess free radical formation. The resulting hyper-thermia could even become severe enough to potentially lead to death. Not a good outcome for long-term weight management.

The next drug class used for weight loss were amphetamines (mar-keted under the trade name Benzedrine in the United States). These were potentially addictive stimulants that suppressed hunger and increased the activity of the sympathetic nervous system, but their use was severely restricted because of their addiction potential in the late 1960s and they were completely eliminated in the over-the-counter market soon after-ward. However, one such amphetamine type drug was approved as a drug in 1959 to be used for a short time period (not exceeding twelve weeks). That drug was phentermine. It is a Class 3-controlled substance meaning it had potential for addiction, but it did suppress appetite. It had the same problems as other amphetamines (increased activation of the sympa-thetic nervous system), but one enterprising doctor thought if he added an approved anti depressive drug (fenfluramine) to phentermine he could reduce the jitters caused by the phentermine to permit longer term use. Hence was born the drug combination known as phen-fen. It should be noted there was no drug approval required because any physician could combine the two drugs for off-label use. Furthermore, all the clinical studies were basically the personal observations of one physician. None of these facts prevented the extraordinary rapid rise of using phen-fen in any weight-loss clinic that had a physician associated with it. Phen-fen weight loss was all the rage. The only trouble was, it wasn't patentable, therefore drug companies couldn't make any money on it since both drugs combined into the phen-fen combination were generic drugs.

That problem was potentially solved when a new drug called dexfen-fluramine (marketed as Redux) was approved by the FDA in 1996. Now you could make some real money with a patented drug. The only problem was that significant health problems were beginning to emerge with the growing use of both phen-fen and Redux; in particular heart valve problems and primary pulmonary hypertension that would require a double transplant of both the lungs and the heart. Obviously, all the necessary requirements for a big class-action lawsuit.

I was asked to be the lead expert on obesity for the plaintiffs in that suit. After giving days of depositions to the lawyers for the drug companies, their best legal defense was to declare me a "junk scientist" and therefore my testimony should not be allowed. Since the country's leading expert in primary pulmonary hypertension was also declared a "junk scientist," I felt I was in good company. Nonetheless, I had to go before the master court judge in Philadelphia to defend myself as an obesity expert. Armed only with a flip chart and a black marking pen (those were the days before PowerPoint), I outlined the reasons why Redux was not working. It did cause weight loss, but in about half the patients in the clinical trial used for its drug approval, they had actually gained body fat. That fact was not disclosed to the FDA in the drug application. The master judge decided I was an expert, and the case settled three days later with an $18 billion settlement by the drug company in 1997.

The next development for weight loss was not a drug, but an extract from the plant (Ephedra sinica), that contained several alkaloids including the stimulant ephedrine and the thermogenic agent, pseudoephedrine. Since it wasn't a drug, it could be sold in health food stores. The growing reports of adverse side effects and death caused the FDA to ban it in 2004.

By this time, the drug industry had a new weight-loss candidate, rimonabant. This was a drug that inhibited the binding of a group of eicosanoids known as endocannabinoids to their receptors in the brain. Endocannabinoids cause hunger. Tetrahydrocannabinol (THC), one of the active ingredients in marijuana also bind to the same receptors. This is why one of the first reactions to smoking marijuana is increased hunger (i.e., the munchies). It was approved as a weight-loss drug in Europe in 2006. However, it was never approved in the United States because of concerns about depression and mood disorders as a well as an increased risk for suicide. In 2008, the drug was banned in Europe.

A number of new drugs have been developed, but none of them have had commercial success. Perhaps, the answer is not looking for new drugs that poison the mitochondria, cause the overstimulation of the sympathetic nervous system, or cause mood disorders in the brain. A better choice would be to look for a new pathway that reduces elevated insulin resistance in obese individuals. That agent already exists and it's not a drug, but the Zone Pro-Resolution Nutrition system for optimizing the Resolution Response.

UNBLOCKING THE RESOLUTION RESPONSE TO ACCOMPLISH LIFE-LONG WEIGHT MANAGEMENT

Weight management becomes more difficult as you age for two reasons. One is increased insulin resistance caused by increasing cellular inflammation. The other is your mitochondria becomes less efficient in converting fatty acids and/or glucose into ATP. Optimizing your Resolution Response helps address both problems. First it reduces insulin resistance by reducing residual cellular inflammation through the increased production of resolvins. Second, it can increase mitochondrial efficiency via the activation of AMP kinase by polyphenols so even though your total muscle mass may decrease with age, the efficiency of the mitochondria within your remaining muscles can increase their ATP production although you are consuming fewer calories following the Zone Diet.

SUMMARY ▸

Calories do count, but the hormonal responses generated by those calories count even more when it comes to reducing insulin resistance, the obligatory first step toward losing excess body fat. The Zone Diet is based on calorie restriction coupled with an accompanying hormonal balance throughout the day that prevents hunger and fatigue. You will experience the benefits of reduced hunger and greater energy in just a few days. To maintain those benefits, you have to practice this dietary lifestyle for a lifetime. However, you will still need to fully complete the Resolution Response by combining the Zone Diet with high-dose EPA and DHA to resolve inflammation in the brain that reduces both insulin resistance and leptin resistance in the hypothalamus and also using high-dose polyphenols to activate AMP kinase to increase the production of new efficient mitochondria needed for successful lifelong weight management.

19

Why Do We Get Sick?

THE BEST WAY to stay well is not developing a chronic disease in the first place. This is why Hippocrates stated some 2,500 years ago that "I will prevent disease whenever I can, for prevention is preferable to cure." That simply means maintaining your wellness for as long as possible. This begins with controlling cellular inflammation as early in life as possible and maintaining yourself in the Zone to optimize the Resolution Response for a lifetime.

WHAT IS WELLNESS?

The goal of medicine should be maintaining wellness. However, defining wellness is a slippery slope, because most people will say if they don't have a chronic disease, then they must be well. That is often a false assumption. Although we have a lot of clinical tests for describing chronic disease, surprisingly we have few markers or even a clinical definition for wellness. I firmly believe the clinical markers that define the Zone that I outlined earlier are also the clinical markers that can be used to define wellness. Once those markers are in their appropriate ranges, then you know you have done everything possible using your diet to optimize the Resolution Response that is the key to maintaining wellness. If you are not in the Zone, although you may not yet have developed a chronic disease, this means your Resolution Response is already partially blocked, which means you have a decreased ability to combat growing levels of cellular inflammation that is constantly amplified by diet-induced inflammation. This combination ensures that you will accelerate your development of some type of chronic disease in the future.

Since injuries that generate inflammation are random, you need to maintain each stage of the Resolution Response at peak efficiency to invoke a strong and robust Resolution Response when needed.

Make no mistake about it, reaching the Zone is necessary to maintain a robust Resolution Response. It requires dietary discipline to achieve the optimal ranges of each of the clinical markers that define wellness. Following the Zone Pro-Resolution Nutrition system, you can bring yourself into the Zone within a relatively short period of time. Staying there is the challenge.

WHAT IS CHRONIC DISEASE?

You can use the figure below to understand the pathway from wellness to chronic disease.

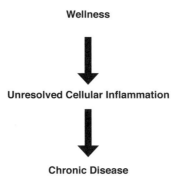

Wellness

↓

Unresolved Cellular Inflammation

↓

Chronic Disease

We all start out in the state of wellness. At the molecular level this means that the inflammation generated by injuries is constantly balanced by your Resolution Response to generate healing. Your pathway toward developing chronic disease starts with increasing cellular inflammation eventually reaching a point that a particular organ is no longer operating at normal efficiency. Furthermore, any unresolved cellular inflammation can be amplified by continued diet-induced inflammation. As I described earlier, the build-up of cellular inflammation is highly dependent on the degree of inhibition of your Resolution Response. The further you are from the Zone, the more your Resolution Response is blocked. Unless your Resolution Response is operating at optimal levels, it is just a matter of time before you develop some type of chronic disorder that will likely require the lifetime use of medication to manage its symptoms. I personally believe that chronic disease is a consequence of long-term blockage of your Resolution Response instead of a drug deficiency condition.

Diseases like heart disease, cancer, and Alzheimer's takes years, if not decades, of constant inflammatory damage to develop. If enough accumulated organ damage caused by scar tissue formation (i.e., fibrosis) develops, then the organ will function at a lower level compromising its performance. Eventually this requires a need for constant medication to manage that chronic condition. This is the loss of function described by Rudolf Virchow in the 19th century as the final stage of unresolved inflammation. It is estimated that 45 percent of all mortality is associated with significant fibrosis.

Once you have a chronic disease, the best you can do is attempt to manage its symptoms for the rest of your life using increasingly higher levels of various medications because you have not eliminated the underlying cause which is increasing levels of cellular inflammation. Today medicine can rarely tell you why you developed a chronic disease (unlike the cause of an infectious disease), only how to manage its symptoms.

On the other hand, a pathway back to an improved state of wellness does exist by optimizing the Resolution Response through the simultaneous reduction of the intensity of diet-induced inflammation coupled with the resolution of as much as possible of the remaining residual cellular inflammation. Only when the residual cellular inflammation is sufficiently reduced, can that be followed by the repair of as much of the damaged tissue as possible. There is no drug for this highly orchestrated biological process, but the Zone Pro-Resolution Nutrition system provides a potential dietary pathway to optimize the efficiency of the Resolution Response. Does optimizing the Resolution Response using the Zone Pro-Resolution Nutrition system completely rectify all the previous long-term existing damage to your organs? Probably not because of prior scar tissue formation (fibrosis), but at least you are moving toward an improved state of wellness that should require the least amount of medication possible in the future to treat the remaining symptoms of an existing chronic disease.

One of the first signs you are moving toward developing a chronic disease is usually the accumulation of excess body fat. So, let's start there to explore how that leads to the eventual development of chronic disease.

Obesity

Once you become obese, your health troubles generally begin to expand along with your waistline. But why? Excess body fat makes your existing fat cells expand in size to accommodate the added fat. A healthy fat cell can do this. If the fat cell is compromised (i.e., it's sick), then it can't expand. This lack of expansion is usually a consequence of fibrosis in the adipose tissue. This reduces oxygen transfer to them making it more difficult to produce adequate levels of ATP and mitochondria in the fat cells and they start producing more free radicals creating oxidative stress. Due to increased oxidative stress, otherwise normally healthy fat cells become sick and with continued oxidative stress they start to die. This uncontrolled cellular death (i.e., necrosis) of the fat cell starts an inflammatory response to remove the damaged tissue and results in a surge of inflammatory macrophages into your adipose tissue. It has been shown that nearly 50 percent of the weight of adipose tissue in obese individuals is composed of these inflammatory cells that keep producing more inflammatory agents (free radicals and cytokines). Without a strong Resolution Response your excess fat becomes a staging area for producing a continuing flow of pro-inflammatory cytokines to other organs that only accelerates growing cellular inflammation throughout the body.

Metabolic syndrome (Pre-diabetes)

Another indication that cellular inflammation is beginning to build-up is the development of insulin resistance. As insulin resistance increases, your pancreas responds by increasing insulin secretion in an attempt to reduce blood glucose levels. This results in constant hyperinsulinemia that distorts insulin's ability to properly manage your metabolism. Developing metabolic syndrome, as the name suggests, indicates that all phases of your metabolism are no longer functioning well. The underlying cause of metabolic syndrome is increased insulin resistance.

According to the Centers for Disease Control more than 86 million Americans have metabolic syndrome. Metabolic syndrome is characterized by increased abdominal obesity, higher triglyceride levels, decreased HDL cholesterol, and increased hypertension caused by sustained hyperinsulinemia. This is also a recipe for making more eicosanoids because the combination of omega-6 fatty acids and elevated insulin increases the reservoir of arachidonic acid (AA) making it easier to generate those eicosanoids, especially leukotrienes. Leukotrienes not only accelerate insulin resistance, but they can also begin attacking the beta cells in the pancreas. The beta cells are responsible for making insulin. Consider metabolic syndrome as a wake-up call that your pancreas is under continuing inflammatory attack. Eventually, your beta cells simply stop producing enough insulin to prevent your blood glucose levels from rising into a danger zone. When that happens, you develop diabetes. The period of time from the beginning development of metabolic syndrome to having full-fledged type 2 diabetes is usually 10-15 years.

Type 2 diabetes

More than 30 million Americans have type 2 diabetes—about 12 percent of the total adult population. However, diabetes is a worldwide epidemic with more than 420 million individuals with this chronic disease. Although type 2 diabetes is a result of an inflammatory attack on the beta cells of the pancreas, it is also indicative that unresolved cellular inflammation has already been metastasizing like a cancer to every organ in the body. This is why once you are a diabetic, you are four times more likely to develop heart disease and almost twice as likely to develop Alzheimer's.

Heart disease

Heart disease remains the #1 cause of death in the United States. Our current diabetic epidemic suggests that heart disease will continue to maintain its top ranking for some time to come. This is because diabetes is ultimately a disease of inflammation characterized by increased glycosylated hemoglobin, elevated insulin, and increased levels of pro-inflammatory cytokines. All of these clinical markers are far more predictive of developing heart disease than is elevated LDL cholesterol. In fact, oxidized LDL is more predictive of future heart disease than is normal LDL cholesterol.

It is now becoming recognized that heart disease is a disease of inflammation, not a disease of elevated cholesterol. In fact, 50 percent of the individuals who develop heart disease have normal cholesterol levels. The recent CANTOS study demonstrated that you can significantly reduce development of heart disease by reducing the levels of pro-inflammatory cytokines with no change in LDL cholesterol levels. The same cytokine that was reduced in the CANTOS study using injections of monoclonal antibodies can also be reduced with high-dose EPA and DHA as reported in the *New England Journal of Medicine* in 1989. Combining the Zone Diet with high-dose EPA and DHA to reduce cytokines and using high-dose polyphenols to reduce oxidized LDL cholesterol seems like a far superior strategy for treating heart disease compared to the current medical love affair that physicians have with statins.

Hypertension is often associated with heart disease because of its strong association with stroke. Both aspirin and statins have little impact on hypertension, but reducing insulin resistance does. This is because one of the first signs of developing metabolic syndrome is often an increase in hypertension. As discussed earlier, the Zone Diet has more potential for reducing hypertension than does the highly recommended Dietary Approaches to Stop Hypertension (DASH) diet. But that is also why the Zone Diet is also more effective than the DASH diet in reducing insulin resistance.

Alzheimer's

It is estimated that 10 percent of all Americans older than 65 have some form of Alzheimer's and this percentage increases to 50 percent by age 85. There is no cure, the current treatments are pathetic at best, and no one knows what causes the condition in the first place. The only area that there is some general agreement is that Alzheimer's is an inflammatory disease and seems to be related to insulin resistance. This is why many neurologists consider Alzheimer's as "type 3 diabetes" because of this strong relationship to insulin resistance. This presents an opportunity for the Zone Pro-Resolution Nutrition system to reduce the likelihood of developing, as well as treating, Alzheimer's.

Since Alzheimer's is an inflammatory condition, then reducing neuroinflammation should be a good starting point for not only its prevention, but also its treatment. This was the goal of the MIND diet described in Chapter 14. As I discussed in that chapter, the Zone Diet has a much better likelihood to reduce neuroinflammation because of its clinically proven results in reducing insulin resistance.

However, that is only part of the equation. It was demonstrated in 2000 that individuals who had Alzheimer's also had an AA/EPA ratio that was 93 percent higher than in age-matched individuals without any cognitive impairment. This is a strong indication that they may also have had more unresolved cellular inflammation in the brain. Drugs have great difficulty passing though the blood-brain barrier, which explains why 99 percent of potential Alzheimer's drugs have failed. On the other hand, EPA and DHA can readily enter the brain if their levels are high enough in the blood. Once in the brain, these omega-3 fatty acids can generate increased levels of resolvins necessary to reduce the neuroinflammation that characterizes Alzheimer's. This is why Alzheimer's can be better understood as a disease caused by a defective Resolution Response. This is also why high-dose EPA and DHA in animal models can also rapidly reduce the development of amyloid plaque precursors in the brain after inducing a concussion injury, as I described in Chapter 17.

Finally, high-dose polyphenols can activate AMP kinase that orchestrates the production of new functional mitochondria to maintain adequate ATP levels for maintaining cognitive brain function. Together, using each of the dietary components of the Zone Pro-Resolution Nutrition system creates a formidable dietary approach to optimize the Resolution Response to potentially prevent Alzheimer's or at least more effectively manage it before it becomes so severe that the patient requires constant supervision.

Cancer

Cancer is often thought of as a genetic disease, yet in 2018 it was shown that healthy individuals have even higher levels of cancer-associated genetic mutations than those with cancer. So, how does one person get cancer and the other doesn't if they have the same, if not a greater number, of cancer-associated mutations? I would suggest it may be differences in the strength of their Resolution Response to respond to the inflammation induced by molecular injuries.

This is why I feel that cancer may be better understood as a metabolic disease than a genetic disease. It is known that cancer is strongly associated with increased production of eicosanoids and increases in NF-κB activity as well as a decrease in AMP kinase activity. The benefit of AMP kinase activation as a cancer prevention strategy is that it also reduces the activity of another gene transcription factor (mTOR), which is strongly implicated in tumor growth.

Another major problem with today's cancer treatment is related to the inability to clean up the cellular debris of dead tumor cells (i.e., necrosis) created by radiation, chemotherapy, or immunotherapy treatments. This cellular debris is the result of necrosis, as opposed to a controlled cell death (i.e., apoptosis) and that debris can become a potent generator of additional inflammation via increased production of pro-inflammatory cytokines. These inflammatory cytokines can act as a feeder system to awaken otherwise dormant tumor cells in distant sites in the body that become resistant to more aggressive chemotherapy. This makes currently practiced cancer treatments a "double-edged sword." Sure, you will kill tumor cells, but the cellular debris left behind sets the body up for new tumor growth in distant sites (metastasis) that may be resistant to all known therapies. Not a very pleasant picture.

It was Charles Serhan at Harvard Medical School who took the lead in demonstrating that resolvins can stop this "cytokine storm" in its tracks by rapidly clearing out the tumor cell debris. The best way to ensure you have adequate levels of EPA and DHA to generate the necessary levels of resolvins is to keep your AA/EPA ratio between 1.5 and 3 before, during, and after your treatment for cancer (like for the rest of your life).

All of these metabolic factors that are major contributing factors for cancer development can be modulated with the Zone Pro-Resolution Nutrition system to enhance your Resolution Response. This doesn't mean that there is not a need for chemotherapy, radiation, or even immunotherapy, but with an optimal Resolution Response it is possible to potentially require a lower intensity of the standard cancer interventions with correspondingly fewer damaging side effects.

AUTOIMMUNE DISORDERS

Autoimmune diseases such as multiple sclerosis, rheumatoid arthritis, type 1 diabetes, and others are considered idiopathic diseases (i.e., diseases of unknown origin). It is very hard to treat a disease if you don't know what causes it. However, we do know that all autoimmune disorders result from an overactive inflammatory response attacking normal tissues. An alternative view of autoimmune disorders might be better understood as a consequence of a blocked Resolution Response. If so, let's look as some common autoimmune conditions.

Multiple sclerosis

Although there is some association of multiple sclerosis with low levels of vitamin D, a stronger association exists with low levels of EPA and DHA in the blood. This is suggested from intervention studies from Norway in subjects with multiple sclerosis that indicated consuming more fruits and vegetables as well as consuming supplemental EPA and DHA resulted in a statistically significant improvement of their disability index after two years compared to the control group who followed the standard Norwegian diet. Those who followed the standard diet became more disabled during the same time period compared to those taking EPA and DHA supplementation who had a reduction of their disability. The primary blood marker that correlated best with this improvement in that time period was a significant decrease in the AA/EPA ratio. As has been suggested for Alzheimer's and cancer, one might consider multiple sclerosis to be the result of a blocked Resolution Response thus making it an ideal chronic disease for an aggressive application of the Zone Pro-Resolution Nutrition system.

Rheumatoid arthritis

Although rheumatoid arthritis affects less than 1 percent of the population, the biological monoclonal antibody drugs to treat it account for more than $25 billion in worldwide sales. These drugs are designed to reduce the pro-inflammatory cytokine, tumor necrosis factor (TNF). Yet in 1989 it was shown that supplementation with 5 grams of EPA and DHA per day would also reduce this same inflammatory cytokine just like the use of injectable monoclonal antibodies drugs. Furthermore, once the EPA and DHA supplementation was discontinued, the levels of TNF and other pro-inflammatory cytokines soon returned to their original levels.

Type 1 diabetes

Unlike type 2 diabetes that usually develops later in life, type 1 diabetes often strikes in childhood and early adulthood. It is known from a 2003 study in Norway that newborn children who took a teaspoon a day of cod liver oil (supplying 0.8 grams of EPA and DHA) for the first year of life had a 26 percent decrease in the development of type 1 diabetes. So, maybe EPA and DHA have a role to play in preventing its development? It is also known that a major driver for the destruction of insulin-producing beta cells in the pancreas is 12-hydroxyeicosatetraenoic acid (12-HETE) derived from AA.

In children with early onset type 1 diabetes, you can begin to see a build-up of circulating diabetes-related antibodies about six months before those antibodies begin to attack and destroy the insulin-producing beta cells in the pancreas. This is called the "honeymoon" period for children with recently diagnosed type 1 diabetes. Recent animal data has indicated that high-dose EPA and DHA could not only reduce the immunological attack on the pancreas, but also potentially increase the survival of the beta cells. The likely mechanism involves the increased resolution of cellular inflammation in the beta cells of the pancreas that blocks the infiltration of immune cells into the islets of the pancreas. Recent case studies have indicated that starting children with early onset type 1 diabetes on high-dose EPA and DHA supplementation reduces their insulin dosage by about 75% if the AA/EPA ratio was reduced to less than 3. There is also an indication that rebuilding of the beta cells was also taking place in these children as measured by the increased levels of C-peptide (a marker of insulin synthesis in the beta cells) as long as the AA/EPA ratio remains less than 3.

It has been my experience working with adult type 1 diabetic patients that they can reduce their levels of insulin once they start following the Zone Pro-Resolution Nutrition system. Whether this is due to a reduction of insulin resistance or an increase in C-peptide production (or a combination of both) remains to be determined.

MIND-BODY DISORDERS

Mind-body disorders are some of the best examples of an idiopathic disease. Since the cause is unknown, the patient's symptoms are all but ignored by the physician who often prescribes antidepressant medication in the hope of better managing their symptoms. Such mind-body idiopathic conditions encompass a great number of chronic disorders such as chronic fatigue syndrome, fibromyalgia, depression, and anxiety. It may be that their underlying cause may actually originate from a dysfunctional gut with the wrong balance of microbes. If so, then the Zone Pro-Resolution Nutrition system has a great potential for managing many mind-body disorders.

The reason why microbes in the gut can potentially affect the brain is because microbes developed a primitive form of communication millions of years ago. It is called "quorum sensing" that allows one microbial species to recognize another and begin working in cooperative actions. Many of these molecules used by microbes are either identical to some of the same neurotransmitters our brain uses, like gamma-aminobutyric acid or GABA, serotonin, and dopamine, or their metabolites that can act as mimics to other neurotransmitters. Because of the direct highway from the gut to the brain via the vagus nerve, the microbes in the gut can be a virtual neurological drug pharmacy (for better or worse) for your brain.

Adding to this complexity is the fact that the gut's bacterial food factories are vastly more sophisticated than our own more-limited digestive enzymes. These bacterial enzymes can breakdown complex carbohydrate polymers (i.e., fermentable fiber), polyphenols, and many synthetic chemicals into a wide array of metabolites that can enter the blood. In fact, nearly 40 percent of the chemicals in the blood come from gut microbial metabolism. These often also have significant metabolic and neurochemical consequences that we simply don't understand yet. Furthermore, many of these mind-body disorders are also characterized by increased neuroinflammation, suggesting that high-dose omega-3 fatty acids will also have a significant role to play in their treatment.

Chronic fatigue syndrome

Chronic fatigue syndrome is usually characterized by profound often incapacitating fatigue. Symptoms include gut problems, impaired memory or thinking as well as anxiety and depression. Not surprisingly, the diagnosis of chronic fatigue syndrome borders on gazing into a crystal ball.

Recent data indicates that the diversity of microbes in the gut is reduced in those individuals with this condition. Reduced microbial diversity is usually associated with the pathway that eventually leads to a leaky gut, and an increase of microbial fragments in the blood causing systemic inflammation. Finally, the newest research indicates that individuals with chronic fatigue syndrome have significant reductions of certain metabolites in their blood. These are the same metabolites that are also decreased in the physiological state known as "dauer" in which the metabolism slows down to essentially minimal life-support status to deal with some undefined environmental stress. That sounds like chronic fatigue to me.

Any environmental stressor (like exposure to toxins, air pollution, or chemicals) acts like an injury that will increase cellular inflammation. If that exposure occurs in the gut, then the increased production of pro-inflammatory cytokines generated by cellular inflammation can travel directly to the brain via the vagus nerve. If that injury is not resolved, then cytokine production continues. Cytokines make you sick and tired. That's another pretty good definition of chronic fatigue syndrome.

Fibromyalgia

Fibromyalgia is characterized by chronic widespread pain that has specific sites or tender points. This is different than the generalized chronic fatigue associated with chronic fatigue syndrome. There also seems to be an age factor involved, as fibromyalgia seems to peak in the age range of 55-65-year-olds compared to a younger age range in the case of chronic fatigue syndrome.

Although there is a lot of confusion between chronic fatigue syndrome and fibromyalgia, the underlying cause of each condition may be related to disturbances in gut biology, which often co-exists with both conditions. Since a leaky gut starts a long process with the end result being increased levels of pro-inflammatory cytokines, it is likely that the diverse pain associated with fibromyalgia may also be related back to gut dysfunction. Of course, the standard treatment for both conditions tends to be antidepressant therapy, which makes no sense if the underlying cause may be gut-induced inflammation.

If this working hypothesis is valid, then the treatment may be relatively simple in principle. Feed the microbes with adequate fermentable fiber and then supplement with more EPA and DHA and polyphenols to rebuild the mucus barrier and repair the integrity of the tight junctions in the gut wall. That's why using the Zone Pro-Resolution Nutrition system seems to make a lot more sense than the standard therapy of taking more antidepressants.

Depression

You can also add depression as another potential mind-body-gut disorder. More than 10 percent of adult Americans take anti depressant drugs. Yet meta-analysis of multiple depression studies using front-line serotonin-selective reuptake inhibitors (SSRI) like Prozac indicate that they are only slightly more effective than a placebo. More detailed analysis indicates that SSRI drugs work in about 25 percent of the patients, make the depression worse in 25 percent of the patients, and for 50 percent of the patients their depression lifts without drugs over time. The fact that anti-depressant drugs take a long time to demonstrate any benefits may be indicative the depression can potentially heal on its own.

However, the treatment of depression can be enhanced with the use of high-dose EPA and DHA. As an example, 10 grams of EPA and DHA per day is effective in treating bipolar as well as treating standard mono-polar depression using slightly lower doses of EPA and DHA. It also appears that high-dose EPA and DHA can also significantly reduce the future occurrence of schizophrenia in high-risk individuals. Although much of that focus has been on the ability of omega-3 free fatty acids to enter the brain to reduce neuroinflammation, their ability to reduce inflammation by improving a leaky gut may be another mechanism to explain their effects. This is especially true since there are reports of higher antibodies to bacterial fragments such as lipopolysaccharide (LPS) in the blood of depressed patients.

Anxiety

Anxiety is an even more diffuse condition to diagnose than depression. Unlike SSRI drugs that take a long time to work, the standard drug treatment for anxiety includes drugs like Valium that work very quickly as a tranquilizer. Unfortunately, these Valium-like drugs are also addictive. Valium interacts with the same receptors in the brain as does the natural neurotransmitter gamma amino butyric acid (GABA). However, it is known that bacteria in the gut can make the neurotransmitters (such as GABA) used for quorum sensing by other microbes. It may be possible that some of the anxiety might be due to lack of GABA being produced by bacteria in the gut. If adequate levels of GABA were being produced in the gut, it could potentially reach the brain via the vagus nerve to act as a Valium-like drug without the addictive properties. This is why current treatment relies on either using anti depressant drugs (probably acting as a placebo) or the use of psychotherapy, like cognitive behavioral therapy, neither of which are that effective in treating anxiety, especially if the problem is related to a deficiency in GABA levels.

It is also known that anxiety is a major cause of relapse in the treatment of addiction. One study using high-dose omega-3 fatty acids demonstrated a statistically significant reduction of relapse in recovering drug addicts. A recent review of the literature has indicated that supplementation with omega-3 fatty acid concentrates containing greater than 2 grams per day of EPA and DHA is required to see any benefits in the treatment of anxiety.

SUMMARY ▶

Hippocrates was correct in stating that prevention is preferable to curing disease. That goal is only possible by optimizing your Resolution Response. You want to maintain your wellness for as long as possible to prevent the development of chronic disease. But to do so, you need an understanding that the ultimate cause for virtually all chronic disease starts with the blocking of your internal Resolution Response. To optimize the Resolution Response requires a dietary program that can easily be followed for a lifetime. The Zone Pro-Resolution Nutrition system provides that dietary approach.

20

Why Do We Age?

AS I DISCUSSED in the last chapter, the primary reason we become sick is increased cellular inflammation caused by the blockage of the Resolution Response. This is also the same reason we get fat. Not surprisingly, when it comes to aging, the usual suspect is the same.

A good definition of aging may be loss of function. Our organs simply don't function as well as they did when we were younger due to unresolved cellular inflammation and the subsequent scar tissue (fibrosis) that forms to cover up the damage. Therefore, it is probably not unexpected that every marker of inflammation increases in the elderly. In fact, no human with authentic medical records has ever lived beyond 122.

Your real goal is not to increase lifespan, but to expand your healthspan. Healthspan is defined as longevity minus years of disability. Consider your healthspan as the number of functional years you live.

Considering that half of all U.S. adults have at least one chronic disease, and by age 65 Americans usually have at least two chronic diseases, a long life of functional health is seemingly harder to achieve. Before you believe the on going hype that medical technology will save you from yourself, the National Center for Health Statistics announced in late 2016 that the life expectancy of Americans fell for the first time since 1993. In fact, the death rates increased in 8 of the 10 top causes of mortality including the #1 cause of death, heart disease. This trend toward decreasing life expectancy has continued. After more than 20 years of unparalleled medical hype (and of course increasing costs), we don't seem to have much to show, especially relative to increasing your healthspan, let alone lifespan.

We age for the same reason you don't find many 40-year-old cars on the road. They wear out. In our case, we wear out by the accumulated damage (like fibrosis) caused by unresolved cellular inflammation. I wrote about this in great detail in my book, *The Anti-Aging Zone*. Although the book was written 20 years ago, its insights on aging still remain relevant today. Rather than simply repeating the concepts that I outlined in that book, let me add some new ones.

Unresolved cellular inflammation is the real driver of weight gain, development of chronic disease, and aging. Without a strong Resolution Response, you have no possible way to reduce unresolved cellular inflammation. Unless increasing levels of unresolved inflammation are reduced by optimizing your Resolution Response, the body is forced to resort to Plan B, which is the development of fibrosis. Fibrosis is scar tissue that encases the unresolved inflammation. It stops the spread of the inflammation, but also causes non-functionality in that damaged part of the organ (and this includes fat cells). The more widespread the fibrosis becomes in your organs, the less functional your body becomes as you age even though you may not have yet developed any chronic disease.

HORMONES AND AGING

We are often led to think of aging as a result of the decreasing levels of the hormones (testosterone, estrogen, and growth hormone) associated with youth. Although it's true that these hormones decrease with age, the negative health consequences of aging are far more associated with the hormones that actually increase with age. These hormones are eicosanoids, insulin, and cortisol. The increases of each of these three hormones are driven by increased cellular inflammation.

Eicosanoids

These are the hormonal mediators of inflammation that are your body's response to injuries (both internal and external). They are needed in small amounts to initiate the inflammatory response to an injury, but beyond the required levels they lead to chronic unresolved cellular inflammation that accelerates the aging process. Their levels are ultimately controlled by the diet. That's why I developed the Zone Diet to keep these eicosanoid levels in a therapeutic zone that is not too high (to cause excess cellular inflammation), but not too low to prevent a necessary inflammatory response to injury.

Insulin

As I have discussed earlier, insulin is central to your metabolism. However, increasing eicosanoid formation generates insulin resistance that not only disturbs your metabolism, but also generates constantly elevated insulin levels in the blood. This is why aging, like virtually every chronic disease, has a strong association with increased insulin resistance. As blood insulin levels rise with increasing insulin resistance, this leads to a further generation of even more eicosanoids especially in the presence of excessive levels of dietary consumption of omega-6 fatty acids. The result of increased eicosanoid production amplifies the effect of any existing chronic unresolved cellular inflammation on the aging process.

Cortisol

As the levels of chronic unresolved cellular inflammation caused by excessive levels of eicosanoids rise, your body's response is to secrete more cortisol to reduce their production because cortisol inhibits their formation. However, increased cortisol levels actually accelerate the rate of aging by the collateral damage it causes. This collateral damage includes increased insulin resistance that makes you gain excess body fat, depressing your immune response that makes you sick, and the loss of cells in the hippocampus that robs you of your memory. All of these lead to a decreased healthspan.

All of these hormonal responses (eicosanoids, insulin, and cortisol) are linked, meaning if one goes up, the others will follow. This is why all roads that decrease your healthspan ultimately lead back to increased chronic unresolved cellular inflammation. Conversely, this is why decreasing the levels of excessive eicosanoids, insulin, and cortisol are the hormonal keys to improving your healthspan. You do these by following the Zone Pro-Resolution Nutrition program.

DEFINING ANTI-AGING MEDICINE

There are no prescription drugs to decrease this potential build-up of eico-sanoids, insulin, and cortisol that occurs as you age. On the other hand, the Zone Pro-Resolution Nutrition system allows you to manipulate each of these hormonal responses in a highly controlled and reproducible manner that results in optimizing your Resolution Response. At the molecular level, you are decreasing the levels of excess eicosanoids, insulin, and cortisol while simultaneously increasing the generation of resolvins (using high-dose omega-3 fatty acids) and activation of AMP kinase (using high-dose polyphenols) that are both critical for healing. The end result is an in-creased healthspan. That's also my definition of anti-aging medicine.

WHY NOT JUST TAKE HORMONES TO SLOW AGING?

There are certain hormones (testosterone, estrogen, and growth hor-mone) that do decrease with aging, so why not just replace them to re-verse the aging process? When you increase these hormones, they also create their own set of unique problems that don't necessarily lead to healthy aging. The sex hormones (testosterone and estrogen) do block the uptake of fat in your fat cells so you will appear younger in the mirror. However, they are called sex hormones for a reason. They are supposed to peak during your most fertile years, and then decrease. This is because hormones are usually multi-tasking molecules. They do several jobs, many of which we are still unaware of. Once you start increasing age-dependent hormones in the body, you run the risk of causing other un-foreseen problems like cancer. This problem first emerged with the early use of estrogen replacement therapy as the first anti-aging drug. It caused cancer. That's a huge price to pay for looking younger. However, those early estrogen hormones were synthetic. Perhaps, if you used exactly the same bioidentical hormones made by the body, you might not have this problem? Unfortunately, the hormones used might be bioidentical in the test tube, but not necessarily in your body, since their metabolism is dif-ferent because they are taken either orally or transdermally as opposed to the natural release from the ovaries . The same is true of testosterone in comparing its fate in the body coming from injections or transdermal patches as opposed to its natural release from the testes.

Likewise, the use of human growth hormone (HGH) will improve the appearance of youth, but once injected, the growth hormone goes directly to the liver where it is converted into another hormone, insulin-like growth factor-1 or IGF-1. IGF-1 is associated with an increased likelihood of cancer development. Nonetheless, since all of these hormones are prescription drugs, they provide a great business opportunity to turn their off-label use into a thriving business, especially if you are a licensed physician running an anti-aging clinic.

WHY ARE WE LIVING LONGER?

The primary reason we are living longer than a century ago is not because of new drug breakthroughs. In fact, the vast majority of the drugs used today (especially for cancer treatment) were developed decades ago. Moreover, the primary cause of our increased lifespan in the 20th century was not drugs, but improvements in public health. This would include clean water coming into the house, improved sanitation of waste water coming out of the home, as well as antibiotics to treat infectious bacterial disease and vaccines to prevent viral disease. Among the largest decreases in mortality were those coming from early childhood mortality and the reduction of mortality associated with childbirth. If you reached age 45 in 1900, the extension of your remaining lifespan would have been only about three years longer by the late 20th century. As I mentioned earlier in this chapter, the lifespan of Americans dropped for the first time in the 21st century in 2015 and has continued to decline. Furthermore, an article published in the *New England Journal of Medicine* in 2005 indicated that our current generation of children may be the first in American history to have a shorter lifespan than their parents due to increased obesity and diabetes. Both conditions are driven by increased insulin resistance caused by unresolved cellular inflammation.

WHY WE LOSE FUNCTION AS WE AGE

Loss of function is caused by increasing fibrosis due to unresolved cellular inflammation as well as just plain losing cells that are not replaced in a timely fashion. The end result is fewer functional cells in the organ resulting in decreased organ function. This is the reason why we become weaker as we age. We lose muscle cells at a faster rate than we can renew them and this is why strength reaches a maximum at age 25 and declines thereafter. In every organ we have organ-specific stem cells that are called upon to make new functional cells to replace the lost cells. Chronic unresolved cellular inflammation can also inhibit the ability of organ-specific stem cells to replace damaged cells for that particular organ. Furthermore, inflammation also ages the stem cells so they can no longer function effectively. So, as we age, increasing cellular inflammation decreases our ability to replace damaged cells in various organs. This results in loss of function. But how fast do different cells in the body actually age? As I have discussed earlier, it is highly variable between the cells in different organs.

Organ	Typical Cell Lifetime
Gut	5 days
Skin	30 days
Heart	10 years
Skeletal muscle	10 years
Fat cells	10 years
Brain	
Hippocampus	25 years
Frontal cortex	Never

You can see there are striking differences found in different organs. The cells that compose your gut lining and outer skin turn over very rapidly, whereas those cells that compose most of your internal organs turn over much more slowly. However, for the cells in the brain, what you start out with is pretty much what you have for life. The cells in the brain are the ones you want to protect from unresolved cellular inflammation.

The pathway to a longer healthspan ultimately lies not with hormone injections, but with changing gene expression that leads to the optimization of your Resolution Response. Specifically, you want to reduce the activation of NF-κB to decrease inflammation, while improving your metabolism with the simultaneous activation of AMP kinase. Both genetic actions can be modulated in the appropriate directions following the Zone Pro-Resolution Nutrition system to optimize your Resolution Response.

There are two dietary ways to activate AMP kinase: calorie restriction and supplementation with high-dose polyphenols. Seems like a lot of work? Can't some non-hormonal anti-aging drug do the same thing? Actually, one such drug potentially exists. It is called metformin, and it is usually the first drug of choice to treat type 2 diabetes. Epidemiological studies have indicated that diabetics who take metformin appear to have less cancer. Animal studies indicate that it may have some anti-aging benefits. So why not just take a metformin pill every day? The reason metformin works is because it increases AMP kinase activity by initially inhibiting the ability of mitochondria to make ATP. As ATP levels decrease, this action can initially activate AMP kinase, but with time this drug-induced inhibition of your mitochondria greatly overwhelms the initial short-term benefits. This is why most diabetics who start on metformin soon graduate to more powerful diabetic drugs as their condition worsens. There is also another class of more powerful diabetic drugs called thiazolidinediones (TZDs) that also activate AMP kinase. Unfortunately, their use is also associated with increased liver toxicity, bladder cancer, and heart disease. Call me crazy, but somehow poisoning your mitochondria or accelerating chronic disease doesn't seem to be like a good way to increase your healthspan.

INCREASING YOUR HEALTHSPAN USING CALORIE RESTRICTION

It is known that in every animal model tested, calorie restriction extends both longevity and prolongs wellness by decreasing the advent of chronic diseases including diabetes, heart disease, and cancer. But what about humans?

The healthiest aging population with legitimate medical records are the Okinawans. Even those Okinawans who reach very advanced age seem to have little evidence of chronic disease. So why do they eventually die? They simply die of old age (think of the example of the 40-year-old car) rather than dying from chronic disease. This is why both the lifespan and healthspan of the Okinawans are the longest in the world.

Recent studies have indicated that when Japanese centenarians (age greater than 100) and super-centenarians (age greater than 105) are compared to the elderly Japanese (greater than age 80) the best predictor of their longevity is not the length of their telomeres. Telomeres are caps at the end of your chromosomes that allow genetic replication to continue. The shorter the telomere length, the less likely the genes in the chromosome can be activated to replace damaged tissue. However, the clinical parameter that correlates best with living to extreme old age in these Japanese subjects was not the length of one's telomeres, but the lack of cellular inflammation. And that's why the goal of the Zone Pro-Resolution Nutrition system is to reduce and resolve excess cellular inflammation for as long as possible by maintaining an optimal Resolution Response. This is also why the Zone Diet is the foundation of the Zone Pro-Resolution Nutrition system because it is a calorie-restricted diet that can be followed indefinitely without hunger or fatigue.

BEYOND CALORIE RESTRICTION

The Zone Pro-Resolution Nutrition system is far more powerful than simply restricting calories. Without adequate levels of omega-3 fatty acids in the diet, you simply can't make adequate levels of resolvins to resolve the chronic cellular inflammation. That's why the Zone Diet is a great start toward an increased healthspan, but using therapeutic levels of omega-3 fatty acids can accelerate the process. Furthermore, it is known that omega-3 fatty acids also can increase the length of telomeres, which only can be to your benefit in increasing your healthspan.

But there is also the need for therapeutic levels of polyphenols if healthy aging is your goal. This information comes from another population who have been studied extensively for their extended healthspan. These are the elderly Italians living in remote sections of Tuscany. The In-Chianti study has demonstrated that the best indicator of reduced mortality and frailty in these elderly individuals is not the total levels of polyphenols they consume, but the levels of polyphenols in their urine. The only way to get levels of polyphenols in the urine is to have high levels of polyphenols in the blood. And what do high levels of polyphenols do if they get into the blood? They activate the gene transcription factor AMP kinase needed to complete the healing of damaged tissue, while simultaneously reducing the activity of the gene transcription factor for inflammation, NF-κB, that causes tissue damage.

There is no single magic bullet for slowing your rate of aging and thus increasing your healthspan to maintain healthy aging, but the Zone Pro-Resolution Nutrition system provides a comprehensive dietary strategy that is strongly supported by existing medical research. The Zone Diet is a calorie-restricted diet without hunger or fatigue. High-dose omega-3 fatty acids not only resolve existing cellular inflammation, but also increase telomere length. Finally, high-dose polyphenols significantly reduce mortality most likely by activating AMP kinase. They are all needed to optimize your Resolution Response. With that optimization of the Resolution Response comes a longer healthspan.

SUMMARY ▷

We all want to enjoy healthy aging where we are more easily able to handle our physical struggles that will occur later in life. Unfortunately for many of us, that hope is cut short with the acceleration of the aging process caused by the growing inability to mount a strong Resolution Response as you age. This can be significantly modified using the Zone Pro-Resolution Nutrition system to reach the Zone so you can enhance your internal Resolution Response and realize your ultimate goal of a longer healthspan.

21

The Future of Medicine

TODAY WE ARE at the crossroads for the future of medicine. Health care costs currently account for more than 18 percent of the American economy. When the #1 industry in your country is devoted to taking care of sick people, that doesn't bode well for the future. Furthermore, we don't seem to get a very good return on investment since by nearly every standard used to measure health status, the overall quality of America's health system is pretty abysmal compared to the rest of the industrialized world.

IDIOPATHIC MEDICINE

We are constantly told that modern medicine is making great strides in curing one chronic disease after another. We are also told that cures for chronic diseases that are currently untreatable such as Alzheimer's will soon be possible. Then why are health care costs spiraling out of control? This is especially true in America, where we spend more money on medical research than all the countries in the world combined. We also have the most modern equipment and the best medical specialists in the world. Yet we spend more on health care per capita than every country in the world, but have very little to show for it.

The definition of an idiopathic medical condition is that it has an unknown origin. That's a nice way of saying "I don't know." What causes cancer? "I don't know." What causes depression? "I don't know." What cause autoimmune diseases like type 1 diabetes, rheumatoid arthritis, and multiple sclerosis? "I don't know." What causes Alzheimer's? "I don't know."

Since modern medicine doesn't know the causes of chronic disease, it simply treats the symptoms without ever knowing what actually caused the disease in the first place. That is equivalent to saying, "fake it until you understand it."

WHY CHRONIC DISEASE IS DIFFERENT THAN INFECTIOUS DISEASE

The great success of medicine in the past has come from its victories over infectious disease. For an acute infectious disease, you can identify the real cause of the disease and then develop a drug to stop it. Vaccines to prevent viral infections and antibiotics to treat bacterial infections are great examples.

Chronic disease is different. The initial event that eventually leads to a chronic disease may have occurred at a much earlier period in time and actually may no longer be present in the body. Such an example might be constant exposure to sun as a teenager, and then having skin cancer develop decades later. However, not every teenager who went to the beach develops skin cancer. Why? I don't know. That's why chronic diseases are idiopathic diseases. We tend to make up stories about why they develop, but unlike acute infectious diseases there is often no clear reason. However, I feel that chronic disease may be a consequence of the body's failure to mount a strong Resolution Response to completely heal the damage caused by any initial injury to the organ. In essence, chronic disease may be better understood as the result of blockage of your Resolution Response. Any unresolved cellular inflammation caused by an initial injury can be further amplified by new factors such as diet- and/or gut-induced inflammation that had nothing to do with the original injury. The damaged cells in the organ are caught in a biological dead end of continuing reinjury and inability to fully heal until eventually there is loss of organ function with increasing fibrosis. That loss of function is then given a name indicating it is a chronic disease. For some it may be diabetes, for others it might be heart disease, for still others it may be Alzheimer's.

Let me give you a personal example that started me on a journey to understand why my family had a history of early mortality from heart disease. Forty-six years ago, my father died of heart disease at age 53 and he was a world-class athlete. What he really died from was a blocked Resolution Response. The initial injury that usually causes the development of an atherosclerotic lesion is the turbulent flow that continually takes place at the branch points of the arteries. Normally a strong Resolution Response would completely heal the injury. However, if the Resolution Response is blocked, the unresolved initial injury can now be amplified by diet-induced inflammation to develop into an atherosclerotic lesion filled with dead (i.e., necrotic) cells. This is known as a soft vulnerable plaque. If that plaque ruptures due to increased cellular inflammation, then the necrotic debris inside the plaque is dumped into the bloodstream initiating a rapid clot formation that usually results in sudden death. The initial cause of the inflammation in my father's artery may likely have been an injury caused by turbulent blood flow amplified by diet-induced inflammation, but the real cause of his death was ultimately a lack of a robust Resolution Response. This is why our current medical thinking of "one cause, one drug" that was so successful in treating acute infectious disease fails to adequately describe the development of chronic disease.

Yes, there are drugs that can manage the symptoms of chronic disease, but those drugs do not cure the disease because they can't activate the Resolution Response essential for healing to take place. Furthermore, those same drugs can now cause numerous side effects (like damage to the mitochondria) that not only further inhibit the Resolution Response, but also can start a new series of injuries that lead to the acceleration of new chronic diseases.

Injuries are random and can occur simultaneously in different parts of your body, but the healing of those injuries requires a highly orchestrated Resolution Response to resolve the inflammation the injury initially generated and then repair the damage caused by that injury. This is why inflammation and the Resolution Response are on-demand responses. Once the injury is healed, both inflammation and the Resolution Response are turned off until the next injury occurs. This is why following the Zone Pro-Resolution Nutrition system must be a constant dietary lifestyle, because the Resolution Response must always be ready to address the inflammation caused by the random injury. The clinical markers that define the Zone indicate your ability to activate each stage of the Resolution Response when needed.

Furthermore, as you age your Resolution Response becomes less efficient, so you must even work harder on the dietary factors that can maintain your Resolution Response at full strength. Consider maintaining an optimal Resolution Response as your ultimate health insurance policy.

DEFINITION OF A CURE

Hippocrates stated that the primary responsibility of a physician is to prevent disease. Failing that goal, then the physician should cure the disease. And if that isn't possible, then the physician should reduce the pain.

The best way to prevent a chronic disease is to maintain a state of wellness supported by an optimal Resolution Response. The end result is healthy aging with an increased healthspan. Unfortunately for many, "healthy aging" has come to mean managing chronic diseases with a lifetime use of drugs. Obviously, that reality is a far cry from Hippocrates' original vision of how medicine should operate.

How do you know if your Resolution Response is working at optimal levels? One definition might be the lack of any chronic disease. You might have some unresolved cellular inflammation, but there is not enough organ damage that results in having to take a medication for a lifetime to manage its symptoms. Nonetheless, this is how most people would define wellness. However, my definition of wellness is stricter. To be well you have to have a robust Resolution Response always on alert to reduce the inflammation caused by random injuries. This is only possible if all three clinical markers of the Zone are in their appropriate ranges. By that criteria, I estimate about 1 percent of Americans are probably well.

Then if you can't prevent a disease, how do you know if you are cured? The definition of a cure might be having no symptoms of the chronic disease for an extended period of time without the use of any drug to manage those symptoms. But for how long? A classic case might be type 2 diabetes where very aggressive dietary therapy can normalize blood sugar levels and maintain them. If your blood sugar levels (and really your HbA_{1c} levels) are normal for at least two years without any drugs, then it would be a reasonable assumption that you no longer have diabetes. Five years is even better, and ten years more so. However, the stabilization of blood glucose levels can only occur if your beta cells in the pancreas have healed and are now working more effectively.

The same is true of hypertension. You should be able state confidently that you are cured of hypertension if your blood pressure remains normal for at least five years without the use of any drugs. Thirty million Americans have diabetes and 75 million Americans have hypertension. It doesn't look like either chronic disease will be cured in the foreseeable future.

At least diabetes and hypertension are chronic diseases defined by numbers. Healing other chronic diseases are not so easy to determine, so rather than curing them, you should be able to manage them without drugs. If you have rheumatoid arthritis and the pain is absent for more than five years without using a drug, you probably have managed the disease. If you have macular degeneration or optical nerve damage and your eyesight improves significantly over the next two years without using a drug, you have probably successfully managed macular degeneration or optical nerve damage. Cancer is trickier since cancer drugs and radiation are known to cause new cancers that may take a decade to develop, so in my opinion you would need at least ten years (not the standard five years) of cancer-free life without any drug intervention to be considered truly managing the disease. Regaining cognitive skills or not having depression are even more subjective, but they can be assessed by standard testing. Heart disease is even more difficult since surrogate markers like cholesterol levels don't count since half of the people who have normal cholesterol levels die of heart disease. Bottom line, we are a long way from managing most chronic diseases without the need for constant drug therapy.

The reason may be that the wild card in curing or managing many chronic diseases is the levels of fibrosis that may have developed from lack of a robust Resolution Response in the past. If that area of the organ is covered by scar tissue, then the function in that area of the organ is probably never coming back. If enough of the organ has fibrosis, it's function will be permanently compromised. Even under those conditions of extensive existing fibrosis, the use of the Zone Pro-Resolution Nutrition system should be able to significantly reduce the current levels of medication to the minimum required to better manage that chronic disease.

A POTENTIAL SOLUTION

Is there a solution to our current medical morass? I think there is, but it requires rebooting medicine and going back to the earliest beginning of medicine that started with Hippocrates.

Let's start with three more of his statements that still echo clearly today.

- Do the patient no harm
- Let food be your medicine, let medicine be your food
- Disease begins in the gut

The power of the Zone Diet is that it can do no harm. You have to eat, but you should also eat smart. By that I mean understanding how the food we eat affects our hormones and the expression of our genes that control the Resolution Response.

Let's face it, drugs have side effects. That's why they have what is called a therapeutic zone. If you give the patient too little of the drug, it has no benefits. It's essentially a placebo. Above some upper level, a drug has toxic effects. Between those two ranges is the drug's therapeutic zone. The benefit of a drug is that patient compliance is usually better than with a diet. Just pop a pill into your mouth or have the doctor give you an injection and you don't have to change your diet (of course that's what probably got you into the problem in the first place).

However, the Zone Pro-Resolution Nutrition system also uses concentrated nutrients to enhance the resolution and repair of cellular inflammation. Any concentrated nutrient can have side effects, this is why you have to have them extremely purified to reduce any such possibility. This can now be done with purified supplements such as ultra-refined omega-3 concentrates and refined polyphenol extracts. Nonetheless, the extent of their use is governed by maintaining the clinical markers for the Zone, which ensures that the use of supplementation with high-purity omega-3 fatty acid concentrates and polyphenol extracts will have no toxicity. The appropriate ultimate dosage with such supplements is determined by the clinical markers of the Zone because the ranges of those markers are known to be strongly associated with a longer healthspan.

Usually the only thing that stops dietary compliance of such purified omega-3 fatty acid concentrates and refined polyphenol extracts is their cost (they aren't reimbursed like drugs) or lack of results (as you would expect when you take a placebo dose of either omega-3 fatty acids or polyphenols). This is why the levels of supplementation using highly refined omega-3 fatty acids and polyphenols you need to optimize the Zone Pro-Resolution Nutrition system is ultimately determined by your blood levels, thus taking into account genetic and biochemical diversity.

This brings me to the second point made by Hippocrates about letting food be your medicine. Diet has the largest therapeutic zone of any medical intervention, but you have to be very compliant to get consistent results. The reason that diet is a good starting point for treating virtually all chronic disease starts with the reduction of the intensity of diet-induced inflammation that is usually the major factor that blocks the Resolution Response. If that first stage of the Resolution Response (i.e., reduction of diet-induced inflammation) is complete, then you have a greater opportunity to resolve and then repair the tissue damage before fibrosis occurs. That is the molecular definition of healing. Since I believe unresolved cellular inflammation is the underlying cause of all chronic disease, then dietary programs to better reduce, resolve, and repair the damage caused by cellular inflammation should be the primary foundation for all medicine in the future.

Finally, our growing understanding of the complexity of the diet and its effect on generating inflammation in the body reinforces the third point made by Hippocrates that disease begins in the gut. If you expand the definition of the gut to include the food we consume, then this makes perfect sense. This means the reduction of the diet- and/or gut-induced inflammation caused by your diet must be the first obligatory step in treating any chronic disease as well as preventing it from developing in the first place.

A NEW VISION

This is why I believe the future of medicine will eventually have to embrace the basic principles articulated by Hippocrates to optimize the Resolution Response through understanding how hormones and gene expression can be controlled by the diet. This can be visualized below.

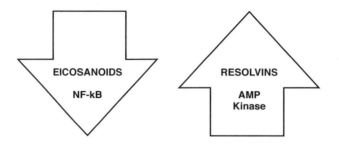

Changing the levels of hormones (eicosanoids and resolvins) and gene transcription factors (NF-κB and AMP kinase) that control the Resolution Response is under your dietary control. Your success balancing these hormones and gene transcription factors are determined by the clinical markers of the Zone. If each of the markers of the Zone are in their appropriate ranges, then each step of the healing process is not likely to be inhibited. This balance cannot be accomplished with drugs, but it can be accomplished with the consistent use of the Zone Pro-Resolution Nutrition system.

REDUCING DRUG USE

Combining the Zone Pro-Resolution Nutrition system with existing drugs is likely to significantly reduce the amounts of any drug currently required to manage the symptoms of any chronic disease. A basic rule of pharmacology is that every time you reduce the dose of a drug by one-half, you will also reduce the side effects of that drug by a factor of four. That's a great return on investment for simply following the Zone Pro-Resolution Nutrition system.

The Zone Pro-Resolution Nutrition system has three distinct dietary components to reduce drug use to manage existing chronic disease: (1) the Zone Diet to *reduce* the intensity of cellular inflammation, (2) omega-3 fatty acids to *resolve* the remaining cellular inflammation, and (3) polyphenols to accelerate the *repair* of the tissue damage. Each dietary component of the Zone Pro-Resolution Nutrition system has its own unique role in the Resolution Response, but to be totally effective they must be used in a biological systems-based approach to develop a highly personalized, but comprehensive strategy for addressing unresolved cellular inflammation based the on the 3 R's of *Reduce, Resolve,* and *Repair* described in this book. Current drug technology simply doesn't have that potential to achieve these necessary outcomes. That's because the Zone Pro-Resolution Nutrition system operates at a different level than drugs. In particular, it's your ability to constantly balance that biological gyroscope consisting of gene transcription factors and hormones controlled by the diet and specifically by the Zone Pro-Resolution Nutrition system without toxicity.

EVIDENCE-BASED WELLNESS VERSUS EVIDENCE-BASED MEDICINE

The drug industry has made the mantra "evidence-based medicine" their calling card for justifying ever-increasing drug costs. The true "drug" you are looking for is a dietary strategy that can control the appropriate gene transcription factors and hormones needed for optimizing your internal Resolution Response. This is my definition of "evidence-based" wellness.

Furthermore, the drugs developed as a result of today's "evidence-based medicine" always seem to work better in clinical trials than real life. This is because drug trials cherry pick their patients by using rigid exclusion criteria often representing only a small fraction of the general population who are then led to believe (primarily by TV advertising) that the newest "breakthrough" drug will solve their problems. Furthermore, randomized controlled trials (RCT) are extolled as the only way to test a drug to find a therapeutic dose somewhere between a placebo level and toxic dose. The result is a very narrow therapeutic zone of the drug that must be taken for the rest of one's life to treat the symptoms of a chronic disease based on the assumption that everyone is genetically and biochemically the same.

In the real world, few drugs work as well as their advertising because they are not addressing the true underlying cause of the symptoms, which is the continuing buildup of chronic unresolved cellular inflammation that constantly blocks the Resolution Response. As a result, the patient takes increasingly complex "cocktails" of different drugs to hopefully manage a chronic condition. Eventually these multi-drug mixtures for one chronic condition cause new complications requiring more drugs from different drug classes until the patient becomes a walking poly pharmacy. The real clinical end result is that the quality of life for the patient usually decreases as their number of medications increase and their healthspan decreases.

Evidence-based wellness presents a totally different perspective. It starts with the premise that there is significant genetic variability between individuals and the goal is to bring their blood markers into appropriate ranges to optimize the Resolution Response so that cellular inflammation can be effectively managed.

Evidence-based wellness can be considered a cellular inflammation clamp. You follow the Zone Pro-Resolution Nutrition system to reach optimal ranges of the clinical markers that define the Zone. It is your blood that tells you what the correct levels of each dietary intervention should be. Although there will be some adjustments (especially the omega-3 fatty acids and polyphenols) with time to take into account the aging process, you are constantly maintaining the same ranges that define the clinical makers of the Zone. Rather than finding different drugs for different chronic diseases, evidence-based wellness has one approach (reaching the Zone to optimize the Resolution Response) that is applicable for every chronic disease.

In the following table, I further compare the differences between evidence-based wellness and evidence-based medicine.

	Evidence-based wellness	Evidence-based medicine
Side effects	Titrating to goal has no toxic side effects	Therapeutic drug dose always has side effects
Choosing the right dose	Titrate to the same goals for everyone	Use RCTs to find appropriate drug dose for highly screened populations
Genetic diversity	Considers genetic diversity	Ignores genetic diversity
Focus	Seeking hormonal and genetic modulation using nutrition	Seeking "druggable" targets for new patentable drugs
Reimbursement	Not reimbursable by insurance companies	Reimbursement by insurance companies

The last point of comparison indicates why the pharmaceutical industry will continue to embrace "evidence-based medicine"—they make a lot of money. Insurance companies reimburse their drugs, letting you think you are getting a great deal on health care even though you are paying a significant portion of your income taxes for Medicare in addition to probably purchasing additional medical insurance to get that "great deal."

However, virtually all of the easy druggable targets were found decades ago. This is why current drug development costs are so high. This is also why the drug industry continues to play a shell game of constantly increasing the price of older generic drugs to maintain their profits while telling the public that new drug discovery is incredibly expensive to justify the extraordinary prices of new drugs. As an example, the price of insulin actually decreased from 2002 to 2006, then dramatically increased by 300 percent from 2007 to 2013.

RETHINKING CHRONIC DISEASE

I often use the analogy of an iceberg when describing chronic disease. Although you see an iceberg floating in the ocean, 90 percent of its mass is below the surface. The same is true of chronic disease. The tips of the iceberg represent chronic diseases we can observe like cancer, heart disease, autoimmune disorders, neurological diseases, and even the aging process. We think of each chronic disease as separate from the other, but they are all interconnected by unresolved cellular inflammation that represents the vast mass of the iceberg below the water that remains out of sight.

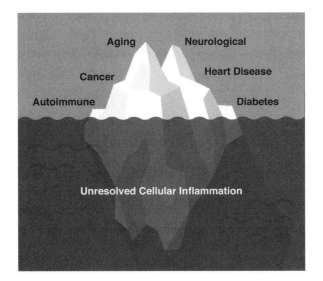

Each of those chronic diseases begins with some type of injury (external or internal) that was not sufficiently healed by the body's natural Resolution Response. As a result, unresolved cellular inflammation is created and can be amplified by continuing diet-induced inflammation. With time (usually measured in decades), organ function is decreased to the extent that we call it chronic disease and try to manage its symptoms with drugs. Chronic diseases are not the result of a drug deficiency, but are the result of a continuing build-up of chronic unresolved cellular inflammation caused by a blocked Resolution Response.

The more you reduce the levels of cellular inflammation following the Zone Pro-Resolution Nutrition system, the size of the remaining peaks, the various chronic diseases, begin to significantly decrease. Furthermore, by following the Zone Pro-Resolution Nutrition system you are applying the basic principles first articulated by Hippocrates to practice a lifetime of hormonal and gene therapy in your kitchen.

This doesn't mean that the Zone Pro-Resolution Nutrition system will completely replace drug therapy in the future. On the contrary, there will always be a place for drugs that have a long-standing track record of relative safety as back-up support to help manage any remaining symptoms of a particular chronic disease.

On the other hand, unless we begin to reduce the underlying cause of chronic disease (i.e., unresolved cellular inflammation) by optimizing your natural Resolution Response, we will continue to watch medical expenditures rise uncontrollably. Unfortunately, that is the direction we are headed for, and we simply do not have the money to pay for such "evidence-based medicine" in the future.

THE ANSWER WAS HIDING IN PLAIN SIGHT

More than 35 years ago, I had my "aha" moment with the discoveries of the role that eicosanoids played in the inflammatory process. This provided me with my initial insight that inflammation was a likely driving force behind virtually all chronic disease. I reasoned that if you could control inflammation in the body, you would get to the ultimate cause of chronic disease.

My journey was far more complicated than I anticipated, but as a result my thinking has become more refined over time. It wasn't inflammation per se, but the blockage of the Resolution Response that results in the growing levels of unresolved cellular inflammation that causes chronic disease. The real destination of my journey was hiding in plain sight for more than 35 years, but the existing scientific knowledge needed to understand the molecular complexity of the Resolution Response was not sufficiently developed until recently. It was the optimization of the Resolution Response, not the reduction of inflammation, that is the key to the future of medicine. It just took me a long time to realize it.

There are more than 7,000 chronic diseases and the vast majority of those diseases are driven by excess cellular inflammation caused by blocking your natural Resolution Response. Yet we have drugs that only treat 500 of them. Even more disturbing, we still don't know how many of these drugs really work. The Zone Pro-Resolution Nutrition system allows you to better manage all 7,000 chronic diseases with a single dietary intervention. What I have tried to demonstrate in this book is that while the molecular events that constitute the Resolution Response in your body are incredibly complex, your diet can help keep that complex system running smoothly and with relative ease in your kitchen.

If the continued increase in unresolved cellular inflammation caused by the continual blocking of the Resolution Response is indeed the driving force for the development of chronic disease, then optimizing your internal Resolution Response should be the critical first step in any treatment process. If you are diagnosed with a chronic disease, your first step should be the immediate implementation of the Zone Pro-Resolution Nutrition system with consistent blood testing to determine your dietary compliance in addition to using any drug therapy that might be suggested by your physician. This allows you to simultaneously address the acute symptoms of the disease with the drug, but also begin addressing the real underlying cause of your condition, which is unresolved cellular inflammation caused by a blocked Resolution Response. Simply taking drugs without optimizing your internal Resolution Response is a surefire prescription to require more medication in the future, not only for managing your current condition, but also increasing the likelihood that other chronic conditions (it's called co-morbidity) are likely to emerge since you are doing nothing to reduce chronic unresolved cellular inflammation in the body. As you move toward the Zone and start to optimize your internal Resolution Response, you now have the potential to use the least amount of proven "older" drugs to manage the remaining symptoms of any chronic disease.

The Zone Pro-Resolution Nutrition system means you must use a systems-based dietary approach and not place all your bets on a single dietary intervention. Only this type of a comprehensive diet working as a finely tuned system will allow you to potentially achieve more meaningful therapeutic results.

The good thing about working with the Zone Pro-Resolution Nutrition system and its inherent non-toxicity is you can begin to immediately reduce unresolved cellular inflammation that has been driven by the worldwide epidemic rise of diet-induced inflammation. The Zone Pro-Resolution Nutrition system provides an alternative approach to usher in a new way of not only more effectively managing chronic disease, but also maintaining wellness for a longer period of time if you don't have an existing chronic disease. This increases your healthspan. Unlike current processed food technology that causes diet-induced inflammation, the Zone Pro-Resolution Nutrition system *reduces, resolves*, and *repairs* the damage caused by diet-induced inflammation by enhancing your Resolution Response to reduce existing unresolved cellular inflammation.

DEVELOPING A ZONE LIFESTYLE

There is obviously more to a longer and better life than simply following the Zone Pro-Resolution Nutrition system. That's why I use the 80-15-5 rule as a general guideline for assessing the impact of various lifestyle components that also help reduce unresolved cellular inflammation to maintain wellness for as long as possible. The lifestyle components that you have total control over are diet, exercise, and stress reduction.

Diet

Eighty percent of your ability to maintain wellness and achieve a longer healthspan is the consistent use of the Zone Pro-Resolution Nutrition system that I have outlined. It takes effort and consistent discipline to reap the health and performance benefits. Is it worth it? I think it is. The longer excess cellular inflammation exists in different organs, the more structural damage you can expect. Following the Zone Pro-Resolution Nutrition system at any stage of life allows you to have better control of hormonal responses and gene expression. The sooner you reduce cellular inflammation to prevent new structural damage caused by fibrosis, the greater your likelihood of moving back toward a higher state of wellness and enjoy a longer and better healthspan.

Exercise

About 15 percent of your eventual wellness will come from consistent exercise. The percentage isn't higher because even the best exercise program will never overcome a poor diet that constantly generates diet-induced inflammation. You can run, but you can't hide from the overwhelming impact of diet-induced cellular inflammation.

It is often said that if you put exercise into a pill, it would be a wonder drug. Why? Because exercise increases the activity of AMP kinase.

So, what is the best exercise program where you get your greatest return on investment? The answer is simply not sitting. The more you reduce the effect of gravity on your body by sitting, the more rapidly the benefits of any exercise or dietary program are eroded. You can see this plainly in the old newsreels of the Mercury astronauts getting out of their space capsules after a limited time in a zero-gravity environment. They were so thoroughly weakened, they had to be physically assisted walking on the deck of the ship after their water landing. It was the ultimate example of physical de-training. The same physiological effects happen, but to a lesser degree, when you sit. The data is quite clear that the longer you sit during the course of the day, the greater your chances of an early death. In particular, it appears the reason why sitting increases mortality may be related to a breakdown in the heart muscle as measured by the increase of the protein troponin in the blood. This is the same protein also released in high amounts during a heart attack.

What's a realistic solution? Try to stand up every 20 minutes and walk around for two minutes then return to your desk. In an eight-hour day, this would account for 48 minutes of walking. This simple exercise change will result in your greatest return on exercise investment. For an additional exercise benefit, park your car or get off public transportation about 15 minutes away from your destination so you are forced to engage in another 30 minutes of walking every day. Another helpful hint is to use the stairs whenever possible. The more you work against gravity, the greater the benefits.

Unfortunately, such a relatively small change will have little impact on reducing insulin resistance or increasing mitochondrial efficiency by activating AMP kinase activity. The most effective exercise to achieve both those goals is high intensity interval training (HIIT). This type of exercise induces higher energy demands, reducing the levels of ATP in that particular muscle group used, resulting in a significant increase in AMP kinase activity that promotes new mitochondrial biogenesis. HIIT is hard work because you are trying to fatigue all the cells in a particular muscle group, but the return on investment for improving wellness is immense.

Stress Reduction

Finally, about 5 percent of your future health can be enhanced with stress reduction. Stress reduction is actually the reduction of long-term chronic activation of the sympathetic nervous system that results in an increased release of cortisol into the blood from the adrenal glands. Cortisol is actually an anti-inflammatory hormone that reduces the formation of eicosanoids. However, it creates significant collateral damage if cortisol remains constantly elevated during periods of long-term chronic stress. This is because elevated cortisol also increases insulin resistance, causes immune suppression, and destroys memory cells in the hippocampus. It is far more effective to reduce unresolved cellular inflammation and its associated insulin resistance by following the Zone Pro-Resolution Nutrition system than using standard stress reduction activities such as meditation. That's why I give stress reduction only 5 percent, but even that small percentage can be a lot in today's world.

One way for relieving stress is sitting in a comfortable chair for 20 minutes every day and trying not to think of anything. It's actually hard work because you are consuming large amounts of blood glucose for the brain to keep yourself focused on thinking of nothing. Another good way of reducing stress is developing a philosophy of life that allows you to remain resilient when adversity arises. That usually takes a lifetime of constant awareness and practice just like following the Zone Pro-Resolution Nutrition system.

SUMMARY ▶

As Hippocrates stated 2,500 years ago, the primary task of medicine should be to prevent disease. Today this means maintaining your wellness to increase your healthspan. This is a lifetime process. Lifestyle is important, but realize that your diet will be the major contributor to your success. In particular, it means reaching the Zone, and more importantly, staying in the Zone to optimize your Resolution Response. The Zone Pro-Resolution Nutrition system provides you with a clinically proven dietary pathway to continuously control both the hormones and the expression of key genes that are both necessary for optimization of the Resolution Response, but it also requires a consistent effort on your part. Likewise, you want to apply the same dietary discipline with regard to exercise and stress reduction for consistent results. The ancients understood the need for being strong in mind and body. Today, this means using diet, exercise, and stress reduction as powerful "drugs" that can significantly influence our hormones and gene expression that optimize the Resolution Response. The only question is if you have the will and discipline to tap into these readily available reservoirs of proven pathways to maintain wellness.

Hopefully this book provides you a new dietary pathway out of the current inflammatory mess we have gotten ourselves into. It is the story of unresolved cellular inflammation: How you increase it by your diet, but also how you can also reduce it by your diet. Equally important is how we can repair the damage caused by increasing cellular inflammation by unblocking the highly orchestrated internal Resolution Response that leads to healing. The more inhibited your internal Resolution Response becomes, the more likely that unresolved cellular inflammation will accelerate the development of any chronic disease especially if amplified by diet-induced inflammation. On the other hand, if you are successful in using the Zone Pro-Resolution Nutrition system, you have the potential to cut the Gordian knot of chronic disease by going to its core to simultaneously reduce excess unresolved cellular inflammation while simultaneously increasing the strength of your Resolution Response. That combination leads to a longer healthspan. That's the promise of the Zone Pro-Resolution Nutrition system and its ability to optimize the Resolution Response. I hope you agree.

Further Support

THE SCIENCE OF the Resolution Response is evolving at a rapid rate. To stay on top of this new knowledge, I can offer you several resources.

The first is www.DrSears.com, which is the science site for the Zone and the Resolution Response. For products and the dietary support to help you optimize your Resolution Response, I would recommend going to www.ZoneLiving.com or call our customer support team at 1-800-404-8171.

A percentage of every product sold on www.ZoneLiving.com goes to support continuing educational and clinical research at my 501c non-profit foundation, the Inflammation Research Foundation (IRF). Published research supported by the IRF as well as upcoming national and international educational conferences on the Resolution Response can be found at www.inflammationresearchfoundation.org.

Glossary of Terms

IT IS DIFFICULT to understand any science if you don't have the definitions to describe it. This is especially true of the Resolution Response. The more you understand the terminology used to describe inflammation and the Resolution Response, the more likely you are able to change your life for the better.

AMP KINASE: The gene transcription factor that can be activated by calorie-restriction, intense exercise, and/or high-dose polyphenols. Once activated, this gene transcription factor orchestrates a broad range of metabolic activities including the production of new mitochondria essential to producing the energy for the repair of damaged tissue.

ARACHIDONIC ACID (AA): The omega-6 fatty acid that is the building block for all pro-inflammatory eicosanoids.

CELLULAR INFLAMMATION: The mismatch between the two distinct phases of inflammation: (1) turning it on (i.e., initiation) and (2) turning it off (i.e., resolution). When the strength of the Resolution Response is not sufficient to completely turn off the intensity of inflammation induced by injury or diet, it results in unresolved cellular inflammation, defined as ongoing inflammation below the perception of pain. Unresolved cellular inflammation is the underlying cause of weight gain, development of chronic disease, and acceleration of the aging process.

CYCLO-OXYGENASE (COX): The enzyme critical for converting AA and EPA into eicosanoids. There are two forms of COX enzymes. One (COX-1) is constantly present in your cells and the other (COX-2) is upregulated as a consequence of increased inflammation by the activation of the master genetic switch of inflammation (NF-κB).

CYTOKINES: Pro-inflammatory proteins released by the activation of NF-κB in response to inflammatory mediators. The primary pro-inflammatory cytokines include tumor necrosis factor (TNF), interleukin-1 (IL-1), and interleukin-6 (IL-6). Cytokines can leave the cell to interact with cytokine receptors embedded on the surface of nearby cells to activate their inflammatory responses.

DIET-INDUCED INFLAMMATION: Any food ingredient or combination of food ingredients in the diet that have the potential to cause increased inflammation by activating the inflammatory gene transcription factor NF-κB. The Resolution Response is inhibited by increased levels of diet-induced inflammation. Diet-induced inflammation also includes inflammatory responses mediated by a leaky gut leading to gut-induced inflammation.

ECTOPIC FAT: A type of fat that is not safely stored in fat cells. This type of fat is commonly called visceral fat and is strongly associated with increased inflammatory damage. An example of ectopic fat is the marbling found in fatty cuts of red meat.

EICOSANOIDS: Hormones derived from 20-carbon essential fatty acids that are the primary drivers of the initiation phase of inflammation. Pro-inflammatory eicosanoids include prostaglandins, thromboxanes, and leukotrienes and these constitute the vast majority of all eicosanoids. Eicosanoids derived from EPA are weakly pro-inflammatory compared to those derived from AA. A limited number of eicosanoids such as PGE_1 and oxylipins have anti-inflammatory effects.

EPIGENETICS: The ability of environmental factors (such as the diet) to affect the final synthesis of proteins coded by your DNA by leaving chemical markers on the DNA such as methylation that prevent that section of the DNA from being expressed. Epigenetic marks also include acetylation of the histones that surround the DHA that also prevent parts of your

DNA from being expressed as well. Epigenetics also includes the ability of non-coding RNA that can inhibit the synthesis of certain proteins expressed by your DNA. The non-coding RNA can also be influenced by diet. Consider the relationship of epigenetics to your DNA to be similar to the relationship of software to your computer. Epigenetic marks on the DNA can also be transmitted to future generations.

FERMENTABLE FIBER: A special type of dietary fiber that can be used as a nutrient source for the bacteria that inhibit the gut. The metabolism of fermentable fiber in the gut produces a number of unique molecules including short-chain fatty acids. These short-chain fatty acids are important to help prevent the formation of a leaky gut, enhance immune responses at the gut wall, and induce favorable neurological changes. Only about 10–15 percent of total dietary fiber content contains fermentable fiber. Non-starchy vegetables are the richest sources of fermentable fiber providing the least amount of carbohydrates.

FIBROSIS: The body's response that limits tissue damage caused by unresolved cellular inflammation. If the injury site is not sufficiently healed, scar tissue forms around the injury site. If enough scar tissue has accumulated in an organ then its function may be compromised enough to be considered a chronic disease.

GENE TRANSCRIPTION FACTORS: These are complex proteins within a cell that when activated by external mediators will direct the cell's DNA to either increase or decrease the synthesis of specific proteins or enzymes related to certain biological functions. Gene transcription factors (especially AMP kinase) often work in networks so that activating one will often affect other gene transcription factors.

GLUCAGON: This is the hormone produced by the pancreas and is generated by the amount of protein in a meal. Glucagon causes the release of stored glycogen in the liver to help stabilize blood glucose levels between meals.

GLYCEMIC LOAD: The total impact of all carbohydrates consumed in a meal that determines the rate that blood glucose levels rise after that meal. The higher the glycemic load of a meal, the more insulin that is secreted to reduce the excess blood glucose. Non-starchy vegetables have the lowest glycemic load while fruits have a higher glycemic load because of their increased sugar content. Grains and starches have the highest glycemic loads because glucose polymers in those foods are rapidly broken down to glucose in the mouth. The balance of the protein-to-the-glycemic load at each meal determines the balance of glucagon and insulin in the blood for the next four to five hours to maintain satiety and reduces mental fatigue by stabilizing blood glucose levels.

GUT: The gut is a complex organ that encompasses every aspect of the digestion, absorption, and elimination of the intake of food. It starts in the mouth and continues through the stomach to the small intestine and eventually to the colon where the resident bacteria finalize the digestion process of fermentable fiber.

GUT-INDUCED INFLAMMATION: Dietary factors that can increase the permeability of the gut wall that allow large protein or microbial fragments to enter into the blood and cause an inflammatory response. The primary food ingredients that increase gut-induced inflammation are excess saturated fats (especially palmitic acid) and the lack of fermentable fiber and polyphenols in the diet.

HORMONE RECEPTORS: Proteins usually on the surface of a cell that bind to a specific hormone. For cell surface receptors, the binding of the hormone starts a signaling cascade inside the cell that results in the final cellular action via second messengers found within the cell.

HORMONES: Molecules that carry a distinct metabolic message to stimulate distant target cells. Most hormones interact with specific receptors on the cell surface, which in turn activate second messengers to activate internal pathways in the cell to carry out the final metabolic action. Hormones are either protein-based (such as insulin or glucagon) or fat-based (eicosanoids, resolvins, and cortisol) molecules.

INFLAMMATION: The body's initial immune response to defend itself against microbial invasion or as a response to tissue damage due to an internal or external injury. Chronic over-activation of the initial inflammatory response or increasing levels of unresolved cellular inflammation will cause tissue damage resulting in the potential loss of organ function.

INSULIN: The key hormone produced by the pancreas in response to blood glucose levels that distributes incoming nutrients to the appropriate organs for immediate use, storage, and release for later use, and also orchestrates a wide variety of other metabolic functions.

INSULIN RESISTANCE: This occurs when the body doesn't properly respond to the levels of circulating insulin. Although insulin binds to its receptor on the surface of the cell, the transmission of the metabolic message to the inside of the cell is attenuated. The underlying cause of insulin resistance is increased levels of unresolved cellular inflammation within the target cell. This causes disturbances in the signaling within the cell after insulin binds to its hormone receptor. Insulin resistance leads to hyperinsulinemia in the blood as the pancreas continues to secrete additional insulin in an effort to reduce excess blood glucose.

LEAKY GUT: A popular description used to describe the breakdown of the various barriers in the gut that increase the permeability of the gut wall. With the development of a leaky gut, large protein or microbial fragments can enter into the blood to cause systemic inflammatory responses.

LIPO-OXYGENASE (LOX): Enzymes that convert 20-carbon omega-6 fatty acids and omega-3 fatty acids into leukotrienes. There are three distinct LOX enzymes (5-LOX, 12-LOX, and 15-LOX). The LOX enzymes in the presence of inflammatory cells like neutrophils are also used in the synthesis of resolvins.

NF-κB: The gene transcription factor that causes the expression of the pro-inflammatory enzyme (COX-2) and pro-inflammatory cytokines from the DNA. These inflammatory mediators are instrumental in causing the further amplification of the inflammation response in nearby cells. This gene transcription factor is under dietary control since it can be activated by leukotrienes or through the activation of the TLR or RAGE receptors by microbial fragments entering from the gut or glycosylated proteins in the blood.

OMEGA-3 FATTY ACIDS: Long-chain omega-3 fatty acids eicosapentaenoic (EPA) and docosahexaenoic acid (DHA) are the molecular building blocks for the generation of resolvins that are directly responsible for the resolution of cellular inflammation. Unlike eicosanoid synthesis in which only EPA can be used, both EPA and DHA can be used to make resolvins. The eicosanoids generated from EPA are 10–100 times less inflammatory that those generated from AA thereby reducing the intensity of the inflammatory response.

OMEGA-6 FATTY ACIDS: The building blocks for generating eicosanoids. Excess levels of omega-6 fatty acids in the diet coupled with the presence of increased insulin levels in the blood due to insulin resistance will increase the production of arachidonic acid (AA) and increase the intensity of the inflammatory response making it more difficult to resolve. The consequence is the build-up of increasing levels of unresolved cellular inflammation in every organ.

POLYPHENOLS: Chemicals found in plants that are defensive compounds to repeal microbial invaders. They are essential for optimal gut health in humans because they help reduce gut wall permeability and dissolve biofilms of pathogenic bacteria. Polyphenols encourage the growth of friendly microbes and inhibit the growth of pathogenic microbes. Polyphenols that enter the blood can also activate specific gene transcription factors such as AMP kinase to synthesize proteins important for reducing excess free radicals, slowing the aging process, and accelerating tissue repair.

RECEPTORS: Binding molecules usually embedded in the outer membrane of a cell. Once activated by hormones or other signaling molecules, they transmit the biological message into the interior of the cell via secondary signaling molecules. Unresolved cellular inflammation can disrupt these internal signaling pathways.

REPAIR: The consequence of optimal activation of the gene transcription factor AMP kinase to increase mitochondrial biogenesis and orchestrate the body's metabolic pathways for the repair of damaged tissue.

RESOLUTION RESPONSE: A natural coordinated orchestration of reducing diet-induced inflammation, followed by its resolution, and then the repair of the damaged tissue that leads to healing. The Resolution Response is controlled by the diet and can be optimized by following the Zone Pro-Resolution Nutrition system. Your success in optimizing your internal Resolution Response can be determined by the three clinical markers that define the Zone.

RESOLVINS: Hormones also known as specialized pro-resolution mediators or SPM. These are the hormones derived from dietary omega-3 fatty acids that turn off inflammatory responses initiated by eicosanoids. Pro-resolution hormones include resolvins, protectins, and maresins. Their mode of action initially reduces the infiltration of neutrophils into the inflamed area and then activate the macrophages in the area to clear out the cellular debris caused by the inflammatory damage.

SECOND MESSENGERS: Molecules generated after a hormone or other molecule interacts with its appropriate receptor on the surface of a cell. Second messengers activate signaling pathways within the cell to carry out the metabolic instructions contained within the hormone or other molecules that initially interacted with the receptor on the cell surface. Unresolved cellular inflammation can disturb the signaling pathways used by second messengers.

TIGHT JUNCTIONS: The cells that form the barriers between the gut and the blood as well as between the brain and the blood, which are held together by specialized proteins known as occludins. The higher the concentration of occludins, the less likely that large protein or microbial fragments can enter the blood from the gut or enter the brain from the blood.

ZONE DIET: A defined dietary program to reduce the intensity of diet-induced inflammation and to enhance the Resolution Response.

ZONE MEAL: A meal that reduces diet-induced inflammation in the body. A Zone meal should contain approximately 400 total calories to reduce inflammation in the brain caused by excess calorie intake. Those calories should contain at least 25 grams of low-fat protein, less than 12 grams of fat, and the rest of the carbohydrates selected from low-glycemic choices (primarily non-starchy vegetables with a limited amount of fruits). These carbohydrates should ideally be rich in fermentable fiber and high in polyphenol content for gut health and activation of AMP kinase. The calorie percentages of a typical Zone meal should be approximately 40 percent carbohydrates, 30 percent protein, and 30 percent fat. A perfectly balanced Zone meal should control hunger and fatigue for four to five hours by stabilizing blood sugar levels based on the hormonal balance of insulin and glucagon levels in the blood.

ZONE PRO-RESOLUTION NUTRITION SYSTEM: The combination of the Zone Diet to reduce diet-induced inflammation coupled with adequate levels of omega-3 fatty acids to resolve cellular inflammation plus adequate levels of polyphenols to activate AMP kinase to repair tissue damaged by cellular inflammation. All components of the Zone Pro-Resolution Nutrition system are needed to optimize the Resolution Response and reduce unresolved cellular inflammation, which is the underlying cause of the development of chronic disease. The success of following the Zone Pro-Resolution Nutrition system is monitored by the clinical markers that determine the Zone.

ZONE PROTEIN: Products derived from a patented flour that can change the location of the protein absorption in the small intestine thereby increasing appetite suppression and reducing insulin resistance.

ZONE SNACK: A mini-Zone meal that contains about 100-200 calories. A balanced Zone snack should control hunger and fatigue for 2-3 hours by maintaining hormonal balance until your next Zone meal.

Inflammation:
The Slightly Longer Course

OUR CELLS ARE constantly prepared for potential microbial attacks and random injuries. Both events can be sensed by the cell via receptors either located on its surface or within its interior. Once any of these receptors are activated, the cell can immediately transmit a message (mediated by gene transcription factors) to release the inflammatory mediators (proteins known as cytokines or hormones such as eicosanoids) to protect itself, to alert neighboring cells that danger is imminent and that they must start to defend themselves or self-destruct by a process known as apoptosis for the good of the other cells in the organ.

We really have two immune systems. The more sophisticated one you hear a lot about is the adaptive immune system. It remembers the bad guys, so when they come back, the cells of the adaptive immune system can make unique weapons (like antibodies) that attack the invaders and target them for destruction. This is how our adaptive immune system keeps tumors under control, at least when the immune system is working efficiently. However, the adaptive immune system is slow to react to danger and there is very little you can do using your diet to affect its activity.

The other part of our immune system, known as the innate immune system, is far more primitive. In fact, we share this immune system with primitive organisms such as invertebrates. You would think that such a primitive part of our immune system would be easy to understand. It's just the opposite. In fact, the 2011 Nobel Prize in Medicine was awarded for the early research into understanding how the innate immune system works.

The innate immune system has no memory and is based only on pattern recognition. However, the innate immune system is the first re-sponder to microbial attacks, physical injuries, or cellular death. More importantly, it is strongly affected by your diet, and in particular by the Zone Pro-Resolution Nutrition system.

TURNING ON THE INNATE IMMUNE SYSTEM

Your innate immune system stands ready to attack at a moment's notice because it is designed to protect against random microbial invasions or physical injuries external or internal to the body. The most likely source of this microbial invasion comes from the trillions of microbes located in your gut. Microbes contain many distinct molecular markers that allow our cells to recognize that the alien organisms have arrived.

Usually the first step in the inflammatory process is the recognition of microbial fragments by receptors on the surface of every cell. These sensors are known as toll-like receptors (TLR). The toll-like receptors (there are 10 different types in humans and 13 in mice) are proteins embedded in the surface of the cell membrane that recognize distinct microbial fragments as an indication that you are under microbial attack. Once a toll-like receptor is activated, it will initiate the release of powerful inflammatory responses via the innate immune system. Unfortunately, these biological sentinels on your cell surface aren't very discriminating, and as a result, food molecules can also interact with them. As an example, toll-like receptor 4 (TLR-4) can interact with saturated fatty acids (especially palmitic acid) mistakenly thinking it is a component of the bacterial wall thus inducing an inflammatory response believing that microbes are invading the body.

Physical injuries generate damaged molecules (usually glycosylated proteins) that interact with a different type of receptor that recognizes damaged cells that should be destroyed usually by the presence of glycosylated proteins. These are known as advanced glycosylated end products or AGE. AGE proteins can activate unique receptors known as RAGE. Like the TLR, once RAGE are activated, they can also send signals via second messengers to your DNA to ramp up the inflammatory response.

However, to initiate an inflammatory response, the signals generated by interaction with their respective receptors (TLR and RAGE) must first awaken the master genetic switch of inflammation.

NF-κB: THE MASTER GENETIC SWITCH OF INFLAMMATION

The key to activating the innate immune system is a protein called nuclear factor-kappaB (NF-κB). This is a gene transcription factor that was only discovered in 1986. There are probably hundreds of different gene transcription factors in every cell, many of which remain undiscovered. Think of them like short cuts on your computer. Once a particular gene transcription factor is activated, it moves into the nucleus of the cell and causes the expression of a very select number of proteins from your DNA to perform a specific task. In the case of NF-κB, the proteins generated are inflammatory enzymes needed to make eicosanoids and inflammatory cytokines. These newly generated inflammatory proteins are the infantry of your innate immune army. The inflammatory enzymes (primarily COX-2) convert the omega-6 fatty acid arachidonic acid (AA) into a wide variety of powerful pro-inflammatory eicosanoids. The pro-inflammatory cytokines generated by this "master switch of inflammation" can also leave the cell to alert nearby cells they will soon be under attack and should begin to ramp up the activation of NF-κB in their own cells. This starts a chain reaction resulting in the initiation of inflammation. It is like pressing the pedal to the metal for the innate immune system.

The eicosanoids cause immediate pain by interacting with pain receptors on the surface of nerves in the tissue and also cause swelling by opening your blood vessels. These are the reasons you feel pain and swelling when you cut your hand. Once they reach the bloodstream, these eicosanoids also transform your normally benign white blood cells into biological killing machines (called neutrophils and macrophages) that can now easily leave the blood to enter onto the area of the ongoing immunological battle. Specific eicosanoids (i.e., leukotrienes) also act as molecular flares to light the pathway for neutrophils and macrophages to reach the site of the battle. In particular, the neutrophils are indiscriminate killers generating incredible amounts of free radicals as well as releasing digestive enzymes that kill any alien microbial organisms including innocent bystanders such as nearby cells. This results in the tissue damage that must eventually be repaired.

The first attack wave by the neutrophils is not long as they have a limited lifetime. But they are followed into this inflammatory battle by long-lived macrophages that continue the destruction although at a slightly attenuated level. For example, obesity can be considered an ongoing chronic inflammatory condition. This is why nearly 50 percent of the cells in the stored fat (i.e., adipose tissue) of obese individuals are composed of inflammatory macrophages due to the lack of an appropriate Resolution Response in that tissue. Their continuous presence generates even more inflammation making it very difficult to lose excess body fat. This means the initiation stage for inflammation where the inflammatory attack started will continue unless turned off by the presence of sufficient levels of resolvins. This represents the middle phase of the Resolution Response. The good news is that you can *reduce* the intensity of the initiation phase with the Zone Diet. The bad news is the wrong dietary choices can also *increase* the intensity of the initiation phase and keep it going by ensuring you will continue generating even more unresolved cellular inflammation caused by diet-induced inflammation. Unfortunately, the latter is taking place on a worldwide basis.

As I stated earlier, the innate immune system can easily be fooled by our diet, especially by saturated fatty acids such as palmitic acid that interacts with toll-like receptors that will in turn activate NF-κB. However, the most powerful activator of NF-κB is stimulated by a distinct group of eicosanoids derived from arachidonic acid (AA). The more you lower AA levels in your cell membranes to decrease the production of these eicosanoids, the less likely you are to activate NF-κB, and this will dramatically reduce the potential intensity of the initiation of inflammation. The best way to do that is to follow the Zone Diet.

Another activator of NF-κB is oxidative stress. Oxidative stress is the scientific term that describes excess free radical formation, either generated by damaged mitochrondria that produce most of the energy in our cells or by neutrophils and macrophages involved in the initiation of inflammation. There are other surprising sources of oxidative stress induced by your diet. One common source is the consumption of excess calories at a meal, which forces the body to process those excess calories by generating stress on the organelle (the endoplasmic reticulum or ER) that is responsible for protein synthesis. Another activator of NF-κB is a consequence of excess glucose in the blood. The chemical reactivity of glucose often results in its covalent binding to proteins in the blood generating advanced glycosylated end products (AGE), which are mistakenly recognized as damaged tissue fragments by your innate immune system. One of these AGE products is glycosylated hemoglobin (HbA_{1c}) that is used as the primary clinical marker to determine whether or not you have diabetes. It also a good marker of oxidative stress. Once these RAGE receptors on the cell surface bind to an AGE product circulating in the blood, NF-κB is also activated.

THE RESOLUTION RESPONSE TO THE RESCUE

Fortunately, there is a separate phase of the inflammatory process that enables us to call back these biological foot soldiers of the ongoing inflammatory wars so that we don't live in a state of constant cellular inflammation and are unable to repair tissue damage caused by inflammation. This phase of the inflammatory process is called resolution.

Although the concept of resolution was first discussed nearly 1,000 years ago, we are only now beginning to understand how it works at the molecular level to heal the damage caused by inflammation to return the cells back to equilibrium to await their next inflammatory assault. The obligatory first step starts with the Zone Diet that reduces diet-induced inflammation that inhibits the Resolution Response as well as decreasing the activation of NF-κB. The next step of the Resolution Response requires adequate levels of omega-3 fatty acids.

Omega-3 fatty acids are critical for the successful resolution of inflammation because they are the building blocks for resolvins. Without adequate levels of these hormones, the turning off or resolution of the inflammatory response can't be totally completed. The result is increased levels of unresolved cellular inflammation.

However, even generating adequate levels of resolvins is not sufficient to repair the tissue damage caused by inflammation. For that you must activate the gene transcription factor AMP kinase so you can begin the repair of damaged tissue.

AMP KINASE: THE MASTER GENETIC SWITCH OF REPAIR

Just as NF-κB is the major gene transcription factor required for the initiation of inflammation caused by an injury, AMP kinase is the gene transcription factor that controls the repair of damaged tissue necessary for the final step of the Resolution Response that leads to healing of that injury. AMP kinase does this by controlling your metabolism and providing the energy production necessary to repair damaged tissue. Without activating AMP kinase, it is difficult to repair the tissue damaged by any unresolved cellular inflammation. Just as adequate levels of dietary omega-3 fatty acids are required to produce resolvins; AMP kinase can be activated by adequate levels of dietary polyphenols. Polyphenols are complex phytochemicals which naturally occur in fruits and vegetables, but unfortunately they are found at only very low concentrations. Fortunately, they can be concentrated to much higher concentrations to produce purified polyphenol extracts that make them excellent agents to activate AMP kinase on a continuous basis. Activation of AMP kinase is the final step of the Resolution Response that initiates the repair of damaged tissue that is necessary for healing.

However, unless you reduce the intensity of diet-induced inflammation sufficiently by following the Zone Diet, it will overwhelm the ability of the Resolution Response to successfully complete the healing process. This is why following the Zone Diet is the first and most important step for optimizing the Resolution Response.

Metabolism of Essential Fatty Acids, Eicosanoids, and Resolvins

DIET IS EXTREMELY complex, especially when discussing essential fatty acids and their eventual metabolism into the specific hormones that turn on and turn off inflammation. I think you will find it worth your effort, if you are willing to follow this complex rabbit hole of essential fatty acid metabolism and the formation of both eicosanoids and resolvins.

METABOLIC PATHWAYS OF OMEGA-6 AND OMEGA-3 FATTY ACIDS

The eicosanoids that control the initiation phase of the inflammatory process can only be synthesized from longer chain essential fatty acids (20 carbon atoms in length). This is why the Greek root for twenty (*eico*) is used to describe eicosanoids. On the other hand, resolvins can be made from both 20 and 22-carbon length essential fatty acids. Of the omega-3 fatty acids, EPA contains 20 carbon atoms, where DHA contains 22 carbon atoms. This is why you can't make eicosanoids from DHA, but you can from EPA. (I will discuss the implications of that statement later in this Appendix.)

However, the vast majority of essential fatty acids (both omega-6 and omega-3) consist of a shorter chain (18 carbon atoms in length), which means they have no direct role in inflammation except as basic building blocks to potentially be made into longer chain essential fatty acids that are the actual substrates to make either eicosanoids or resolvins.

The metabolic conversion of short-chain essential fatty acids (18 carbons in length into the longer-chain essential fatty acids (20-22 carbons in length) is normally a slow and inefficient process. This is why it is difficult for vegetarians to make adequate levels of EPA and DHA to generate resolvins since these longer chain omega-3 fatty acids are not found in plants.

This metabolic conversion is inefficient because it consists of several rate-limiting steps controlled by enzymes ultimately under dietary control. These enzymes are the "gate keepers" of inflammation. Specifically, the rate-limiting steps are controlled by the delta-5-desaturase and delta-6 desaturase enzymes. These enzymes insert distinct double bonds into the essential fatty acid molecule until it reaches the correct spatial configuration that can be converted into distinct eicosanoids and resolvins that turn on and turn off the inflammatory process respectively. Furthermore, these gate-keeping enzymes are controlled to a great extent by the balance of the hormones generated by the Zone Diet.

EICOSANOIDS

Only three essential fatty acids can be made into eicosanoids. These are arachidonic acid (AA), eicosapentaenoic acid (EPA), and dihomo gamma linolenic acid (DGLA). AA and DGLA are omega-6 fatty acids and EPA is an omega-3 fatty acid. To add to the complexity, eicosanoids generated from AA are strongly pro-inflammatory whereas those from EPA are weakly pro-inflammatory, and those from DGLA are strongly anti-inflammatory. Wait a minute, you were probably thinking that EPA was always considered to be an anti-inflammatory fatty acid? It should be noted that the eicosanoids derived from EPA are about 10-100 times less pro-inflammatory than those derived from AA, so in comparison the eicosanoids generated from EPA cause potentially far less inflammatory damage to a particular organ than the eicosanoids derived from AA. But there is one eicosanoid derived from DGLA that is the kingpin of anti-inflammatory eicosanoids. It is called PGE_1. Unfortunately, as I have found out over the past 35 years, it is very difficult to consistently control its production.

The metabolic conversion of the primary dietary short-chain omega-6 (linoleic acid) and omega-3 (alpha linolenic acid) fatty acids into the three long-chain essential fatty acids (AA, EPA, and DGLA) required for eicosanoid formation use the same enzymes including the rate-limiting desaturase enzymes. Thus, the balance of the shorter-chain omega-6 and omega-3 fatty acid levels in the diet will a have significant impact on the types of inflammatory hormones that are eventually synthesized because the omega-6 and omega-3 fatty acids are competing for the same enzymes. This means the more omega-6 fatty acids in your diet, the more AA you will produce compared to EPA. Furthermore, both the rate-limiting enzymes (delta-5- and delta-6-desaturase) are also under dietary control. In particular, both desaturase enzymes are stimulated by increased blood levels of the hormone insulin (stimulated by the levels of carbohydrate in the diet as well your severity of insulin resistance), but also inhibited by the hormone glucagon (stimulated by the levels of protein in the diet). Now you can begin to see why the Zone Diet has such a strong relevance for controlling the balance of eicosanoids by determining the balance of insulin and glucagon. By controlling the balance of insulin-to-glucagon levels in the blood and especially by reducing insulin resistance, you can change the levels of AA, DGLA, and EPA in the body that control the activities of the key desaturase enzymes as well as the balance of the omega-6 and omega-3 fatty acids in the diet. The end result will provide a significantly better control of the intensity of the initiation of inflammation and therefore require fewer resolvins to put out the inflammatory fire.

The metabolic pathways leading to AA and EPA are essentially the same since they use the same enzymes as shown in Figure 1.

You can see by this figure that the more EPA you have in the diet, the more you can inhibit the enzyme (delta-5-desaturase) needed to make AA. So here was my "clever" thinking (although very elementary in hindsight) in 1982. If I could find a suitable plant source of GLA and extract the oil (borage was the best choice once my brother and I learned how to grow it in Saskatchewan), then supplement the diet with GLA it would be rapidly transformed into DGLA. If I then inhibited its further metabolism into AA by adding enough fish oil rich in EPA to inhibit the activity of the delta-5-desaturase enzyme, then the levels of DGLA would rise and we would be off to fame and fortune because DGLA is the omega-6 fatty acid that eventually generates PGE_1. Sometimes, reality gets in the way. I didn't count upon the powerful effect of insulin to activate the enzyme that converts DGLA into AA and thus overwhelm the rather puny amounts of EPA I was supplying at the time. Hence, I needed to create

Figure 1. Metabolic Pathways for the Synthesis of Arachidonic Acid (AA)
and Eicosapentaenoic Acid (EPA)

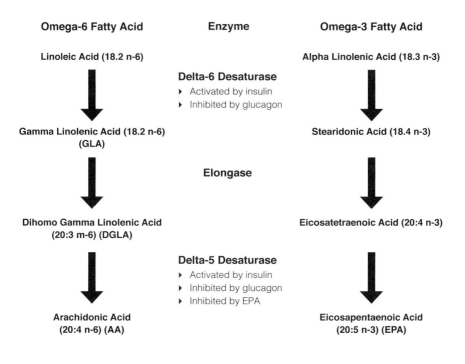

the Zone Diet if I ever wanted to truly reduce the intensity of the initiation of inflammation caused by eicosanoids generated from AA.

But what about the omega-3 fatty acid, docosahexaenoic acid (DHA)? It can't be made into eicosanoids, but it has plenty of other roles to play because of its ability to generate resolvins. DHA can be made from EPA, although through a more complicated pathway as shown in Figure 2.

Although there are additional steps in the metabolic conversion of EPA into DHA, it is an ongoing process so that DHA levels are always greater than EPA levels in the blood and your organs. Although DHA is not very important for eicosanoid formation, the presence of both DHA and EPA are critical for making resolvins.

Thus, the balance of omega-6 and omega-3 fatty acids in the diet plus the balance of protein and the glycemic load in the Zone Diet will have a powerful impact on the eventual balance of inflammatory eicosanoids (derived from AA) and equally powerful resolvins (derived from EPA and DHA).

Figure 2. Metabolic Pathways for the Conversion of EPA into DHA

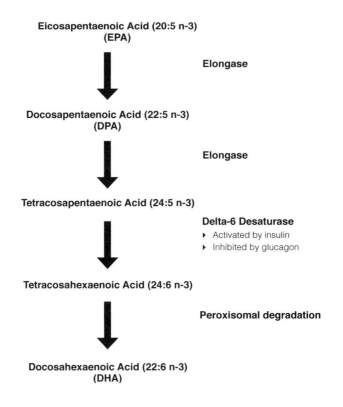

There are two ways to change the balance of resolvins relative to eicosanoids in your body. The first is following the Zone Diet, which will not only lower the intake of omega-6 fatty acids but also stabilizes insulin to prevent the stimulation of the delta-5-desaturase enzyme that would accelerate the conversion of omega-6 fatty acids into AA. The other way is to supplement with EPA and DHA using high-dose ultra-refined omega-3 concentrates to increase their levels in the blood to generate adequate levels of the precursor necessary to make resolvins to resolve cellular inflammation. Ideally, you want to do both to optimize the Resolution Response.

METABOLISM OF ARACHIDONIC ACID INTO EICOSANOIDS

Unbound fatty acids are potentially toxic because they can act as biological detergents to dissolve membranes if they are freely roaming around in the cell. This is why the essential fatty acids used for the production of both eicosanoids and resolvins are safely stored in the membranes of every cell as phospholipids that can be released on demand.

What controls that release of those fatty acids are a group of enzymes known as phospholipases. If these enzymes were not active, then you would be unable to release stored fatty acids and therefore never able to generate either eicosanoids or resolvins. What activates the phospholipase enzymes are metabolic changes caused by injuries. This is why inflammation is also produced on demand and is normally inactive unless you have constant injuries or high levels of unresolved cellular inflammation.

Furthermore, these phospholipase enzymes are pretty dumb. They can't distinguish arachidonic acid (AA) from omega-3 fatty acids such as EPA and DHA. The phospholipase enzyme just reaches into the membrane of the cell and whichever one of the three fatty acids is most abundant in the membrane will be the one that gets released to be made into either eicosanoids or resolvins. It is like a biological lottery. Unfortunately, most of us have a far greater abundance of AA sitting in the membranes than EPA or DHA. As a result, AA will be the most likely essential fatty acid released.

Once AA is released it will be immediately synthesized into an eicosanoid. But which one? It depends on which enzyme grabs it first as shown in Figure 3.

Figure 3. Synthesis of Eicosanoids

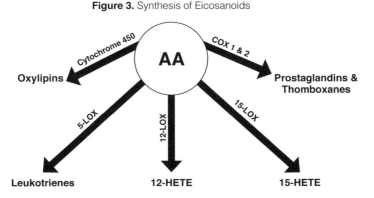

To make this diagram simpler, just remember that prostaglandins cause pain, thromboxanes cause your platelets to clot, leukotrienes activate NF-κB, and 12-HETE causes insulin resistance and encourages cancer cells to metastasize. These are all pretty good reasons not to have excess AA in your cell membranes. If you have more EPA and less AA in the cell membrane, then the eicosanoids from EPA will lower the level of intensity for the initiation of inflammation because they have weaker inflammatory actions than those eicosanoids generated from AA. This is why maintaining the AA/EPA ratio in an appropriate range (i.e., a 1.5 to 3 ratio as opposed to the average American who has a 20:1 ratio) to reduce the intensity of the initiation phase of inflammation is so important for optimizing the Resolution Response. Otherwise, you will have a continuing tsunami of cellular inflammation that will be impossible to completely resolve, thus creating chronic unresolved cellular inflammation.

METABOLISM OF RESOLVINS

Even if you turn down the intensity of inflammation, you still must eventually turn it off. For that you need the resolvins generated primarily from EPA and DHA. If you thought eicosanoid formation was difficult to follow, it gets even more complex for the generation of resolvins because there are a lot of additional enzymatic steps in their formation as shown in Figure 4.

Figure 4. Synthesis of Resolvins

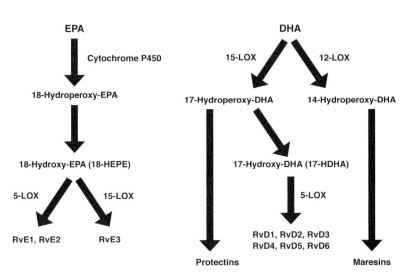

Yet all of these complex eicosanoid and resolvin pathways can readily be modified using the Zone Pro-Resolution Nutrition system as long as you follow the Zone Diet coupled with adequate supplementation with EPA and DHA.

WHY ANTI-INFLAMMATORY DRUGS HAVE SIDE EFFECTS

All anti-inflammatory drugs have side effects. These drugs include aspirin, non-steroidal anti-inflammatory drugs (NSAIDs), and corticosteroids. How these side effects manifest is actually quite varied depending on the drug.

To make prostaglandins, thromboxanes, or leukotrienes from AA requires the enzymes known as cyclo-oxygenase (COX) and lipo-oxygenase (LOX) as shown below.

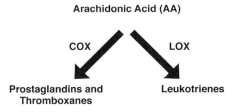

Most of the common anti-inflammatory drugs only inhibit the COX enzymes that make prostaglandins or thromboxanes. Aspirin is an irreversible inhibitor of COX enzymes thereby reducing both pain and excessive clotting, whereas over the counter (OTC) drugs such as Aleve and Motrin are competitive inhibitors of the same enzymes, but primarily affect the prostaglandins that cause pain. This is why your physician recommends taking an aspirin to prevent a heart attack instead of other anti-inflammatory drugs. All this may appear to be good news, but there is a catch. None of these common anti-inflammatory drugs will inhibit the production of leukotrienes. Leukotrienes are the true "bad boys" of eicosanoids. First, by inhibiting the COX enzymes, you are forcing more AA into the leukotriene pathway. Since leukotrienes are the most pro-inflammatory of the eicosanoids, they generate more inflammatory damage in other organs than do other eicosanoids. The second reason is that leukotrienes are powerful promoters of insulin resistance that causes many of your problems in the first place by constantly elevating insulin levels that stimulate the overproduction of AA. To add insult to injury, leukotrienes also activate the gene transcription factor (NF-κB) that turns on inflammation, as well as their ability to promote cancer metastasis, cause leakiness in the blood-brain-barrier, and are intimately involved in a lot of other chronic diseases like asthma.

The only anti-inflammatory drug that can consistently inhibit leukotriene synthesis as well as other eicosanoids are powerful synthetic corti-costeroids like prednisone. The natural hormone cortisol can also inhibit leukotriene synthesis, but it is not nearly as powerful as synthetic cortico-steroids. Cortisol and corticosteroids work through a different mechanism than simply inhibiting enzymes that make eicosanoids. They prevent the release of AA (as well as other fatty acids such as EPA and DHA) from their storage sites in the cell membrane. This will not only stop leukotriene synthesis, but it will also inhibit resolvin synthesis. Furthermore, the side effects of synthetic corticosteroids are severe; they depress the immune system, increase insulin resistance leading to weight gain and diabetes, cause thinning of the skin, promote bone loss as well as causing mood swings and other associated neurological problems. These side effects be-come quite pronounced especially with long-term use. This is why these drugs are used as the last resort to treat inflammation.

MORE BAD NEWS ABOUT ANTI-INFLAMMATORY DRUGS

However, even with the right levels of omega-3 fatty acids in the body, their conversion into resolvins requires the presence of inflammatory cells (neutrophils) to start the oxidation of these omega-3 fatty acids as the first step toward making resolvins. If these inflammatory cells are not present due to chronic use of anti-inflammatory drugs, then the gen-eration of pro-resolving hormones grinds to a halt regardless of the omega-3 fatty acid levels in the blood. This is the other reason that anti-inflammatory drugs are also anti-resolution drugs. This is also why all anti-inflammatory drugs have side effects. The more powerful the an-ti-inflammatory drug, the greater its anti-resolution side effects. Without adequate levels of resolvins, the Resolution Response remains blocked.

WHY AREN'T THERE ANY PRO-RESOLUTION DRUGS?

You might initially think resolvins would be easy to synthesize in the lab, so why are there no resolvin drugs on the market? The answer is because their stereochemistry (i.e., structure in three-dimensional space) is so complex. This is the same reason they can't make EPA and DHA econom-ically in a lab or a factory. At a medical conference on resolvins, I asked one of the leading producers of lipids as prescription drugs what the projected cost of synthetically produced resolvins for use as a pharmaceutical might be? His answer was about $50 million per kilogram. That's a lot of money. At another resolvin conference, I learned about new potential synthetic pathways that were being proposed that could potentially reduce the cost of resolvins to only $5-10 million per kilogram. That is still a lot of money. Even if it became economically feasible to synthesize resolvins, they have a very short lifespan in the body measured in minutes and they have to be injected. Furthermore, you have no idea when an injury may strike and since the cellular inflammation those injuries generate is often below the perception of pain you don't realize the need for immediate resolvin formation.

Fortunately, there is another way to make resolvins so they can be made on-demand when injury-induced inflammation starts. Simply consume enough omega-3 fatty acids in the diet to maintain adequate levels so the body can make resolvins on demand when needed. The amount you need is determined by the AA/EPA ratio in the blood. Furthermore, the more you reduce the intensity of diet-induced inflammation by following the Zone Diet, the fewer omega-3 fatty acids you will need to complete the resolution process and set the final stage for the Resolution Response, which is the repair of damaged tissue.

Energy-Sensing Gene Transcription Factors

IF YOU THOUGHT that eicosanoid and resolvin metabolism was complex, then you are in for a treat learning about energy-sensing gene transcription factors. These specific gene transcription factors are the proteins responsible for alerting the body that it is running low on fuel and better shift its metabolism to rebuild its energy stores. Since most of the energy used in the body comes from the production of ATP, you might expect there would be various intermediates in its synthesis that activate the energy-sensing gene transcription factors.

Energy-sensing gene transcription factors evolved earlier in time than did inflammation-inducing gene transcription factors such as NF-κB. This makes sense because if an organism can't make enough ATP, it will die before it will be attacked by microbial invasion.

There are two primary energy-sensing gene transcription factors. One is the *silent information regulator T* (SIRT) system that senses any decrease in nicotinamide adenine dinucleotide (NAD) levels and the other is AMP kinase that senses any decrease in ATP. Not surprisingly they both regulate each other. NAD is required for the synthesis of ATP in the mitochondria. Conversely, any drop in ATP levels causes an increase in NAD production by the activation of the enzyme (nicotinamide phosphoribosyltransferase or Nampt) to increase NAD levels. There are seven different SIRT gene transcription factors that are activated by increased NAD. Once activated, they in turn increase the production of serine-threonine liver kinase B1 (LKB1), which in turn activates AMP kinase. As complicated as it seems, this is a very elegant feedback system to make sure the cell is constantly sensing key metabolites needed for the production of ATP as shown below.

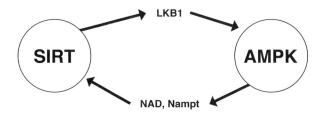

AMP kinase is rapidly activated by anything that decreases ATP levels, such as calorie restriction, intense exercise, or poisoning of the mito-chondrial production of ATP (such as using drugs like metformin). On the other hand, the activation of SIRT by polyphenols is a slower process.

The SIRT system can continually be activated by the dietary intake of polyphenols that occupy an allosteric site in the various SIRT gene tran-scription factors. Allosteric sites are distinct from the actual catalytic site in complex proteins such as SIRT. Polyphenols that bind to the allosteric site of the SIRT gene transcription factor induce a conformational change that allows it to start its necessary catalytic activities. Delphinidins are among the most effective polyphenols to activate such sites in the various SIRT gene transcription factors. As long as SIRT is activated, it in turns keeps AMP kinase in a constantly activated state that affects a wide range of other gene transcription factors that control virtually every aspect of your metabolism as shown below.

Metabolic Actions Increased	Metabolic Actions Decreased
Mitochondria biogenesis	Fatty acid synthesis
Glucose uptake	Cholesterol synthesis
Fatty acid uptake	Glycogen synthesis
Blood flow	Insulin resistance
Fatty acid oxidation	Tumor growth
Autophagy and mitophagy	Inflammation

What does this mean for you? Let's first look at the metabolic actions that are increased once you activate AMP kinase. If you make more mitochondria, you have more energy. If your glucose uptake increases, you treat diabetes. If you are an athlete and you make more mitochondria, then you have more energy. If you increase the uptake of fatty acids into the muscle and increase fatty acid oxidation to make ATP, you lose excess body fat. If your blood flow increases, you treat hypertension, and if you don't have hypertension, you will transfer more oxygen to your muscle cells to produce more energy. If you increase autophagy and mitophagy, you are cleaning up the garbage in your cells.

The benefits of depressing other metabolic actions by increased activation of AMP kinase are just as impressive. If you decrease fatty acid synthesis, your levels of triglycerides in blood go down. If you decrease cholesterol synthesis, your cholesterol levels go down. If you reduce glycogen synthesis, you retain less water. If you reduce insulin resistance, you lose weight and have gone a long way towards treating any chronic disease. If tumor growth rates are reduced, that's the most effective way to treat cancer. Finally, if you optimize the final step of your Resolution Response, you maintain wellness creating a longer healthspan.

These gene transcription-signaling networks that orchestrate all of these metabolic benefits are incredibly complex, but all require the activation of AMP kinase. Bottom line, anything that activates AMP kinase (and doesn't poison your mitochondria in the process) increases your healthspan. That's one of the benefits of following the Zone Diet. It's a calorie-restricted diet that can activate AMP kinase. On the other hand, excess calorie intake (especially glucose) inhibits the activity of AMP kinase. That's why the Zone Diet is a calorie-restricted diet with a balanced protein-to-glycemic load ratio. You can further enhance the Zone Diet by supplementing with large amounts of purified water-soluble polyphenols (like delphinidins) that will activate the various SIRT gene transcription factors without increasing calorie intake. Once you combine the Zone Diet and water-soluble polyphenols (such as delphindins) you have a highly sophisticated dietary intervention to maintain AMP kinase activation. Add to this dietary intervention periods of high-intensity interval training (HIIT), and you have now done everything possible to keep the "enzyme of life" (AMP kinase) constantly on alert to complete the final step of the healing process, which is the repair of damaged tissue.

AMP KINASE AND GUT FUNCTION

Just as the activation of AMP kinase has multiple actions for optimizing your metabolism, it is also critical for improved gut health. Short-chain fatty acids (SCFA) that are one of the by-products of fermentable fiber metabolism activate AMP kinase in the gut wall. This increase in AMP kinase activity not only increases the assembly of tight junctions in the gut wall that reduce the likelihood of developing a leaky gut, but AMP kinase also increases the activity of the goblet cells in the gut wall to produce more mucus to maintain your first line of defense (the mucus barrier) that prevents both microbial fragments and large proteins from interacting with the gut wall. Activation of AMP kinase by delphinidins also inhibits the action of the sodium-glucose transporter 1 (SGLT1) that reduces the entry of glucose into the blood and thus reduces insulin secretion.

Discovering drugs that activate AMP kinase without significant side effects has been one of the great failures of modern medicine. The use of the Zone Pro-Resolution Nutrition system using purified maqui polyphenol extracts (rich in delphinidins) provides a potential solution to control the genetic master switch of your metabolism.

AMP Kinase and Mitochondria

THROUGHOUT THIS BOOK I have emphasized the critical role that mitochondria play in the production of ATP. Without adequate levels of ATP, the repair of damaged tissue will never be complete, and the final stage of the Resolution Response will remain inhibited. Yet as critical as mitochondria are to our survival, we are just beginning to understand how they orchestrate metabolism and ultimately control our healthspan.

AMP KINASE: MASTER GENETIC SWITCH FOR YOUR MITOCHONDRIA

Your metabolism is how you convert food into energy and then use that energy to keep you alive. This task ultimately involves AMP kinase Once you activate AMP kinase, you set in motion a wide network of other gene transcription factors that results in the repair of damaged tissue. Some of these gene transcription factors (like Nrf2) increase the synthesis of anti-oxidative enzymes that reduce excess free radicals, others (like PPARɣ) reduce inflammation, and still others (like PGC-1α) increase the generation of new mitochondria leading to better energy generation. It is your mitochondria that provide the necessary energy needed to ultimately repair the damage caused by inflammation and thus complete the Resolution Response. In essence, your ability to heal inflammatory damage is ultimately determined by the health of your mitochondria.

MITOCHONDRIA

Mitochondria are the engines of life producing nearly 90 percent of all the chemical energy (primarily adenosine triphosphate or ATP) generated by a cell. Without their appearance about 800 million years ago there would not be any multi-cellular life (including us) existing on the planet.

Today mitochondria are only an afterthought as they are considered to be small organelles inside every living cell. An organelle is simply a "little organ" inside the cell that does something necessary for the cell to survive. The primary job of mitochondria is to convert fatty acids and glucose into chemical energy (ATP) that makes life possible. They also act as quality control agents that determine whether or not a damaged cell will be destroyed by apoptosis (i.e., programmed cell death) for the good of the organ. However, understanding the complexity of mitochondria may also provide significant answers as to why we get sick and why we age. Without adequate ATP production you can't finish the repair process and thus complete the Resolution Response. Of course, the longer that the inflammation caused by the initial injury has been amplified by diet-induced inflammation, the more difficult it becomes to repair the damage because of fibrosis.

Unfortunately, in the process of making ATP your mitochondria also generate a lot of free radicals. Mitochondria are easily damaged because they are at ground zero of a constant generation of free radicals. Think of mitochondria as living inside an X-ray machine that is constantly turned on. When their DNA is damaged, they go rogue and begin making less ATP and more free radicals to attack everything in the cell. So not only does a cell have to be constantly making new mitochondria (this is called mitochondrial biogenesis), but also it has to select out the damaged ones for destruction (this is called mitophagy). This is more difficult than it appears. A cell can't store more than 10 seconds worth of ATP. This is because ATP is made on demand. A typical muscle cell may have 2,000 mitochondria. So, picking out a damaged one, removing it, as well as making its replacement to take its spot without a drop off of ATP production is pretty complex. This job is made a lot easier if the gene transcription factor AMP kinase is constantly activated.

AMP KINASE ACTIONS

Perhaps the greatest benefit from the constant activation of AMP kinase is slowing the aging process by improving the efficiency of your metabolism. This results in an increase in your healthspan. At the molecular level, slowing the aging process can be better understood as an acceleration of the repair of damaged tissue that requires massive amounts of energy as well as the continual clean-up of accumulated garbage in the cell through a process known as autophagy. AMP kinase controls both processes.

   Here are just a small number of the metabolic actions controlled by AMP kinase.

Antioxidant activity

One factor in the aging process is the increase of oxidative stress caused by the excess production of free radicals. Increased AMP kinase activity results in the activation of another gene transcription factor known as Nrf2. This gene transcription factor goes directly into the nucleus of the cell to cause the increased synthesis of anti-oxidative enzymes such as glutathione peroxidase (GPX), superoxide dismutase (SOD), and catalase. Unlike classical dietary antioxidant vitamins (such as vitamins A, E, and C), these antioxidative enzymes can reduce thousands of times more free radicals than can vitamins. The reduction of excess free radicals and their associated decrease of oxidative stress is strongly associated with decreased mortality.

Anti-inflammatory activity

Another benefit of AMP kinase activation is its stimulation of another gene transcription factor known as peroxisome proliferator-activated receptor gamma (PPAR-γ) that has anti-inflammatory actions as well as inhibiting the activation of the gene transcription factor nuclear factor kappaB (NF-κB), the master genetic switch for turning on inflammatory responses. So, by activating AMP kinase you are significantly modulating the intensity of inflammation by turning down NF-κB while simultaneously increasing PPAR-γ activity.

Gut health activity

If you can activate AMP kinase, then you also dramatically improve gut health especially in combination with fermentable fiber. The goblet cells in the gut wall are activated by AMP kinase to increase mucus production. With this increase, the mucus barrier is strengthened and the population of *Akkermansia muciniphila* increases since they reside primarily in the outer layer of the mucus barrier. There are other ways to increase *Akkermansia* in the gut, such as gastric bypass surgery (it also activates AMP kinase activity due to calorie restriction), but polyphenol activation of AMP kinase remains your most powerful and desirable approach.

Even more importantly for gut health, AMP kinase acts as the master architect that orchestrates the assembly of tight junctions in the gut wall thereby decreasing the formation of a leaky gut. The end result is that the combinations of increased AMP kinase activity and increased *Akkermansia* growth in the gut reduces the penetration of bacterial fragments such as lipopolysaccharide (LPS) into the blood that would otherwise interact with toll-like receptors (TLR) to generate low-level chronic inflammation that leads to metabolic endotoxemia with a corresponding increase in obesity and diabetes. Although the short-chain fatty acids (primarily butyrate) are key fermentation by-products of fermentable fiber and are important for gut health, without AMP kinase activation to orchestrate the building of new tight junctions in the cell wall, the short-chain fatty acids will not be utilized to their maximum potential to optimize gut health.

AMP KINASE ACTIVATION WITH DRUGS

With all these great benefits associated with activating AMP kinase, isn't there some drug that will do all the work for you? Unfortunately, not without some serious side effects. The primary drugs used to activate AMP kinase also poison your mitochondria. Remember that AMP kinase is an energy sensor of ATP levels in the cell. So, if you initially decrease your mitochondria efficiency, ATP levels will drop and that will temporarily increase AMP kinase activity. But this type of drug strategy is not very useful for the long term. Metformin is one such drug that works by this mechanism. Although used as the first line of treatment for managing diabetes, it eventually fails because of its negative long-term impact on mitochondrial energy production as well as its side effects on the gut such as diarrhea, nausea, and vomiting. This is why lifestyle modifications (diet and exercise) that also activate AMP kinase have a significantly greater benefit in the long-term management of diabetes than does metformin. Even with these side effects, metformin is currently being pushed as an anti-aging drug. However, all this can change with the increased intake of dietary polyphenols and even more so with supplementation using high-dose water-soluble polyphenol extracts rich in delphinidins such as purified maqui extracts.

HISTORY OF MITOCHONDRIA

Life on earth began about three billion years ago with bacteria. However, at that time the world was devoid of oxygen (similar to the interior of the gut). The primary source of making ATP by bacteria was the fermentation of any available nutrient available and the generation of methane, hydrogen, and other gases in the process.

Through a lucky break about two billion years ago, certain bacteria that made methane started to hang around other bacteria that made hydrogen because the hydrogen could be used by the methane-producing bacteria as a fuel source to improve their survival. Over the course of the next billion or so years and with lots of gene swapping, a symbiosis developed that allowed the combination of these two bacteria with a potential evolutionary advantage over other bacteria. Only one thing was missing, oxygen. When oxygen began to appear in the atmosphere, this symbiotic union of the two bacteria were in the ideal position to use oxygen to enable the generation of far greater levels of ATP through oxidative phosphorylation. This increased energy supply made it possible for an abundance of new multi-cellular organisms to appear 600 million years ago because of the increased energy demands needed for the specialization of functions. This was known as the Cambrian period in which there was an explosion of different multi-cellular species made possible with the increased ATP production needed for specialization.

MITOCHONDRIA AND CELLULAR QUALITY CONTROL

The efficient functioning of any organ depends on the consistent interaction of the cells within that organ. When a cell is damaged beyond repair, it undergoes a process of programmed cell death known as apoptosis. This type of cellular death is actually good for the organ and safely removes the damaged cell and sets the stage for a new healthy cell to take its place. This highly orchestrated process is initiated by the mitochondria in the cell and carried out by further instructions from AMP kinase. You lose about 50 billion cells on a daily basis to this apoptotic process. That seems like a lot of cells, but your body contains about 10 trillion living cells. This means you are losing about 0.5 percent of your cells on a daily basis. However, if they are not replaced, organ function will eventually decrease with time.

Many of those lost cells are replaced by new stem cells in the organ that are activated to take their place. Unfortunately, you don't have an unlimited number of stem cells in a particular organ (except for your adipose tissue that is exceptionally rich in stem cells), so with time the number of functional cells in that organ will decrease leading to a condition of atrophy. This is especially true for your muscle cells and that's why your peak strength usually occurs around age 25.

When cell death is uncontrolled or cells have been killed by cancer drugs, radiation treatment, or excessive oxidative stress, the result is a different type of cell death called necrosis. This uncontrolled cell death leaves behind a lot of cellular debris that now becomes a constant source of ongoing inflammation. This is why the resolution process is so important in reducing the side effects of cancer chemotherapy and radiation treatments as previously described.

However, mitochondria have their own autophagy program known as mitophagy where damaged mitochondria are targeted for destruction and replaced with new healthy functional mitochondria without the cell being forced to undergo apoptosis. That process of mitophagy and mitochondrial biogenesis is controlled by AMP kinase. The more functional your mitochondria are in a particular cell the less likely that cell will be damaged in the future. This means a greater healthspan.

MITOCHONDRIAL COMMUNICATION

Mitochondria are in constant physical contact with your endoplasmic reticulum (ER) where new proteins are synthesized based on the activation of your DNA by gene transcription factors. The ER is essentially a factory inside the cell where new proteins are made. Like any factory, they need a constant supply of energy provided by your mitochondria. As you increase your calorie intake beyond what is needed, this forces the cell to metabolize those excess calories and puts a greater stress on the ER and the mitochondria that supply the energy for the synthesis of those proteins. The end result is your mitochondria are more likely to become damaged by the excessive production of free radicals as more fuel (fatty acids or glucose) is pushed through them to make enough ATP for the ER to continue the synthesis of new proteins. Reducing calorie intake reduces ER stress and also decreases the likelihood of mitochondrial damage.

DRUGS THAT INHIBIT MITOCHONDRIAL FUNCTION

There are a great number of common drugs that inhibit mitochondria. These include drugs commonly used to treat diabetes (metformin and thiazolidinediones), depression (SSRI drugs), neurological disorders (anti-psychotic medications), inflammation (aspirin and corticosteroids), cardiovascular disease (statins and beta blockers), cancer drugs for the treatment of HIV, and anesthetics. Many of their side-effects can be attributed to their inhibition of ATP production by poisoning your mitochondria. This is why following the Zone Pro-Resolution Nutrition system is so important when you are taking any of these drugs.

IMPROVING MITOCHONDRIAL FUNCTION

A primary dietary goal of the Zone Pro-Resolution Nutrition program is the activation of AMP kinase to maintain optimal mitochondrial function. This can be targeted with precision using high-dose polyphenols (especially water-soluble delphinidins that can enter the blood) to activate AMP kinase indirectly by increasing the activity of the SIRT genes described in Appendix E. Your secondary "drugs" are calorie restriction (like the Zone Diet) and high-intensity interval training (HIIT). Any intervention that improves mitochondrial function will automatically extend your healthspan. The more you combine polyphenols, calorie restriction, and HIIT, the greater the benefits on extending your healthspan.

.

Gut Physiology

TO BETTER UNDERSTAND the role of fermentable fiber in the Zone Diet, a good place to start would be to understand what really happens in the gut when you consume food. It's quite an odyssey starting with our sense of smell and taste, continuing with the digestion and absorption of nutrients we need in the small intestine, and finally ending in the colon where much of the complex action of this organ takes place because that is where the bulk of bacteria in the gut resides. It's also a long journey. The total transit time from when you eat something and its final exit in the stool is about 30 hours and many complex events happen along the way.

Before this journey even starts, the body does some advance planning starting with the smell of food. This is your first defense against potential toxicity since you can smell rancid food because microbes are digesting the remains of the day (or the week). If food smells bad, that means it is usually rich in microbial fermentation products, and the brain immediately tells you not to eat it. At the same time, the smell of food can activate the dopamine reward centers in the brain to instruct you that you are making the right choice.

Once you decide to put food in your mouth, you still have another defense system to protect you, your taste buds. There are five distinct tastes that these receptors in the tongue can recognize. One of them is a bitter taste. This is usually an indication of plant toxins (like alkaloids) or microbial toxins. In either case, these taste receptors can alert you to spit the unsuitable food choice out before it enters your digestive system. This is why deep frying poor-quality meat or fish is a great way to ensure its consumption because deep frying in combination with the flour coating can cover up any rancid taste.

This same system of taste receptors can also affect your dopamine reward system in the brain. This is especially true of sweet taste receptors. A sweet taste usually indicates glucose, and that is actually the nutrient the brain needs to function optimally. Other tastes can trigger embedded memories of that particular food and, if they are favorable, give you the go-ahead signal to eat. This is also why the processed food industry has mastered the use of sugar, fat, and salt to make their otherwise tasteless products into irresistible foods by hijacking your brain's dopamine reward system that starts with the taste receptors in the tongue.

Not everyone has the same number of taste receptors. Some individuals known as supertasters have higher concentrations of taste receptors in the tongue and are more easily affected (positively or negatively) by a particular food source. On the other hand, cancer chemotherapy or the aging process will reduce the number of your taste receptors. Without adequate levels of taste receptors, food has little taste and therefore little reward, so you are less likely to have any desire to eat. Surprisingly, taste receptors are also distributed throughout the gut but primarily in the small intestine. Now they are multi-tasking by sending hormonal signals to the brain indicating the presence of food at different locations of its journey through the gut.

Before the food actually enters the digestion tract, you usually chew it. This will not only increase the absorption of nutrients by increasing the surface area of the food, but more importantly gives time for hormonal signals to begin reaching the appetite and reward centers in the brain. This is why the first bite of food is usually the best, especially from those foods rich in sugar and fat (i.e., desserts). Your saliva contains the enzyme amylase that can break down refined sugar into glucose and fructose as well as doing the same to starches and grain-based products (such as pasta, pizza, and pastries) that interact with your taste receptors sending a loud and clear signal to the brain that this is good stuff to eat.

It is often said that everything above the neck tells you to eat, and everything below the neck tells you to stop eating. This is why you should chew your food thoroughly in order to give the digested food some time to get below the neck and start sending hormonal signals to the brain that enough is enough. This is also why smoothies don't control your appetite as well as eating solid food.

Obviously chewing can be taken to the extreme as it was in the early 20th century with idea of Fletcherism. This was the dietary philosophy of Horace Fletcher that suggested you should chew each bite of food 25 times before swallowing. Somewhere between Fletcherism and drinking smoothies is a good compromise to activate your dopamine reward center, and to reduce calorie consumption in the process.

STOMACH: YOUR INTERNAL FOOD PROCESSOR

If bacteria make it past your odor and taste receptors, they still face many formidable changes before they can try to invade your bloodstream.

Even if you inhale your meal, your stomach will still do much of the "chewing" for you. This is because once food enters the stomach it also enters into a world of acid. This acid has two tasks to accomplish. The first is to activate the protein-digesting enzymes needed to begin breaking down dietary protein. The second is to kill bacteria contained in the food you have just put into your mouth. Strong acid is a very effective killer of live bacteria and that includes probiotics. This is why 99.9 percent of probiotics are destroyed outright in the stomach. The reason the strong acid doesn't also destroy your stomach wall lining is because of two things. The first is because the epithelial cells that line the stomach are constantly secreting bicarbonate to neutralize the acid before it reaches the surface of the stomach. The second reason is that the cells lining the gut are the most rapidly dividing cells in the body and are replaced every few days. This is also why they are very prone to destruction by cancer drugs, which are designed to kill rapidly dividing cells of any type including those that protect the gut lining.

Besides being a vat of acid, the stomach is also a remarkable blender. It can take a wide variety of food formats and put them through an intense muscular churning combined with stomach enzymes that turn ingested food into the equivalent of a partially digested smoothie. The technical term for this "smoothie" is chyme.

SMALL INTESTINE: ABSORPTION CENTRAL

Once the chyme is prepared in the stomach, it's time to begin the absorption process, which is the real reason that you eat. This is done in the small intestine. The small intestine is composed of three segments (duodenum, jejunum, and ileum). These three segments represent approximately a 20-foot section of your gut that gets first crack at the easy-to-absorb nutrients. This is a sophisticated process as it prevents large fragments of undigested protein from getting close to the surface of the gut wall where they can provoke significant immunological and inflammatory responses. This is the underlying cause of food allergies. This is why maintenance of the integrity of the mucus barrier that lines the entire gut is a key for gut health.

Mucus is actually a complex polymer of carbohydrates made by specialized cells (i.e., goblet cells) located throughout your digestive system. This is the primary barrier to prevent undigested food as well as pathological microbes that may bypass the stomach's acid vat from interacting with the cell wall of the gut causing inflammatory damage. There are two parts to this mucus barrier. The loose outer layer allows friendly bacteria (especially *Akkermansia*) to attach to it and their presence helps to prevent pathogenic microbes from reaching the gut wall. The very dense inner layer of the mucus barrier acts as a trap to prevent even friendly bacteria and large protein fragments access to the cells that line the gut. The word "friendly" is not quite correct. There are about 1,000 to 1,500 microbes that have adapted to exist in our gut. Actually, your gut has adapted to make a home for them. In return, they provide useful metabolic services such as the production of various metabolites derived from fermentable fiber necessary to maintain gut health as well as neurotransmitters and vitamins produced by the same bacteria. These friendly bacteria also secrete unique antibiotics to prevent their truly pathogenic cousins from gaining a foothold in the gut. However, if these "friendly" microbes or their fragments get into the blood, they can then become a powerful source of inflammation. Just as you can cause diet-induced inflammation by making the wrong food choices, you can also cause gut-induced inflammation if you don't have enough fermentable fiber (both in quantity and diversity) to maintain a healthy gut wall and a robust mucus barrier to protect it. Finally, the mucus barrier also lubricates the flow of food through the digestive process preventing the bloating and abdominal pain usually associated with gut disorders.

Once the chyme begins to move from the stomach into the first part of the small intestine, or duodenum, the complexity of the digestion process begins to unfold. The first step of this journey requires a dramatic increase of the pH of the chyme back to neutral. Like the locks of the Panama Canal, the acid environment of the stomach is blocked out and the pH rises back to normal levels in the duodenum. This change in pH ensures that when the pancreas starts pumping a wide array of digestive enzymes needed to break down the crude chyme into a further digested format that these enzymes will not be denatured by the low pH found in the stomach.

The lining of the gut wall of the small intestine is composed of tight junctions between cells so that only very small molecules can pass through it and into the blood. Nutrient flow into the blood is only possible because pancreatic enzymes finish breaking down complex sugars and starches into single glucose molecules (monosaccharides) that can be absorbed directly into the blood via transporters on the gut wall. Other pancreatic enzymes digest proteins into small fragments containing from one to three amino acids that can also be easily absorbed. This is important since any peptide length greater than three amino acids has the potential to induce an immunological response by the immune cells lined up behind the inner skin that lines your gut. This is why a healthy gut wall in addition to a functional mucus barrier is critical to prevent protein-based allergies. The likely candidates includes nut, dairy, egg, soy, wheat, and fish allergies. We can also add gluten to that collection of proteins. Finally, the pancreas also secretes still another group of enzymes into this section of the small intestine to break down complex fats into fragments and with the help of bile salts can also enter the body and then be reassembled by the liver into lipoproteins that then enter directly into the blood.

The actual absorption of much of your meal that has been broken down into simple sugars (glucose and fructose), small protein fragments, and the fatty acids takes place primarily in the jejunum, which is the mid-section of the small intestine.

The final absorption of the more difficult to digest nutrients such as those in harder to digest proteins (like casein found in milk) and non-starchy vegetables takes place in the ileum, which is the last section of the small intestine.

It's a pretty precise operation that must be completed in a relatively short period of time (3-5 hours) as powerful contraction waves powered by the release of serotonin from the gut wall are constantly pushing the digested food mass through the small intestine.

Surprisingly, the vast majority of serotonin in the body is not in your brain, but your gut. Not only are large amounts of serotonin required to maintain the contraction waves to move the chyme along the gut, but also if for some reason a truly toxic microbe or toxin gets into the gut, there will be a massive release of serotonin to either cause vomiting or severe diarrhea (or both) in an effort to get these microbes or toxins out of the body before they can potentially enter your blood.

To add even more complexity to this inner skin, the small intestine is constantly sending hormonal signals directly to the brain via the vagus nerve to provide information on the progress of the meal. Only about one percent of the cells (called L-cells) that line the gut will have the ability to secrete such hormones. Upon receiving these hormonal signals from the L-cells, the hypothalamus in the brain decides to either stop eating or continue to eat. Most of those hormone-secreting L-cells are located in the last leg of the journey in the ileum. The two primary "stop-eating" hormones are PYY and GLP-1. The levels of these secreted hormones respond to protein levels still remaining in the last segment of the gut. As long as these hormones are being secreted and reach the brain, they tell the brain that we are full because they signal satiety. This is why consuming adequate protein at each meal is key to avoiding over consuming calories. The secret of gastric bypass surgery is the increased production of satiety hormones because much of the limited amounts of food (including protein) that the patient can eat after their gastric bypass surgery is now dumped directly on those hormone-secreting L-cells located primarily in the ileum sending powerful satiety signals to the brain that tells you to stop eating.

COLON: FERMENTATION CENTRAL

So far, it's been a fairly fast ride from the mouth to the end of the small intestine. Now the journey slows down considerably, and finally fermentable fiber begins to play a dominant role in gut health. Up to this point, all the easy-to-digest nutrients have been extracted by the small intestine for use by our human cells. What is left is the indigestible part of our meal. Although leaving the small intestine might be the last call for nutrient extraction for human cells, it becomes the first call for the microbes in your gut to start getting fed. The vast majority of all gut bacteria are located in the large intestine, also known as the colon. This is because the massive and rapid contractions that had pushed the food rapidly through the small intestine slow down considerably, otherwise microbes in the colon couldn't undertake the slow process to break down fermentable fiber because it is their primary food source. The large intestine or colon is essentially a large fermentation tank that uses enzymes secreted from the bacteria to break down the carbohydrate polymers that comprise fermentable fiber into individual monosaccharides that the bacteria in the gut use as its energy source. Our human cells can't make those enzymes. That's why we can't digest fermentable fiber. Remember virtually all the easily absorbed nutrients that can be digested to smaller components have already been absorbed in the small intestine for our own body's needs, meaning the digestion of fermentable fiber becomes the primary source of nutrition for the bacteria in the gut. The more extensive genetic diversity of bacteria in the gut enables them to make the necessary enzymes needed for the job. This is why you must maintain a significant bacterial diversity in the colon to ensure they ultimately get fed. The absence of adequate fermentable fiber in the diet or not having a wide diversity of bacterial DNA to make the enzymes necessary to breakdown the fermentable fiber to monosaccharides that feed the bacteria in your colon will generate the same result, your gut health will be compromised.

Without fermentable fiber as a nutrition source, the bacteria in the gut will not be very happy because they are going to be constantly hungry. When your friendly gut bacteria (especially *Akkermansia muciniphila*) get hungry, they start digesting your mucus barrier, which itself can be used as a source of fermentable fiber. This is the first step toward the development of a leaky gut.

You need about five to six grams a day of fermentable fiber to supply adequate nutrition to your gut microbes (assuming you have a good bacterial diversity to ferment the fiber). Only about 10–15 percent of your total fiber intake is usually fermentable, this means you must eat a lot of total fiber (at least 30 grams) per day.

Currently, there is no good definition of fermentable fiber issued by the FDA. Therefore, you don't have any way of finding out the levels of fermentable fiber that are actually in a food product. The FDA has recently issued some strange new definitions relative to carbohydrates and fiber. To even begin understanding these definitions you need some background on the FDA terminology. According to the FDA if a food ingredient contains a single carbohydrate (like fructose) or two carbohydrates linked together (like table sugar which contains fructose and glucose), then it is called a sugar on the nutritional label. That's simple enough. Now here comes the hard part. If a food ingredient contains more than three or more carbohydrates, it is called "other carbohydrates." The new guidelines issued by the FDA now defines dietary fiber as:

> "non-digestible soluble and insoluble carbohydrates (with three or more monomeric units) and lignin that intrinsic and intact in plant; isolated or synthetic non-digestible carbohydrates (with three or more monomeric units) determined by the FDA to have physiological effects that have physiological effects that are beneficial to humans."

Kudos to the FDA for such a concise clarification of fermentable fiber. For example, are the complex carbohydrates of human breast milk considered a fiber or just "other carbohydrates"? It doesn't come from a plant, so it must be "other carbohydrates" even though it is critical for initially establishing the correct bacterial composition in the infant's gut. Likewise, dairy milk has very interesting complex carbohydrates more similar to those in human breast milk and are far more complex than those found in plant fibers, and yet they also fall under the listing of "other carbohydrates" because there is no listing for fiber on dairy milk. However, the FDA does include cellulose as a dietary fiber even though humans can't break it down to the monosaccharides that the microbes in our gut need to survive.

Nonetheless, we know that there are several food sources that seem to be rich in fermentable fiber. These would include non-starchy vegetables (broccoli, cauliflower, onions, asparagus, and artichoke hearts), selected fruits (like berries, apples, and pears), legumes (like beans and lentils), as well as mushrooms and garlic. This is important since it is the diversity and amount of fermentable fiber in the diet that determines the diversity of the bacterial composition in the colon and ultimately the health of your gut.

Regardless of the FDA definitions, the best source of fermentable fiber remains human breast milk. Unfortunately, it is hard to find human breast milk in your local supermarket. Even in plants that contain fermentable fiber, there are many differences. For example, fermentable fiber could be polymers of fructose (i.e., fructans), which are the best plant sources for nourishing the microbes in your colon. Non-starchy vegetables, selected fruits, and garlic fall into this class. Then there are polymers of galatose (i.e., galactans) which include legumes (beans and lentils). Finally, there are polymers of unique carbohydrates from marine sources (like sea weeds) and mushrooms. It is only from the polymers of glucose (i.e., grains and starches) that our human DNA can make the necessary enzymes for their rapid breakdown into glucose, but this glucose gets rapidly absorbed in the small intestine before they ever reach the colon thus providing virtually no nutrition to the bacteria in the colon.

The best sources of fermentable fiber for the Zone Pro-Resolution Nutrition system will be non-starchy vegetables since they contain the least amount of carbohydrates with the maximum amount of fermentable fiber, thereby allowing you to better control blood insulin levels. Equally important they provide the best source of nutrients to enable the bacteria in your colon to produce short-chain fatty acids (SCFA) as metabolites of the fermentation process that are the keys to true gut health.

The rest of the fiber you eat is essentially useless for the bacteria in your colon, however it does have some benefit as a bulking agent for your stool to make its eventual exit easier from the colon. Since there is essentially no oxygen in the colon, some of the other fermentation metabolites of monosaccharides from fermentable fiber are gases like methane, hydrogen, and trace amounts of others such as hydrogen sulfide (methane and hydrogen are odorless, but hydrogen sulfide is not). These gases are the source of flatulence. Not surprisingly, good sources of fermentable fiber are also good sources of flatulence. This is why there is virtually no flatulence when you eat large amounts of refined carbohydrates because they have no fermentable fibers.

Since there is no test for the levels and types of fermentable fiber in carbohydrates, it really becomes a guessing game as to the amounts you are consuming other than levels of flatulence and quality of your stool. However, as I said above, the key products of bacterial fermentation are short-chain fatty acids (SCFA) that keep you alive by not only maintaining the integrity of the gut lining in the colon, but also by supplying the energy for the immune cells that line the gut wall to maintain a constant alert for microbial invasions. These SCFA have specific receptors in the target immunological cells. These SCFA have a wide range of actions from its effect on the central nervous system including anti-depressant action as well as enhancing the satiety effects of PYY and GLP-1 coming from the L-cells in the gut.

If these SCFA were so important, why not give them as a supplement and forget about fermentable fiber and flatulence? First, they wouldn't work very well because the SCFA would be rapidly absorbed in the small intestine and never reach the colon where they are needed by the bacteria. Second, the most important of these SCFA produced from the fermentation of fermentable fiber is butyric acid, which is the primary component of vomit, which makes dietary supplementation less likely.

THE END OF THE JOURNEY

At the end of your meal's 30-hour journey (most of that time spent in the colon), the residue of that meal has been extracted of virtually all of its potential nutrition for both you and the bacteria in the colon and is now ready for exit. This is the stool. More than half the weight of the stool is live bacteria (this is why you can analyze it for bacterial DNA to determine the microbial diversity in your gut). This is also why it smells. Along with those bacteria the stool also includes non-fermentable fiber (like cellulose), and possibly some undigested food, and trapped gases from fermentation (this is why your stool sometime floats).

In fact, in the earliest days of medicine, analyzing the stool was an indication of a patient's health. Stool inspection can still be used to indicate if your colon is working well. In fact, there is even a visual standard (the Bristol Stool Chart) that is used to identify seven different classes of stool shape and density. The more your stool is like a snake easily exiting your body, the healthier your gut is. The healthier your gut is, the healthier you will be.

References

PROLOGUE

Oates JA. "The 1982 Nobel Prize in Physiology or Medicine." Science 218: 765–766 (1982)

Sears B. *The Zone*. Regan Books. New York, NY (1995)

Sears B. *The OmegaRx Zone*. Regan Books. New York, NY (2001)

Sears B. *The Mediterranean Zone*. Ballantine Books. New York, NY (2014)

Serhan CN. "Pro-resolving lipid mediators are leads for resolution physiology." Nature 510: 92–101 (2014)

CHAPTER 1: WHAT IS THE ZONE?

Sears B. *The Zone*. Regan Books. New York, NY (1995)

CHAPTER 4: OVERVIEW OF THE ZONE PRO-RESOLUTION NUTRITION SYSTEM: A DEFINED DIETARY PATHWAY TO THE ZONE

Arai Y, Martin-Ruiz CM, Takayama M, Abe Y, Takebayashi T, Koyasu S, Suematsu M, Hirose N, and von Zglinicki T. "Inflammation, but not telomere length, predicts successful ageing at extreme old age." EBioMedicine 2:1549–1558 (2015)

Brickman AM, Khan UA, Provenzano FA, Yeung LK, Suzuki W, Schroeter H, Wall M, Sloan RP, and Small SA. "Enhancing dentate gyrus function with dietary flavanols improves cognition in older adults." Nat Neurosci 17:11798–1803 (2014)

Das SK, Gilhooly CH, Golden JK, Pittas AG, Fuss PJ, Cheatham RA, Tyler S, Tsay M, McCrory MA, Lichtenstein AH, Dallal GE, Dutta C, Bhapkar MV, Delany

JP, Saltzman E, and Roberts SB. "Long-term effects of 2 energy-restricted diets differing in glycemic load on dietary adherence, body composition, and metabolism in CALERIE: A 1-y randomized controlled trial." Am J Clin Nutr 85:1023–1030 (2007)

Davinelli S, Bertoglio JC, Zarrelli A, Pina R, and Scapagnini G. "A randomized clinical trial evaluating the efficacy of an anthocyanin-maqui berry extract on oxidative stress biomarkers." J Am Coll Nutr 34: Suppl 1:28–33 (2015)

Endres S, Ghorbani R, Kelley VE, Georgilis K, Lonnemann G, van der Meer JW, Cannon JG, Rogers TS, Klempner MS, and Weber PC, Schaeffer EJ, Wolff SM, and Dinarello CA. "The effect of dietary supplementation with n-3 polyunsaturated fatty acids on the synthesis of interleukin-1 and tumor necrosis factor by mononuclear cells." N Engl J Med 320:265–271 (1989)

Fontana L, Villareal DT, Das SK, Smith SR, Meydani SN, Pittas AG, Klein S, Bhapkar M, Rochon J, Ravussin E, and Holloszy JO. "Effects of 2-year calorie restriction on circulating levels of IGF-1, IGF-binding proteins and cortisol in nonobese men and women: A randomized clinical trial." Aging Cell 15: 22–27 (2016)

Georgiou T, Neokleous A, Nikolaou D, and Sears B. "Pilot study for treating dry age-related macular degeneration (AMD) with high-dose omega-3 fatty acids." PharmaNutrition 2:8–11 (2014)

Martin CK, Bhapkar M, Pittas AG, Pieper CF, Das SK, Williamson DA, Scott T, Redman LM, Stein R, Gilhooly CH, Stewart T, Robinson L, and Roberts SB. "Effect of calorie restriction on mood, quality of life, sleep, and sexual function in healthy nonobese adults: The CALERIE 2 randomized clinical trial." JAMA Intern Med 176: 743–752 (2016)

McNamara RK, Perry M, and Sears, B. "Dissociation of C-reactive protein levels from long-chain omega-3 fatty acid status and anti-depressant response in adolescents with major depressive disorder: An open-label dose-ranging trial." J Nutr Therapeutics 2:235–243 (2013)

Meydani M, Das S, Band M, Epstein S, and Roberts S. "The effect of caloric restriction and glycemic load on measures of oxidative stress and antioxidants in humans: Results from the CALERIE trial of human caloric restriction." J Nutr Health Aging 15:456–60 (2011)

Pittas AG, Das SK, Hajduk CL, Golden J, Saltzman E, Stark PC, Greenberg AS, and Roberts SB. "A low-glycemic load diet facilitates greater weight loss in overweight adults with high insulin secretion but not in overweight adults with low insulin secretion in the CALERIE trial." Diabetes Care 28:2939–41 (2005)

Rabassa M, Cherubini A, Zamora-Ros R, Urpi-Sarda M, Bandinelli S, Ferrucci L, and Andres-Lacueva C. "Low levels of a urinary biomarker of dietary polyphenol are associated with substantial cognitive decline over a 3-year period in older adults: The Invecchiare in Chianti study." J Am Geriatr Soc 63:938–946 (2015)

Rabassa M, Zamora-Ros R, Andres-Lacueva C, Urpi-Sarda M, Bandinelli S, Ferrucci L, and Cherubini A. "Association between both total baseline urinary and dietary polyphenols and substantial physical performance decline risk in older adults: A 9-year follow-up of the InCHIANTI study." J Nutr Health Aging 20:478–485 (2016)

Ravussin E, Redman LM, Rochon J, Das SK, Fontana L, Kraus WE, Romashkan S, Williamson DA, Meydani SN, Villareal DT, Smith SR, Stein RI, Scott TM, Stewart TM, Saltzman E, Klein S, Bhapkar M, Martin CK, Gilhooly CH, Holloszy JO, Hadley EC, and Roberts SB. "A 2-year randomized controlled trial of human caloric restriction: Feasibility and effects on predictors of healthspan and longevity." J Gerontol A Biol Sci Med Sci. 70:1097–104 (2015)

Romashkan SV, Das SK, Villareal DT, Ravussin E, Redman LM, Rochon J, Bhapkar M, and Kraus WE. "Safety of two-year caloric restriction in non-obese healthy individuals." Oncotarget 7: 19124–19133 (2016)

Sears, B. *The Zone*. Regan Books. New York, NY (1995)

Sears B, Bailes J, and Asselin B. "Therapeutic uses of high-dose omega-3 fatty acids to treat comatose patients with severe brain injury." PharmaNutrition 1: 86–89 (2013)

Sorgi PJ, Hallowell EM, Hutchins HL, and Sears B. "Effects of an open-label pilot study with high-dose EPA/DHA concentrates on plasma phospholipids and behavior in children with attention deficit hyperactivity disorder Nutr J 13: 16 (2007)

Urpi-Sarda M, Andres-Lacueva C, Rabassa M, Ruggiero C, Zamora-Ros R, Bandinelli S, Ferrucci L, and Cherubini A. "The relationship between urinary total polyphenols and the frailty phenotype in a community-dwelling older population: The InCHIANTI study." J Gerontol A Biol Sci Med Sci 70: 1141–1147 (2015)

Willcox BJ, Willcox DC, Todoriki H, Fujiyoshi A, Yano K, He Q, Curb JD, and Suzuki M. "Caloric restriction, the traditional Okinawan diet, and healthy aging: The diet of the world's longest-lived people and its potential impact on morbidity and life span." Ann N Y Acad Sci 1114:434–455 (2007

Willcox DC, Willcox BJ, Todoriki H, Curb JD, and Suzuki M. "Caloric restriction and human longevity: What can we learn from the Okinawans?" Biogerontology 7:173–177 (2006)

Zamora-Ros R, Rabassa M, Cherubini A, Urpí-Sardà M, Bandinelli S, Ferrucci L, and Andres-Lacueva C. "High concentrations of a urinary biomarker of polyphenol intake are associated with decreased mortality in older adults." J Nutr 143:1445–1450 (2013)

CHAPTER 5: HOW INFLAMMATION KEEPS YOU ALIVE AND THE RESOLUTION RESPONSE KEEPS YOU WELL

Afonso PV, Janka-Junttila M, Lee YJ, McCann CP, Oliver CM, Aamer KA, Losert W, Cicerone MT, and Parent CA. "LTB4 is a signal-relay molecule during neutrophil chemotaxis." Dev Cell 22: 1079–1091 (2012)

Baker RG, Hayden MS, and Ghosh S. "NF-κB, inflammation, and metabolic disease." Cell Metab 13: 11–22 (2011)

Bierhaus A, Stern DM, and Nawroth PP. "RAGE in inflammation: A new therapeutic target?" Curr Opin Investig Drugs 7: 985–991 (2006)

Cai D. "Neuroinflammation and neurodegeneration in overnutrition-induced diseases." Trends Endocrinol Metab 24: 40–47 (2013)

Camandola S, Leonarduzzi G, Musso T, Varesio L, Carini R, Scavazza A, Chiarpotto E, Baeuerle PA, and Poli G. "Nuclear factor-κB is activated by arachidonic acid but not by eicosapentaenoic acid." Biochem Biophys Res Commun 229: 643–647 (1996)

Canetti C, Silva JS, Ferreira SH, and Cunha FQ. "Tumour necrosis factor-alpha and leukotriene B(4) mediate the neutrophil migration in immune inflammation." Br J Pharmacol 134:1619–28 (2001)

Crofts CAP, Zinn C, Wheldon MC, and Schofield GM. "Hyperinsulinemia: A unifying theory of chronic disease?" Diabesity 1: 34–43 (2015)

Fielding CA, Jones GW, McLoughlin RM, McLeod L, Hammond VJ, Uceda J, Williams AS, Lambie M, Foster TL, Liao CT, Rice CM, Greenhill CJ, Colmont CS, Hams E, Coles B, Kift-Morgan A, Newton Z, Craig KJ, Williams JD, Williams GT, Davies SJ, Humphreys IR, O'Donnell VB, Taylor PR, Jenkins BJ, Topley N, and Jones SA. "Interleukin-6 signaling drives fibrosis in unresolved inflammation." Immunity 40: 40–50 (2014)

Gloire G, Legrand-Poels S, and Piette J. "NF-κB activation by reactive oxygen species: Fifteen years later." Biochem Pharmacol 72: 1493–1505 (2006)

Guo H, Callaway JB, and Ting J. "Inflammasomes: Mechanism of action, role in disease and therapeutics." Nat Med 21: 677–687 (2015)

Hardie DG. "Keeping the home fires burning: AMP-activated protein kinase." J Royal Society Interface 15:20170774 (2018)

Hardie DG, Ross FA, and Hawley SA. "AMP-activated protein kinase: A target for drugs both ancient and modern." Chem Bio 19: 1222–1236 (2012)

Huang S, Rutkowsky JM, Snodgrass RG, Ono-Moore KD, Schneider DA, Newman JW, Adams SH, and Hwang DH. "Saturated fatty acids activate TLR-mediated proinflammatory signaling pathways." J Lipid Res 53: 2002–2013 (2012)

Iwasaki A and Medzhitov R. "Control of adaptive immunity by the innate immune system." Nat Immunol 16: 343–353 (2015)

Kawai T and Akira S. "The role of pattern-recognition receptors in innate immunity: Update on Toll-like receptors." Nat Immunol 11: 373–384 (2010)

Sanchez-Galan E, Gomez-Hernandez A, Vidal C, Martin-Ventura JL, Blanco-Colio LM, Munoz-Garcia B, Ortega L, Egido J, and Tunón J. "Leukotriene B4 enhances the activity of nuclear factor-kappaB pathway through BLT1 and BLT2 receptors in atherosclerosis." Cardiovasc Res 81: 216–225 (2009)

Sen R and Baltimore D. "Multiple nuclear factors interact with the immunoglobulin enhancer sequences." Cell 46: 705–716 (1986)

Serhan CN, Ward PA, and Gilroy DW, and Samir S. *Fundamentals of Inflammation.* Cambridge University Press. Cambridge, UK (2010)

Serhan CN. "Pro-resolving lipid mediators are leads for resolution physiology." Nature 510: 92–101 (2014)

Tobon-Velasco JC, Cuevas E, and Torres-Ramos MA. "Receptor for AGEs (RAGE) as mediator of NF-κB pathway activation in neuroinflammation and oxidative stress." CNS Neurol Disord Drug Targets 13: 1615–1626 (2014)

Trowbridge HO and Emling RC. *Inflammation: A Review of the Process*. Quintessence Publising. Chicago, IL (1997)

Volchenkov R, Sprater F, Vogelsang P, and Appel S. "The 2011 Nobel Prize in physiology or medicine." Scand J Immunol 75: 1–4 (2012)

Weisberg SP, McCann D, Desai M, Rosenbaum M, Leibel RL, and Ferrante AW. "Obesity is associated with macrophage accumulation in adipose tissue." J Clin Invest 112: 1796–1808 (2003)

Wick G, Grundtman C, Mayerl C, Wimpissinger TF, Feichtinger J, Zelger B, Sgonc R, and Wolfram D. "The immunology of fibrosis." Annu Rev Immunol 31: 107–135 (2013)

Yan SF, Ramasamy R, and Schmidt AM. "Mechanisms of disease: Advanced glycation end-products and their receptor in inflammation and diabetes complications." Nat Clin Pract Endocrinol Metab 4: 285–293 (2008)

Zang M, Xu S, Maitland-Toolan KA, Zuccollo A, Hou X, Jiang B, Wierzbicki M, Verbeuren TJ, and Cohen RA. "Polyphenols stimulate AMP-activated protein kinase, lower lipids, and inhibit accelerated atherosclerosis in diabetic LDL-receptor-deficient mice." Diabetes 55: 2180–2191 (2006)

Zhang Q, Lenardo MJ, and Baltimore D. "30 years of NF-κB: A blossoming of relevance to human pathobiology." Cell 168: 37–57 (2017)

Zhang X, Zhang G, Zhang H, Karin M, Bai H, and Cai D. "Hypothalamic IKKbeta/NF-κB and ER stress link overnutrition to energy imbalance and obesity." Cell 135: 61–73 (2008)

CHAPTER 6: DIET-INDUCED INFLAMMATION

Brenner RR. "Nutritional and hormonal factors influencing desaturation of essential fatty acids." Prog Lipid Res 20: 41–47 (1981)

De Fina LF. Vega GL. Leonard D. and Grundy SM. "Fasting glucose, obesity, and metabolic syndrome as predictors of type 2 diabetes: The Cooper Center longitudinal study." J Investig Med 60: 1164–1168 (2012)

Ebbeling CB, Swain JF, Feldman HA, Wong WW, Hachey DL, Garcia-Lago E, and Ludwig DS. "Effects of dietary composition on energy expenditure during weight-loss maintenance." JAMA 307: 2627–2634 (2012)

Endres S, Ghorbani R, Kelley VE, Georgilis K, Lonnemann G, van der Meer JW, Cannon JG, Rogers TS, Klempner MS, Weber PC, Schaeffer EJ, Wolff SM, and Dinarello CA. The effect of dietary supplementation with n-3 polyunsaturated fatty acids on the synthesis of interleukin-1 and tumor necrosis factor by mononuclear cells." N Engl J Med 320: 265–271 (1989)

Foster-Powell K, Holt SH, and Brand-Miller JC. "International table of glycemic index and glycemic load values: 2002." Am J Clin Nutr 76: 5–56 (2002)

Harris WS, Pottala JV, Varvel SA, Borowski JJ, Ward JN, and McConnell JP. "Erythrocyte omega-3 fatty acids increase and linoleic acid decreases with age: Observations from 160,000 patients." Prostaglandins Leukot Essent Fatty Acids 88:257–263 (2013)

Levitan EB, Liu S, Stampfer MJ, Cook NR, Rexrode KM, Ridker PM, Buring JE, and Manson JE. "HbA$_{1c}$ measured in stored erythrocytes and mortality rate among middle-aged and older women." Diabetologia 51: 267–275 (2008)

Ludwig DS, Majzoub JA, Al-Zahrani A, Dallal GE, Blanco I, and Roberts SB. "High glycemic index foods, overeating, and obesity." Pediatrics 103: E26 (1999)

McLaughlin T, Reaven G, Abbasi F, Lamendola C, Saad M, Waters D, Simon J, and Krauss RM. "Is there a simple way to identify insulin-resistant individuals at increased risk of cardiovascular disease?" Am J Cardiol 96: 399–404 (2005)

Moss M. *Salt Sugar Fat: How the Food Giants Hooked Us*. Random House. New York (2014)

Ohnishi H and Saito Y. "Eicosapentaenoic acid (EPA) reduces cardiovascular events: Relationship with the EPA/arachidonic acid ratio." J Atheroscler Thromb 20: 861–877 (2013)

Rahman I, Biswas SK, and Kirkham PA. "Regulation of inflammation and redox signaling by dietary polyphenols." Biochem Pharmacol 72: 1439–52 (2006)

Salazar MR, Carbajal HA, Espeche WG, Leiva Sisnieguez CE, March CE, Balbin E, Dulbecco CA, Aizpurúa M, Marillet AG, and Reaven GM. "Comparison of the abilities of the plasma triglyceride/high-density lipoprotein cholesterol ratio and the metabolic syndrome to identify insulin resistance." Diab Vasc Dis Res 10: 346–52 (2013)

Sánchez-Galán E, Gómez-Hernández A, Vidal C, Martín-Ventura JL, Blanco-Colio LM, Muñoz-García B, Ortega L, Egido J, and Tuñón J. "Leukotriene B4 enhances the activity of nuclear factor-kappaB pathway through BLT1 and BLT2 receptors in atherosclerosis." Cardiovasc Res 81: 216–225 (2009)

Sears B. *The Zone*. Regan Books. New York, NY (1995)

Sears B. *OmegaRx Zone*. Regan Books. New York, NY (2001)

Sears B. *The Anti-Inflammation Zone*. Regan Books. New York, NY (2005)

Sears, B. *Toxic Fat*. Thomas Nelson. Knoxville, TN (2008)

Sears B. *The Mediterranean Zone*. Ballantine Books. New York, NY (2014)

Silver MJ, Hoch W, Kocsis JJ, Ingerman CM, and Smith JB. "Arachidonic acid causes sudden death in rabbits." Science 183: 1085–1087 (1974)

Spite M, Claria J, and Serhan CN. "Resolvins, specialized proresolving lipid mediators, and their potential roles in metabolic diseases." Cell Metab 19: 21–36 (2014)

Wei D, Li J, Shen M, Jia W, Chen N, Chen T, Su D, Tian H, Zheng S, Dai Y, and Zhao A. "Cellular production of n-3 PUFAs and reduction of n-6-to-n-3 ratios

274 ∎ **APPENDIX H**

in the pancreatic beta-cells and islets enhance insulin secretion and confer protection against cytokine-induced cell death." Diabetes 59:471–478 (2010)

Yee LD, Lester JL, Cole RM, Richardson JR, Hsu JC, Li Y, Lehman A, Belury MA, and Clinton SK. "Omega-3 fatty acid supplements in women at high risk of breast cancer have dose-dependent effects on breast adipose tissue fatty acid composition." Am J Clin Nutr 91: 1185–1194 (2010)

Yokoyama M, Origasa H, Matsuzaki M, Matsuzawa Y, Saito Y, Ishikawa Y, Oikawa S, Sasaki J, Hishida H, Itakura H, Kita T, Kitabatake A, Nakaya N, Sakata T, Shimada K, and Shirato K. "Effects of eicosapentaenoic acid on major coronary events in hypercholesterolaemic patients (JELIS): A randomised open-label, blinded endpoint analysis." Lancet 369: 1090–1098 (2007)

Zhang X, Zhang G, Zhang H, Karin M, Bai H, and Cai D. "Hypothalamic IKKbeta/ NF-κB and ER stress link overnutrition to energy imbalance and obesity." Cell 135:61–73 (2008)

CHAPTER 7: MARKERS OF THE ZONE

Adams PB, Lawson S, Sanigorski A, and Sinclair AJ. "Arachidonic acid to eicosapentaenoic acid ratio in blood correlates positively with clinical symptoms of depression." Lipids 31 (Suppl): S157–161 (1996)

Aggarwal V, Schneider AL, and Selvin E. "Low hemoglobin A(1c) in nondiabetic adults: An elevated risk state?" Diabetes Care 35: 2055–2060 (2012)

Carson AP, Fox CS, McGuire DK, Levitan EB, Laclaustra M, Mann DM, and Muntner P. "Low hemoglobin A1c and risk of all-cause mortality among US adults without diabetes." Circ Cardiovasc Qual Outcomes. 3: 661–667 (2010)

Chilton FH, Patel M, Fonteh AN, Hubbard WC, and Triggiani M. "Dietary n-3 fatty acid effects on neutrophil lipid composition and mediator production. Influence of duration and dosage." J Clin Invest. 91: 115–22 (1993)

Endres S, Ghorbani R, Kelley VE, Georgilis K, Lonnemann G, van der Meer JW, Cannon JG, Rogers TS, Klempner MS, Weber PC, Schaeffer EJ, Wolff SM, and Dinarello CA. "The effect of dietary supplementation with n-3 polyunsaturated fatty acids on the synthesis of interleukin-1 and tumor necrosis factor by mononuclear cells." N Engl J Med 320: 265–271 (1989)

Fontani G, Corradeschi F, Felici A, Alfatti F, Bugarini R, Fiaschi AI, Cerretani D, Montorfano G, Rizzo AM, and Berra B. "Blood profiles, body fat and mood state in healthy subjects on different diets supplemented with omega-3 polyunsaturated fatty acids." Eur J Clin Invest 35: 499–507 (2005)

Fontani G, Corradeschi F, Felici A, Alfatti F, Migliorini S, and Lodi L. "Cognitive and physiological effects of omega-3 polyunsaturated fatty acid supplementation in healthy subjects." Eur J Clin Invest 35: 691–699 (2005)

Fukuda Y, Hashimoto Y, Hamaguchi M, Fukuda T, Nakamura N, Ohbora A, Kato T, Kojima T, and Fukui M. "Triglycerides to high-density lipoprotein cholesterol ratio is an independent predictor of incident fatty liver; a population-based cohort study." Liver Int 36: 713–720 (2016)

Georgiou T and Prokopiou E. "The new era of omega-3 fatty acids supplementation: Therapeutic effects on dry age-related macular degeneration." J Stem Cells 10: 205–215 (2015)

Harris WS. "The omega-3 index: Clinical utility for therapeutic intervention." Curr Cardiol Rep 12: 503–508 (2010)

Harris WS, Luo J, Pottala JV, Espeland MA, Margolis KL, Manson JE, Wang L, Brasky TM, and Robinson JG. "Red blood cell polyunsaturated fatty acids and mortality in the Women's Health Initiative Memory Study." J Clin Lipidol 11: 250–259 (2017)

Hasegawa T, Otsuka K, Iguchi T, Matsumoto K, Ehara S, Nakata S, Nishimura S, Kataoka T, Shimada K, and Yoshiyama M. "Serum n-3 to n-6 polyunsaturated fatty acids ratio correlates with coronary plaque vulnerability: An optical coherence tomography study." Heart Vessels 29: 596–602 (2014)

Holvoet P, Mertens A, Verhamme P, Bogaerts K, Beyens G, Verhaeghe R, Collen D, Muls E, and Van de Werf F. "Circulating oxidized LDL is a useful marker for identifying patients with coronary artery disease." Arterioscler Thromb Vasc Biol 21: 844–848 (2001)

Holvoet P. "Oxidized LDL and coronary heart disease." Acta Cardiol 59: 479–484 (2004)

Inoue K, Kishida K, Hirata A, Funahashi T, and Shimomura I. "Low serum eicosapentaenoic acid / arachidonic acid ratio in male subjects with visceral obesity." Nutr Metab 10: 25 (2013)

Iwani NA, Jalaludin MY, Zin RM, Fuziah MZ, Hong JY, Abqariyah Y, Mokhtar AH, and Nazaimoon WM. "Triglyceride to HDL-C ratio is associated with insulin resistance in overweight and obese children." Sci Rep 7: 40055 (2017)

Jiang Y, Djuric Z, Sen A, Ren J, Kuklev D, Waters I, Zhao L, Uhlson CL, Hong YH, Murphy RC, Normolle DP, Smith WL, and Brenner DE. "Biomarkers for personalizing omega-3 fatty acid dosing." Cancer Prev Res 7: 1011–22 (2014)

Kawabata T, Hirota S, Hirayama T, Adachi N, Hagiwara C, Iwama N, Kamachi K, Araki E, Kawashima H, and Kiso Y. "Age-related changes of dietary intake and blood eicosapentaenoic acid, docosahexaenoic acid, and arachidonic acid levels in Japanese men and women." Prostaglandins Leukot Essent Fatty Acids 84: 131–137 (2001)

Kitagawa M, Haji S, and Amagai T. "Elevated serum AA/EPA Ratio as a predictor of skeletal muscle depletion in cachexic patients with advanced gastro-intestinal cancers." In Vivo 31: 1003–1009 (2017)

Kondo T, Ogawa K, Satake T, Kitazawa M, Taki K, Sugiyama S, and Ozawa T. "Plasma-free eicosapentaenoic acid/arachidonic acid ratio: A possible new coronary risk factor." Clin Cardiol 9: 413–416 (1986)

McLaughlin T, Allison G, Abbasi F, Lamendola C, and Reaven G. "Prevalence of insulin resistance and associated cardiovascular disease risk factors among normal weight, overweight, and obese individuals." Metabolism 53: 495–499 (2004)

Nagai K, Koshiba H, Shibata S, Matsui T, and Kozaki K. "Correlation between the serum eicosapentaenoic acid-to-arachidonic acid ratio and the severity of cerebral white matter hyperintensities in older adults with memory disorder." Geriatr Gerontol Int 15 (Suppl 1): 48–52 (2015)

Nagata M, Hata J, Hirakawa Y, Mukai N, Yoshida D, Ohara T, Kishimoto H, Kawano H, Kitazono T, Kiyohara Y, and Ninomiya T. "The ratio of serum eicosapentaenoic acid to arachidonic acid and risk of cancer death in a Japanese community: The Hisayama Study." J Epidemiol 27: 578–583 (2017)

Ninomiya T, Nagata M, Hata J, Hirakawa Y, Ozawa M, Yoshida D, Ohara T, Kishimoto H, Mukai N, Fukuhara M, Kitazono T, and Kiyohara Y. "Association between ratio of serum eicosapentaenoic acid to arachidonic acid and risk of cardiovascular disease: The Hisayama Study." Atherosclerosis 231: 261–267 (2013)

Nishihira J, Tokashiki T, Higashiuesato Y, Willcox DC, Mattek N, Shinto L, Ohya Y, and Dodge HH. "Associations between serum omega-3 fatty acid levels and cognitive functions among community-dwelling octogenarians in Okinawa, Japan: The KOCOA study." J Alzheimers Dis 51: 857–866 (2016)

Ohnishi H and Saito Y. "Eicosapentaenoic acid (EPA) reduces cardiovascular events: Relationship with the EPA/arachidonic acid ratio." J Atheroscler Thromb 20: 861–877 (2013)

Rizzo AM, Montorfano G, Negroni M, Adorni L, Berselli P, Corsetto P, Wahle K, and Berra B. "A rapid method for determining arachidonic/eicosapentaenoic acid ratios in whole blood lipids: Correlation with erythrocyte membrane ratios and validation in a large Italian population of various ages and pathologies." Lipids Health Dis 9: 7 (2010)

Rizzo AM, Corsetto PA, Montorfano G, Opizzi A, Faliva M, Giacosa A, Ricevuti G, Pelucchi C, Berra B, and Rondanelli M. "Comparison between the AA/EPA ratio in depressed and non-depressed elderly females: Omega-3 fatty acid supplementation correlates with improved symptoms but does not change immunological parameters." Nutr J 11: 82 (2012)

Salazar MR, Carbajal HA, Espeche WG, Leiva Sisnieguez CE, Balbín E, Dulbecco CA, Aizpurúa M, Marillet AG, and Reaven GM. "Relation among the plasma triglyceride/high-density lipoprotein cholesterol concentration ratio, insulin resistance, and associated cardio-metabolic risk factors in men and women." Am J Cardiol 109: 1749–1753 (2012)

Salazar MR, Carbajal HA, Espeche WG, Aizpurúa M, Dulbecco CA, and Reaven GM. "Comparison of two surrogate estimates of insulin resistance to predict cardiovascular disease in apparently healthy individuals." Nutr Metab Cardiovasc Dis 27: 366–373 (2017)

Sears B. The OmegaRx Zone. Regan Books. New York, NY (2002)

Sears B. "Anti-inflammatory diets." J Am Coll Nutr 34 (Suppl 1): 14–21 (2015)

Shibata M, Ohara T, Yoshida D, Hata J, Mukai N, Kawano H, Kanba S, Kitazono T, and Ninomiya T. "Association between the ratio of serum arachidonic acid to eicosapentaenoic acid and the presence of depressive symptoms in a general Japanese population: The Hisayama Study." J Affect Disord 237: 73–79 (2018)

Sorgi PJ, Hallowell EM, Hutchins HL, and Sears B. "Effects of an open-label pilot study with high-dose EPA/DHA concentrates on plasma phospholipids and behavior in children with attention deficit hyperactivity disorder." Nutr J 6: 16 (2007)

Suwa M, Yamaguchi S, Komori T, Kajimoto S, and Kino M. "The association between cerebral white matter lesions and plasma omega-3 to omega-6 polyunsaturated fatty acids ratio to cognitive impairment development." Biomed Res Int 2015: 153437 (2015)

von Schacky C. "Omega-3 index and cardiovascular health." Nutrients 6: 799–814 (2014)

Wakabayashi Y, Funayama H, Ugata Y, Taniguchi Y, Hoshino H, Ako J, and Momomura S. "Low eicosapentaenoic acid to arachidonic acid ratio is associated with thin-cap fibroatheroma determined by optical coherence tomography." J Cardiol 66: 482–488 (2015)

Yokoyama M, Origasa H, Matsuzaki M, Matsuzawa Y, Saito Y, Ishikawa Y, Oikawa S, Sasaki J, Hishida H, Itakura H, Kita T, Kitabatake A, Nakaya N, Sakata T, Shimada K, and Shirato K. "Effects of eicosapentaenoic acid on major coronary events in hypercholesterolaemic patients (JELIS): A randomised open-label, blinded endpoint analysis." Lancet 369: 1090–1098 (2007)

CHAPTER 8: ZONE DIET: REDUCING DIET-INDUCED INFLAMMATION

Agus MS, Swain JF, Larson CL, Eckert EA, and Ludwig DS. "Dietary composition and physiologic adaptations to energy restriction." Am J Clin Nutr 71: 901–907 (2000)

Barlovic DP, Thomas MC, and Jandeleit-Dahm K. "Cardiovascular disease: What's all the AGE/RAGE about?" Cardiovasc Hematol Disord Drug Targets. 10: 7–15 (2010)

Bierhaus A, Stern DM, and Nawroth PP. "RAGE in inflammation: A new therapeutic target?" Curr Opin Investig Drugs 7: 985–991 (2006)

Brattbakk HR, Arbo I, Aagaard S, Lindseth I, de Soysa AK, Langaas M, Kulseng B, Lindberg F, and Johansen B. "Balanced caloric macronutrient composition downregulates immunological gene expression in human blood cells-adipose tissue diverges." OMICS 17: 41–52 (2013)

Brennan IM, Luscombe-Marsh ND, Seimon RV, Otto B, Horowitz M, Wishart JM, and Feinle-Bisset C. "Effects of fat, protein, and carbohydrate and protein load on appetite, plasma cholecystokinin, peptide YY, and ghrelin, and energy intake in lean and obese men." Am J Physiol Gastrointest Liver Physiol 303: G129–140 (2012)

Brenner RR. "Hormonal modulation of delta-6 and delta-5 desaturases: Case of diabetes." Prostaglandins Leukot Essent Fatty Acids 68: 151–162 (2003)

Bujak AL, Crane JD, Lally JS, Ford RJ, Kang SJ, Rebalka IA, Green AE, Kemp BE, Hawke TJ, Schertzer JD, and Steinberg GR. "AMPK activation of muscle autophagy prevents fasting-induced hypoglycemia and myopathy during aging." Cell Metab 21: 883–890 (2015)

Choquet H and Meyre D. "Genetics of obesity: What have we learned?" Curr Genomics 12: 169–179 (2011)

Civitarese AE, Carling S, Heilbronn LK, Hulver MH, Ukropcova B, Deutsch WA, Smith SR, and Ravussin E. "Calorie restriction increases muscle mitochondrial biogenesis in healthy humans." PLoS Med 4: e76 (2007)

Das SK, Roberts SB, Bhapkar MV, Villareal DT, Fontana L, Martin CK, Racette SB, Fuss PJ, Kraus WE, Wong WW, Saltzman E, Pieper CF, Fielding RA, Schwartz AV, Ravussin E, and Redman LM. "Body-composition changes in the comprehensive assessment of long-term effects of reducing intake of energy (CALERIE)-2 study: A 2-y randomized controlled trial of calorie restriction in nonobese humans." Am J Clin Nutr 105: 913–927 (2017)

Donaldson IJ and Göttgens B. "Evolution of candidate transcriptional regulatory motifs since the human-chimpanzee divergence." Genome Biol 7: R52 (2006)

Dumesnil JG, Turgeon J, Tremblay A, Poirier P, Gilbert M, Gagnon L, St-Pierre S, Garneau C, Lemieux I, Pascot A, Bergeron J, and Despres JP. "Effect of a low-glycaemic index-low-fat-high protein diet on the atherogenic metabolic risk profile of abdominally obese men." Br J Nutr 86: 557–568 (2001)

Eaton SB and Konner M. "Paleolithic nutrition. A consideration of its nature and current implications." N Engl J Med 312: 283–289 (1985)

Ebbeling CB, Leidig MM, Feldman HA, Lovesky MM, and Ludwig DS. "Effects of a low-glycemic load vs. low-fat diet in obese young adults: A randomized trial." JAMA 297: 2092–2102 (2007)

Evangelista LS, Heber D, Li Z, Bowerman S, Hamilton MA, and Fonarow GC. "Reduced body weight and adiposity with a high-protein diet improves functional status, lipid profiles, glycemic control, and quality of life in patients with heart failure: A feasibility study." J Cardiovasc Nurs 24: 207–215 (2009)

Fontana L, Villareal DT, Das SK, Smith SR, Meydani SN, Pittas AG, Klein S, Bhapkar M, Rochon J, Ravussin E, and Holloszy JO. "Effects of 2-year calorie restriction on circulating levels of IGF-1, IGF-binding proteins and cortisol in nonobese men and women: A randomized clinical trial." Aging Cell 15: 22–27 (2016)

Fontani G, Corradeschi F, Felici A, Alfatti F, Bugarini R, Fiaschi AI, Cerretani D, Montorfano G, Rizzo AM, and Berra B. "Blood profiles, body fat and mood state in healthy subjects on different diets supplemented with omega-3 polyunsaturated fatty acids." Eur J Clin Invest 35: 499–507 (2005)

Foster-Powell K, Holt SH, and Brand-Miller JC. "International table of glycemic index and glycemic load values: 2002." Am J Clin Nutr 76: 5–56 (2002)

Gannon MC, Nuttall FQ, Saeed A, Jordan K, and Hoover H. "An increase in dietary protein improves the blood glucose response in persons with type 2 diabetes." Am J Clin Nutr 78: 734–741 (2003)

Gannon MC and Nuttall FQ. "Control of blood glucose in type 2 diabetes without weight loss by modification of diet composition." Nutr Metab 3: 16 (2006)

Hamdy O, Mottalib A, Morsi A, El-Sayed N, Goebel-Fabbri A, Arathuzik G, Shahar J, Kirpitch A, and Zrebiec J. "Long-term effect of intensive lifestyle intervention on cardiovascular risk factors in patients with diabetes in real-world clinical practice: A 5-year longitudinal study." BMJ Open Diabetes Res Care 5:e000259 (2017)

Gilad Y, Oshlack A, Smyth GK, Speed TP, and White KP. "Expression profiling in primates reveals a rapid evolution of human transcription factors." Nature 440: 242–245 (2006)

Hardie DG. "Keeping the home fires burning: AMP-activated protein kinase." J Royal Society Interface 15: 20170774 (2018)

Hardie DG, Ross FA, and Hawley SA. "AMP-activate protein kinase: A target for drugs both ancient and modern." Chem Bio 19: 1222–1236 (2012)

Institute of Medicine: *Dietary Reference Intakes: Energy, Carbohydrate, Fiber, Fat, Fatty Acids, Cholesterol, Protein, and Amino Acids.* Washington, DC, National Academies Press. (2002)

Jenkins DJ, Wong JM, Kendall CW, Esfahani A, Ng VW, Leong TC, Faulkner DA, Vidgen E, Greaves KA, Paul G, and Singer W. "The effect of a plant-based low-carbohydrate diet on body weight and blood lipid concentrations in hyperlipidemic subjects." Arch Intern Med 169: 1046–1054 (2009)

Johnston CS, Tjonn SL, and Swan PD. "High-protein, low-fat diets are effective for weight loss and favorably alter biomarkers in healthy adults." J Nutr 134: 586–591 (2004)

Johnston CS, Tjonn SL, Swan PD, White A, Hutchins H, and Sears B. "Ketogenic low-carbohydrate diets have no metabolic advantage over non-ketogenic low-carbohydrate diets." Am J Clin Nutr 83: 1055–1061 (2006)

Johnston CS, Tjonn SL, Swan PD, White A, and Sears B. "Low-carbohydrate, high-protein diets that restrict potassium-rich fruits and vegetables promote calciuria." Osteoporos Int 17: 1820–1821 (2006)

Kajita K, Mune T, Ikeda T, Matsumoto M, Uno Y, Sugiyama C, Matsubara K, Morita H, Takemura M, Seishima M, Takeda J, and Ishizuka T. "Effect of fasting on PPARγ and AMPK activity in adipocytes." Diabetes Res Clin Pract 81:144–149 (2008)

Katsumata Y, Todoriki H, Higashiuesato Y, Yasura S, Willcox DC, Ohya Y, Willcox BJ, and Dodge HH. "Metabolic syndrome and cognitive decline among the oldest old in Okinawa: In search of a mechanism. The KOCOA project." J Gerontol A Biol Sci Med Sci 67: 126–134 (2012)

Katsumata Y, Todoriki H, Higashiuesato Y, Yasura S, Ohya Y, Willcox DC, and Dodge HH. "Very old adults with better memory function have higher low-density lipoprotein cholesterol levels and lower triglyceride to high-density lipoprotein cholesterol ratios: KOCOA project." J Alzheimers Dis 34: 273–279 (2013)

Kernoff PB, Willis AL, Stone KJ, Davies JA, and McNicol GP. "Antithrombotic potential of dihomo-gamma-linolenic acid in man." Br Med J 3: 1441–1444 (1977)

Kitabchi AE, McDaniel KA, Wan JY, Tylavsky FA, Jacovino CA, Sands CW, Nyenwe EA, and Stentz FB. "Effects of high-protein versus high-carbohydrate diets on markers of beta-cell function, oxidative stress, lipid peroxidation, proinflammatory cytokines, and adipokines in obese, premenopausal women without diabetes: A randomized controlled trial." Diabetes Care 36:1 919–1925 (2013)

Kuipers RS, Luxwolda MF, Dijck-Brouwer DA, Eaton SB, Crawford MA, Cordain L, and Muskiet FA. "Estimated macronutrient and fatty acid intakes from an East African Paleolithic diet." Br J Nutr 104: 1666–1687 (2010)

Lasker DA, Evans EM, and Layman DK. "Moderate carbohydrate, moderate protein weight loss diet reduces cardiovascular disease risk compared to high carbohydrate, low protein diet in obese adults: A randomized clinical trial." Nutr Metab 5: 30 (2008)

Layman DK, Shiue H, Sather C, Erickson DJ, and Baum J. "Increased dietary protein modifies glucose and insulin homeostasis in adult women during weight loss." J Nutr 133: 405–410 (2003)

Layman DK, Boileau RA, Erickson DJ, Painter JE, Shiue H, Sather C, and Christou DD. "A reduced ratio of dietary carbohydrate to protein improves body composition and blood lipid profiles during weight loss in adult women." J Nutr 133: 411–417 (2003)

Layman DK, Anthony TG, Rasmussen BB, Adams SH, Lynch CJ, Brinkworth GD, and Davis TA. "Defining meal requirements for protein to optimize metabolic roles of amino acids." Am J Clin Nutr 101: 1330S–1338S (2015)

Layman DK, Evans EM, Erickson D, Seyler J, Weber J, Bagshaw D, Griel A, Psota T, and Kris-Etherton P. "A moderate-protein diet produces sustained weight loss and long-term changes in body composition and blood lipids in obese adults." J Nutr 139: 514–521 (2009)

Ludwig DS, Majzoub JA, Al-Zahrani A, Dallal GE, Blanco I, and Roberts SB. "High glycemic index foods, overeating, and obesity." Pediatrics 103: E26 (1999)

Ludwig DS. "The glycemic index: Physiological mechanisms relating to obesity, diabetes, and cardiovascular disease." JAMA 287: 2414–2423 (2002)

Liu K, Wang B, Zhou R, Lang HD, Ran L, Wang J, Li L, Kang C, Zhu XH, Zhang QY, Zhu JD, Doucette S, Kang JX, and Mi MT. "Effect of combined use of a low-carbohydrate, high-protein diet with omega-3 polyunsaturated fatty acid supplementation on glycemic control in newly diagnosed type 2 diabetes: A randomized, double-blind, parallel-controlled trial." Am J Clin Nutr 108:256–265 (2018)

Mamerow MM, Mettler JA, English KL, Casperson SL, Arentson-Lantz E, Sheffield-Moore M, Layman DK, and Paddon-Jones D. "Dietary protein distribution positively influences 24-h muscle protein synthesis in healthy adults." J Nutr 144: 876–80 (2014)

Markova M, Pivovarova O, Hornemann S, Sucher S, Frahnow T, Wegner K, Machann J, Petzke KJ, Hierholzer J, Lichtinghagen R, Herder C, Carstensen-Kirberg M, Roden M, Rudovich N, Klaus S, Thomann R, Schneeweiss R, Rohn S, and Pfeiffer AF. "Isocaloric diets high in animal or plant protein reduce liver fat and inflammation in individuals with type 2 diabetes." Gastroenterology 152: 571–585 (2017)

Markovic TP, Jenkins AB, Campbell LV, Furler SM, Kraegen EW, and Chisholm DJ. "The determinants of glycemic responses to diet restriction and weight loss in obesity and NIDDM." Diabetes Care 21:687–694 (1998)

Mattison JA, Colman RJ, Beasley TM, Allison DB, Kemnitz JW, Roth GS, Ingram DK, Weindruch R, de Cabo R, and Anderson RM. "Caloric restriction improves health and survival of rhesus monkeys." Nat Comm 8: 14063 (2017)

McCay CM, Crowell MF, and Maynard LA. "The effect of retarded growth upon the length of life span and upon the ultimate body size." J Nutr 10: 63–79 (1935)

McDonald RB and Ramsey JJ. "Honoring Clive McCay and 75 years of calorie restriction research." J Nutr 140: 1205–1210 (2010)

McLaughlin T, Allison G, Abbasi F, Lamendola C, and Reaven G. "Prevalence of insulin resistance and associated cardiovascular disease risk factors among normal weight, overweight, and obese individuals." Metabolism 53: 495–499 (2004)

Mergenthaler P, Lindauer U, Dienel GA, and Meisel A. "Sugar for the brain: The role of glucose in physiological and pathological brain function." Trends Neurosci 36: 587–597 (2013)

Moosheer SM, Waldschütz W, Itariu BK, Brath H, and Stulnig TM. "A protein-enriched low glycemic index diet with omega-3 polyunsaturated fatty acid supplementation exerts beneficial effects on metabolic control in type 2 diabetes." Prim Care Diabetes. 8: 308–314 (2014)

Mottalib A, Sakr M, Shehabeldin M, and Hamdy O. "Diabetes remission after nonsurgical intensive lifestyle intervention in obese patients with type 2 diabetes." J Diabetes Res 2015: 468704 (2015)

Nowick K, Gernat T, Almaas E, and Stubbs L. "Differences in human and chimpanzee gene expression patterns define an evolving network of transcription factors in brain." Proc Natl Acad Sci U S A. 106: 22358–22363 (2009)

Oates JA. "The 1982 Nobel Prize in Physiology or Medicine." Science 218: 765–768 (1982)

Oeckinghaus A, Hayden MS, and Ghosh S. "Crosstalk in NF-κB signaling pathways." Nat Immunol 12: 695–708 (2011)

Owen OE, Felig P, Morgan AP, Wahren J, and Cahill GF. "Liver and kidney metabolism during prolonged starvation." J Clin Invest 48: 574–583 (1969)

Parker B, Noakes M, Luscombe N and Clifton P. "Effect of a high-protein, high–monounsaturated fat weight loss diet on glycemic control and lipid levels in type 2 diabetes." Diabetes Care 25: 425–430 (2002)

Pearce KL, Clifton PM, and Noakes M. "Egg consumption as part of an energy-restricted high-protein diet improves blood lipid and blood glucose profiles in individuals with type 2 diabetes." Br J Nutr 105: 584–592 (2011)

Pereira MA, Swain J, Goldfine AB, Rifai N, and Ludwig DS. "Effects of a low-glycemic load diet on resting energy expenditure and heart disease risk factors during weight loss." JAMA 292: 2482–2490 (2004)

Pittas AG, Das SK, Hajduk CL, Golden J, Saltzman E, Stark PC, Greenberg AS, and Roberts SB. "A low-glycemic load diet facilitates greater weight loss in overweight adults with high insulin secretion but not in overweight adults with low insulin secretion in the CALERIE trial." Diabetes Care 28: 2939–2941 (2005)

Pittas AG, Roberts SB, Das SK, Gilhooly CH, Saltzman E, Golden J, Stark PC, and Greenberg AS. "The effects of the dietary glycemic load on type 2 diabetes risk factors during weight loss." Obesity 14: 2200–2209 (2006)

Racette SB, Rochon J, Uhrich ML, Villareal DT, DAS SK, Fontana L, Bhapkar M, Martin CK, Redman LM, Fuss PJ, Roberts SB, and Kraus WE. "Effects of two years of calorie restriction on aerobic capacity and muscle strength." Med Sci Sports Exerc 49: 2240–2249 (2017)

Ravussin E, Redman LM, Rochon J, Das SK, Fontana L, Kraus WE, Romashkan S, Williamson DA, Meydani SN, Villareal DT, Smith SR, Stein RI, Scott TM, Stewart TM, Saltzman E, Klein S, Bhapkar M, Martin CK, Gilhooly CH, Holloszy JO, Hadley EC, and Roberts SB. "A 2-year randomized controlled trial of human caloric restriction: Feasibility and effects on predictors of healthspan and longevity." J Gerontol A Biol Sci Med Sci 70: 1097–1104 (2015)

Roth JA, Etzioni R, Waters TM, Pettinger M, Rossouw JE, Anderson GL, Chlebowski RT, Manson JE, Hlatky M, Johnson KC, and Ramsey SD. "Economic return from the Women's Health Initiative estrogen plus progestin clinical trial: A modeling study." Ann Intern Med 160: 594–602 (2014)

Samuel VT and Shulman GI. "Mechanisms for insulin resistance: Common threads and missing links." Cell 148: 852–871 (2012)

Sánchez-Galán E, Gómez-Hernández A, Vidal C, Martín-Ventura JL, Blanco-Colio LM, Muñoz-García B, Ortega L, Egido J, and Tuñón J. "Leukotriene B4 enhances the activity of nuclear factor-kappaB pathway through BLT1 and BLT2 receptors in atherosclerosis." Cardiovasc Res 81: 216–225 (2009)

Sayegh AI. "The role of cholecystokinin receptors in the short-term control of food intake." Prog Mol Biol Transl Sci 114: 277–316 (2013)

Sears B. *The Zone*. Regan Books. New York, NY (1995)

Sears B. *Mastering the Zone*. Regan Books. New York, NY (1997)

Sears B. *The Anti-Aging Zone*. Regan Books. New York, NY (1999)

Sears B. *The OmegaRx Zone*. Regan Books. New York, NY (2002)

Sears B. *The Anti-Inflammation Zone*. Regan Books. New York, NY (2005)

Sears B. *Toxic Fat*. Thomas Nelson. Nashville, TN (2008)

Sears B. *The Mediterranean Zone*. Ballantine Books. New York, NY (2014)

Sears B. "Phosphatidyl quarternary ammonium compounds." U.S. Patent No. 4,086,257 (1978)

Sears B and Yesair DW. "Xenobiotic delivery vehicles." U.S. Patent No. 4,298,594 (1981)

Sears B. "Synthetic phospholipid compounds." U.S. Patent No. 4,426,330 (1984)

Sears B and Perry M. "The role of fatty acids in insulin resistance." Lipids Health Disease 14: 121 (2015)

Stentz FB, Brewer A, Wan J, Garber C, Daniels B, Sands C, and Kitabchi AE. "Remission of pre-diabetes to normal glucose tolerance in obese adults with high protein versus high carbohydrate diet." BMJ Open Diabetes Res Care 4: e000258 (2016)

Stone KJ, Willis AL, Hart WM, Kirtland SJ, Kernoff PB, and McNicol GP. "The metabolism of dihomo-gamma-linolenic acid in man." Lipids 14: 174–180 (1979)

Stulnig TM. "The Zone Diet and metabolic control in type 2 diabetes." J Am Coll Nutr 34 Suppl 1: 39–41 (2015)

van der Klaauw AA, Keogh JM, Henning E, Trowse VM, Dhillo WS, Ghatei MA, and Farooqi IS. "High protein intake stimulates postprandial GLP-1 and PYY release." Obesity 21:1602–1607 (2013)

White AM, Johnston CS, Swan PD, Tjonn SL, and Sears B. "Blood ketones are directly related to fatigue and perceived effort during exercise in overweight adults adhering to low-carbohydrate diets for weight loss: A Pilot study." J Am Diet Assoc 107: 1792–1796 (2007)

Whitten P. "Stanford's secret weapon." Swimming World 34: 1–6 (1993)

CHAPTER 9: FERMENTABLE FIBER: THE KEY TO MAINTAINING GUT HEALTH

Anderson SC. *The Psychobitoic Revolution*. National Geographic Books. Washington DC (2017)

Anhê FF, Roy D, Pilon G, Dudonné S, Matamoros S, Varin TV, Garofalo C, Moine Q, Desjardins Y, Levy E, and Marette A. "A polyphenol-rich cranberry extract protects from diet-induced obesity, insulin resistance and intestinal inflammation in association with increased *Akkermansia* spp. population in gut microbiota of mice." Gut 64: 872–883 (2015)

Asarian L and Bächler T. "Neuroendocrine control of satiation." Horm Mol Biol Clin Investig 19: 163–192 (2014)

Bergmann O, Zdunek S, Felker A, Salehpour M, Alkass K, Bernard S, Sjostrom SL, Szewczykowska M, Jackowska T, Dos Remedios C, Malm T, Andrä M, Jashari R, Nyengaard JR, Possnert G, Jovinge S, Druid H, and Frisén J. "Dynamics of cell generation and turnover in the human heart." Cell 161: 1566–1575 (2015)

Blasser MJ. *Missing Microbes*. Henry Holt. New York, NY (2014)

Bliss ES and Whiteside E. "The gut-brain axis, the human gut microbiota and their integration in the development of obesity." Front Physiol 9: 900 (2018)

Cani PD, Amar J, Iglesias MA, Poggi M, Knauf C, Bastelica D, Neyrinck AM, Fava F, Tuohy KM, Chabo C, Waget A, Delmée E, Cousin B, Sulpice T, Chamontin B, Ferrières J, Tanti JF, Gibson GR, Casteilla L, Delzenne NM, Alessi MC, and Burcelin R. "Metabolic endotoxemia initiates obesity and insulin resistance." Diabetes 56: 1761–1772 (2007)

Cani PD, Amar J, Iglesias MA, Poggi M, Knauf C, and Bastelica D. "Metabolic endotoxemia initiates obesity and insulin resistance." Diabetes 56: 1761–1772 (2007)

Caesasr R, Tremaroli V, Kovatcheva-Datchary P, Cani PD, and Backhed F. "Crosstalk between gut microbiota and dietary lipids aggravates WAT inflammation through TLR signaling." Cell Metabol 22: 1–11 (2015)

Chambers ES, Morrison DJ, and Frost G. "Control of appetite and energy intake by SCFA: What are the potential underlying mechanisms?" Proc Nutr Soc 74: 328–336 (2015)

Chio CC, Baba T, and Black KL. "Selective blood-tumor barrier disruption by leukotrienes." J Neurosurg 77: 407–410 (1992)

Christiansen CB, Gabe MBN, Svendsen B, Dragsted LO, Rosenkilde MM, and Holst JJ. "The impact of short-chain fatty acids on GLP-1 and PYY secretion from the isolated perfused rat colon." Am J Physiol Gastrointest Liver Physiol 315: G53–G65 (2018)

Chronaiou A, Tsoli M, Kehagias I, Leotsinidis M, Kalfarentzos F, and Alexandrides TK. "Lower ghrelin levels and exaggerated postprandial peptide-YY, glucagon-like peptide-1, and insulin responses, after gastric fundus resection, in patients undergoing Roux-en-Y gastric bypass: A randomized clinical trial." Obes Surg 22: 1761–1770 (2012)

Collen A. *10% Human*. Harper Collins. New York, NY (2015)

Cornick S, Tawiah A, and Chadee K. "Roles and regulation of the mucus barrier in the gut." Tissue Barriers 3: e982426 (2015)

Delcour JA, Aman P, Courtin CM, Hamaker BR, and Verbeke K. "Prebiotics, fermentable dietary fiber, and health claims." Adv Nutr 7: 1–4 (2016)

Derrien M. "*Akkermansia muciniphila*, a human intestinal mucin-degrading bacterium." Int J Systematic and Evolutionary Microbiology 54: 1469–1476 (2004)

Daud NM, Ismail NA, Thomas EL, Fitzpatrick JA, Bell JD, Swann JR, Costabile A, Childs CE, Pedersen C, Goldstone AP, and Frost GS. "The impact of oligofructose on stimulation of gut hormones, appetite regulation and adiposity." Obesity 22: 1430–1438 (2014)

de Vogel-van den Bosch HM, Bünger M, de Groot PJ, Bosch-Vermeulen H, Hooiveld GJ, and Müller M. "PPARγ-mediated effects of dietary lipids on intestinal barrier gene expression." BMC Genomics 9: 231 (2008)

Everard A and Cani PD. "Gut microbiota and GLP-1." Rev Endocr Metab Disord 15: 189–196 (2014)

Fasano A. "Zonulin and its regulation of intestinal barrier function: The biological door to inflammation, autoimmunity, and cancer." Physiol Rev 91: 151–175 (2011)

Fredricks D. *The Human Microbiota: How Microbial Communities Affect Health and Disease.* Wiley-Blackwell. New York, NY (2013)

Gershon MD. *The Second Brain.* Harper Collins. New York, NY (1999)

Goodman BE. "Insights into digestion and absorption of major nutrients in humans." Adv Physiol Educ 34: 44–53 (2010)

Greiner TU and Bäckhed F. "Microbial regulation of GLP-1 and L-cell biology." Mol Metab 5: 753–758 (2016)

Grossi E and Pace F eds. *Human Nutrition from the Gastroenterologist's Perspective.* Springer. New York, NY (2016)

Kaliannan K, Wang B, Xiang-Yong L, Kim K-J, and Kang JX. "A host-microbiome interaction mediates the opposing effects of omega-6 and omega-3 fatty acids on metabolic endotoxemia." Sci Reports 5: 112276 (2015)

Kimura R, Takahashi N, Lin S, Goto T, Murota K, Nakata R, Inoue H, and Kawada T. "DHA attenuates postprandial hyperlipidemia via activating PPARγ in intestinal epithelial cells." J Lipid Res 54: 3258–3268 (2013)

Konturek SJ and Brzozowski T. "Role of leukotrienes and platelet activating factor in gastric mucosal damage and repair." J Physiol Pharmacol 42:107–133 (1991)

Larraufie P, Martin-Gallausiaux C, Lapaque N, Dore J, Gribble FM, Reimann F, and Blottiere HM. "SCFAs strongly stimulate PYY production in human enteroendocrine cells." Sci Rep 8: 74 (2018)

Leclercq S, Matamoros S, Cani PD, Neyrinck AM, Jamar F, Stärkel P, Windey K, Tremaroli V, Bäckhed F, Verbeke K, de Timary P, and Delzenne NM. "Intestinal permeability, gut-bacterial dysbiosis, and behavioral markers of alcohol-dependence severity." Proc Natl Acad Sci U S A 111: E4485–4493 (2014)

López-Moreno J, García-Carpintero S, Jimenez-Lucena R, Haro C, Rangel-Zúñiga OA, Blanco-Rojo R, Yubero-Serrano EM, Tinahones FJ, Delgado-Lista J, Pérez-Martínez P, Roche HM, López-Miranda J, and Camargo A. "Effect of dietary lipids on endotoxemia influences postprandial inflammatory response." J Agric Food Chem 65: 7756–7763 (2017)

Lyte M and Cryan JF. *Microbial Endocrinology: The Microbiota-Gut-Brain Axis.* Springer. New York, NY (2014)

Masumoto S, Terao A, Yamamoto Y, Mukai T, Miura T, and Shoji T. "Non-absorbable apple procyandian prevent obesity associated with gut microbial and metabolomics changes." Sci Reports 6: 31208 (2016)

Mayer E. *The Mind-Gut Connection*. Harper Wave. New York, NY (2016)

Nettleton JE, Reimer RA, and Shearer J. "Reshaping the gut microbiota: Impact of low-calorie sweeteners and the link to insulin resistance?" Physiol Behav164 (Pt B): 488–493 (2016)

Pelaseyed T, Bergström JH, Gustafsson JK, Ermund A, Birchenough GM, Schütte A, van der Post S, Svensson F, Rodríguez-Piñeiro AM, Nyström EE, Wising C, Johansson ME, and Hansson GC. "The mucus and mucins of the goblet cells and enterocytes provide the first defense line of the gastrointestinal tract and interact with the immune system." Immunol Rev 260: 8–20 (2014)

Pepino MY, Tiemann CD, Patterson BW, Wice BM, and Klein S. "Sucralose affects glycemic and hormonal responses to an oral glucose load." Diabetes Care 36: 2530–2535 (2013)

Pepino MY. "Metabolic effects of non-nutritive sweeteners." Physiol Behav 152 (Pt B): 450–5 (2016)

Psichas A, Sleeth ML, Murphy KG, Brooks L, Bewick GA, Hanyaloglu AC, Ghatei MA, Bloom SR, and Frost G. "The short chain fatty acid propionate stimulates GLP-1 and PYY secretion via free fatty acid receptor 2 in rodents." Int J Obes 39: 424–429 (2015)

Roach M. *Gulp*. W.W. Norton and Company. New York, NY (2013)

Roopchand DE, Carmody RN, Kuhn P, Moskal K, Rojas-Silva, Turnbaugh PJ, and Raskin I. "Dietary polyphenols promote growth of gut bacterium *Akkermansia muninphila* and attenuate high-fat diet-induced metabolic syndrome." Diabetes 64: 2847–2858 (2015)

Schneeberger M, Everard A, Gómez-Valadés AG, Matamoros S, Ramírez S, Delzenne NM, Gomis R, Claret M, and Cani PD. "*Akkermansia muciniphila* inversely correlates with the onset of inflammation, altered adipose tissue metabolism and metabolic disorders in mice." Sci Reports 5: 16643 (2015)

Schroeder N, Marquart LF, and Gallaher DD. "The role of viscosity and fermentability of dietary fibers on satiety- and adiposity-related hormones in rats." Nutrients 5: 2093–2113 (2013)

Slavin J. "Fiber and prebiotics." Nutrients 5: 1417-1435 (2013)

Sonnenburg ED, Smits SA, Tikhonov M, Higginbottom SK, Wingreen NS, and Sonnenburg JL. "Diet-induced extinctions in the gut microbiota compound over generations." Nature 529: 212–215 (2016)

Sonneburg J and Sonnenburg E. *The Good Gut*. Penguin Books. New York, NY (2016)

Spalding KL, Bhardwaj RD, Buchholz BA, Druid H, and Frisén J. "Retrospective birth dating of cells in humans." Cell 122: 133–143 (2005)

Spalding KL, Arner E, Westermark PO, Bernard S, Buchholz BA, Bergmann O, Blomqvist L, Hoffstedt J, Näslund E, Britton T, Concha H, Hassan M, Rydén M, Frisén J, and Arner P. "Dynamics of fat cell turnover in humans." Nature 453: 783–787 (2008)

Spalding KL, Bergmann O, Alkass K, Bernard S, Salehpour M, Huttner HB, Boström E, Westerlund I, Vial C, Buchholz BA, Possnert G, Mash DC, Druid H, and Frisén J. "Dynamics of hippocampal neurogenesis in adult humans." Cell 153: 1219–1227 (2013)

Spreckley E and Murphy KG. "The L-cell in nutritional sensing and the regulation of appetite." Front Nutr 2: 23 (2015)

Suez J, Korem T, Zeevi D, Zilberman-Schapira G, Thaiss CA, Maza O, Israeli D, Zmora N, Gilad S, Weinberger A, Kuperman Y, Harmelin A, Kolodkin-Gal I, Shapiro H, Halpern Z, Segal E, and Elinav E. "Artificial sweeteners induce glucose intolerance by altering the gut microbiota." Nature 514: 181–186 (2014)

Tuohy K and Del Rio D. *Diet-Microbe Interactions in the Gut.* Academic Press. London, UK (2015)

van der Klaauw AA, Keogh JM, Henning E, Trowse VM, Dhillo WS, Ghatei MA, and Farooqi IS. "High protein intake stimulates postprandial GLP-1 and PYY release." Obesity 21: 1602–1607 (2013)

Vanuytsel T, van Wanrooy S, Vanheel H, Vanormelingen C, Verschueren S, Houben E, Salim Rasoel S, Toth J, Holvoet L, Farré R, Van Oudenhove L, Boeckxstaens G, Verbeke K, and Tack J. "Psychological stress and corticotropin-releasing hormone increase intestinal permeability in humans by a mast cell-dependent mechanism." Gut 63: 1293–1299 (2014)

Wrangham R. *Cooking with Fire.* Basic Books. New York, NY (2010)

Yeomans MR, Tepper BJ, Rietzschel J, and Prescott J. "Human hedonic responses to sweetness: Role of taste genetics and anatomy." Physiol Behav 91: 264–273 (2007)

Zanchi D, Depoorter A, Egloff L, Haller S, Mählmann L, Lang UE, Drewe J, Beglinger C, Schmidt A, and Borgwardt S. "The impact of gut hormones on the neural circuit of appetite and satiety: A systematic review." Neurosci Biobehav Rev 80: 457–475 (2017)

CHAPTER 10: OMEGA-3 FATTY ACIDS: AGENTS OF RESOLUTION

Arsenescu V, Arsenescu RI, King V, Swanson H, and Cassis LA. "Polychlorinated biphenyl-77 induces adipocyte differentiation and proinflammatory adipokines and promotes obesity and atherosclerosis." Environ Health Perspect 116: 761–768 (2008)

Ashley JT, Ward JS, Schafer MW, Stapleton HM, and Velinsky DJ. "Evaluating daily exposure to polychlorinated biphenyls and polybrominated diphenyl ethers in fish oil supplements." Food Addit Contam Part A Chem Anal Control Expo Risk Assess. 8: S1944–1957 (2010)

Bellenger J, Bellenger S, Bataille A, Massey KA, Nicolaou A, Rialland M, Tessier C, Kang JX, and Narce M. "High pancreatic n-3 fatty acids prevent STZ-induced diabetes in fat-1 mice: Inflammatory pathway inhibition. Diabetes 60: 1090–1099 (2011)

Bhatt DL, Steg G, Mill M, Brinton EA, Jacobson TA, Ketchum SB, Doyle RT, Juliano RA, Jiao L, Granowitz G, Tardif JC, and Ballantyne CM. "Cardiovascular risk reduction with icosapent ethyl for hypertriglyceridemia." N Engl J Med 380: 11–22 (2019)

Bhattacharya A, Chandrasekar B, Rahman MM, Banu J, Kang JX, and Fernandes G. "Inhibition of inflammatory response in transgenic fat-1 mice on a calorie-restricted diet." Biochem Biophys Res Commun 349: 925–930 (2006)

Blasbalg TL, Hibbeln JR, Ramsden CE, Majchrzak SF, and Rawlings RR. "Changes in consumption of omega-3 and omega-6 fatty acids in the United States during the 20th century." Am J Clin Nutr 93: 950–962 (2011)

Bonds DE, Harrington M, Worrall BB, Bertoni AG, Eaton CB, Hsia J, Robinson J, Clemons TE, Fine LJ, and Chew EY. "Effect of long-chain n-3 fatty acids and lutein + zeaxanthin supplements on cardiovascular outcomes: Results of the Age-Related Eye Disease Study 2 (AREDS2) randomized clinical trial." JAMA Intern Med 174: 763–771 (2014)

Brenner RR. "Nutritional and hormonal factors influencing desaturation of essential fatty acids." Prog Lipid Res 20: 41–7 (1981)

Brenner RR. "Hormonal modulation of delta 6 and delta 5 desaturases: Case of diabetes." Prostaglandins Leukot Essent Fatty Acids 68: 151–162 (2003)

Calder PC. "Omega-3 fatty acids and inflammatory processes: From molecules to man." Biochem Soc Trans 45: 1105–1115 (2017)

Chen CT and Bazinet RP. "β-oxidation and rapid metabolism, but not uptake regulate brain eicosapentaenoic acid levels." Prostaglandins Leukot Essent Fatty Acids 92: 33–40 (2015)

Elajami TK, Colas RA, Dalli J, Chiang N, Serhan CN, and Welty FK. "Specialized proresolving lipid mediators in patients with coronary artery disease and their potential for clot remodeling." FASEB J 30: 2792-2801 (2016)

el Boustani S, Causse JE, Descomps B, Monnier L, Mendy F, and Crastes de Paulet A. "Direct in vivo characterization of delta 5 desaturase activity in humans by deuterium labeling: Effect of insulin." Metabolism 38: 315–321 (1989)

Endres S, Ghorbani R, Kelley VE, Georgilis K, Lonnemann G, van der Meer JW, Cannon JG, Rogers TS, Klempner MS, Weber PC, Schaeffer EJ, Wolff SM, and Dinarello CA. "The effect of dietary supplementation with n-3 polyunsaturated fatty acids on the synthesis of interleukin-1 and tumor necrosis factor by mononuclear cells." N Engl J Med 320: 265–271 (1989)

Georgiou T, Neokleous A, Nikolaou D, and Sears B. "Pilot study for treating dry age-related macular degeneration (AMD) with high-dose omega-3 fatty acids." PharmaNutrition 2:8–11 (2014)

Georgiou T and Prokopiou E. "The new era of omega-3 fatty acids supplementation: Therapeutic effects on dry age-related macular degeneration." J Stem Cells 10: 205–215 (2015)

Germano M, Meleleo D, Montorfano G, Adorni L, Negroni M, Berra B, and Rizzo AM. "Plasma, red blood cells, phospholipids and clinical evaluation after long chain omega-3 supplementation in children with attention deficit hyperactivity disorder (ADHD)." Nutr Neurosci 10: 1–9 (2007)

Griffitts J, Saunders D, Tesiram YA, Reid GE, Salih A, Liu S, Lydic TA, Busik JV, Kang JX, and Towner RA. "Non-mammalian fat-1 gene prevents neoplasia when introduced to a mouse hepatocarcinogenesis model: Omega-3 fatty acids prevent liver neoplasia." Biochim Biophys Acta 1801: 1133–1144 (2010)

Hansen JB, Olsen JO, Wilsgard L, Lyngmo V, and Svensson B. "Comparative effects of prolonged intake of highly purified fish oils as ethyl ester or triglyceride on lipids, haemostasis and platelet function in normolipaemic men." Eur J Clin Nutr 47: 497–507 (1993)

Harris WS. "The omega-3 index: Clinical utility for therapeutic intervention." Curr Cardiol Rep 12: 503–508 (2010)

Harris WS, Luo J, Pottala JV, Espeland MA, Margolis KL, Manson JE, Wang L, Brasky TM, and Robinson JG. "Red blood cell polyunsaturated fatty acids and mortality in the Women's Health Initiative Memory study." J Clin Lipidol 11: 250–259 (2017)

Harris WS, Pottala JV, Varvel SA, Borowski JJ, Ward JN, and McConnell JP. "Erythrocyte omega-3 fatty acids increase and linoleic acid decreases with age: Observations from 160,000 patients." Prostaglandins Leukot Essent Fatty Acids 88: 257–263 (2013)

Heydari B, Abdullah S, Pottala JV, Shah R, Abbasi S, Mandry D, Francis SA, Lumish H, Ghoshhajra BB, Hoffmann U, Appelbaum E, Feng JH, Blankstein R, Steigner M, McConnell JP, Harris W, Antman EM, Jerosch-Herold M, and Kwong RY. "Effect of omega-3 acid ethyl esters on left ventricular remodeling after acute myocardial infarction: The OMEGA-REMODEL randomized clinical trial." Circulation 134: 378–391 (2016)

Igarashi M, Chang L, Ma K, and Rapoport SI. "Kinetics of eicosapentaenoic acid in brain, heart and liver of conscious rats fed a high n-3 PUFA containing diet." Prostaglandins Leukot Essent Fatty Acids 89: 403–412 (2013)

Innes JK and Calder PC. "Omega-6 fatty acids and inflammation." Prostaglandins Leukot Essent Fatty Acids 132: 41–48 (2018)

Kang JX, Wang J, Wu L, and Kang ZB. "Transgenic mice: Fat-1 mice convert n-6 to n-3 fatty acids." Nature 427: 504 (2004)

Kawabata T, Hirota S, Hirayama T, Adachi N, Kaneko Y, Iwama N, Kamachi K, Araki E, Kawashima H, and Kiso Y. "Associations between dietary n-6 and n-3 fatty acids and arachidonic acid compositions in plasma and erythrocytes in young and elderly Japanese volunteers." Lipids Health Dis 10: 138 (2011)

Krokan HE, Bjerve KS, and Mork E. "The enteral bioavailability of eicosapentaenoic acid and docosahexaenoic acid is as good from ethyl esters as from glyceryl esters in spite of lower hydrolytic rates by pancreatic lipase in vitro." Biochim Biophys Acta 1168: 59–67 (1993)

Kuipers RS, Luxwolda MF, Dijck-Brouwer DA, Eaton SB, Crawford MA, Cordain L, and Muskiet FA. "Estimated macronutrient and fatty acid intakes from an East African Paleolithic diet." Br J Nutr 104: 1666–1687 (2010)

Lebbadi M, Julien C, Phivilay A, Tremblay C, Emond V, Kang JX, and Calon F. "Endogenous conversion of omega-6 into omega-3 fatty acids improve neuropathology in an animal model of Alzheimer's disease." J Alzheimers Dis 27: 853–869 (2011)

Li J, Li FR, Wei D, Jia W, Kang JX, Stefanovic-Racic M, Dai Y, and Zhao AZ. "Endogenous n-3 polyunsaturated fatty acid production confers resistance to obesity, dyslipidisemia, and diabetes in mice." Mol Endocrinol 28: 1316–1328 (2014)

Mason JE, Cook NR, Lee I-M, Christen W, Bassuk SS, Mora S, Gibson H, Albert CM, Gordon D, Copeland T, D'Agostino D, Friedenberg G, Ridge C, Bubes V, Giovannucci EL, Willett WC, and Burning JE. "Marine n-3 fatty acids and prevention of cardiovascular disease and cancer." N Engl J Med 380: 23–32 (2019)

Mayer K, Kiessling A, Ott J, Schaefer MB, Hecker M, Henneke I, Schulz R, Günther A, Wang J, Wu L, Roth J, Seeger W, and Kang JX. "Acute lung injury is reduced in fat-1 mice endogenously synthesizing n-3 fatty acids." Am J Respir Crit Care Med 179: 474–483 (2009)

McNamara RK, Perry M, and Sears, B. "Dissociation of C-reactive protein levels from long-chain omega-3 fatty acid status and anti-depressant response in adolescents with major depressive disorder: An open-label dose-ranging trial." J Nutr Therapeutics 2: 235–243 (2013)

Nordoy A, Barstad L, Connor WE, and Hatcher L. "Absorption of the n-3 eicosapentaenoic and docosahexaenoic acids as ethyl esters and triglycerides by humans." Am J Clin Nutr 53: 1185–1190 (1991)

Norris PC, Skulas-Ray AC, Riley I, Richter CK, Kris-Etherton PM, Jensen GL, Serhan CN, and Maddipati KR. "Identification of specialized pro-resolving mediator clusters from healthy adults after intravenous low-dose endotoxin and omega-3 supplementation: A methodological validation." Sci Rep 8: 18050 (2018)

Papanikolaou Y, Brooks J, Reider C, and Fulgoni VL. "U.S. adults are not meeting recommended levels for fish and omega-3 fatty acid intake: Results of an analysis using observational data from NHANES 2003-2008." Nutr J 13: 31 (2014)

Pelikanova T, Kohout M, Base J, Stefka Z, Kovar J, Kazdova L, and Valek J. "Effect of acute hyperinsulinemia on fatty acid composition of serum lipids in non-insulin-dependent diabetics and healthy men." Clin Chim Acta 203: 329–337 (1991)

Picado C. "Mechanisms of aspirin sensitivity." Curr Allergy Asthma Rep 6: 198–202 (2006)

Rawshani A, Sattar N, Franzén S, Rawshani A, Hattersley AT, Svensson A-M, and Eliasson B. "Excess mortality and cardiovascular disease in young adults with type 1 diabetes in relation to age at onset: A nationwide, register-based cohort study." Lancet 392: 477–486 (2018)

Reis GJ, Silverman DI, Boucher TM, Sipperly ME, Horowitz GL, Sacks FM, and Pasternak RC. "Effects of two types of fish oil supplements on serum lipids and plasma phospholipid fatty acids in coronary artery disease." Am J Cardiol 66: 1171–1175 (1990)

Rita C ed. *Eicosanoids, Inflammation and Chronic Inflammatory Diseases: Pathophysiology, Health Effects and Targets for Therapies.* Nova New Science (2015)

Romanatto T, Fiamoncini J, Wang B, Curi R, and Kang JX. "Elevated tissue omega-3 fatty acid status prevents age-related glucose intolerance in fat-1 transgenic mice." Biochim Biophys Acta 1842: 186–191 (2014)

Sacks FM, Bray GA, Carey VJ, Smith SR, Ryan DH, Anton SD, McManus K, Champagne CM, Bishop LM, Laranjo N, Leboff MS, Rood JC, de Jonge L, Greenway FL, Loria CM, Obarzanek E, and Williamson DA. "Comparison of weight-loss diets with different compositions of fat, protein, and carbohydrates." N Engl J Med 360: 859–873 (2009)

Salem N and Kuratko CN. "A reexamination of krill oil bioavailability studies." Lipids Health Dis 13: 137 (2014)

Sears B. *The Zone.* Regan Books. New York, NY (1995)

Sears B. *The OmegaRx Zone.* Regan Books. New York, NY (2001)

Sears B. *The Anti-Inflammation Zone.* Regan Books. New York, NY (2005)

Sears B, Bailes J, and Asselin B. "Therapeutic uses of high-dose omega-3 fatty acids to treat comatose patients with severe brain injury." PharmaNutrition 1: 86–89 (2013)

Sears B. "High-dose omega-3 fatty acids and vitamin D for preservation of residual beta cell mass in type 1 diabetes." CellR4 4: e2107 (2016)

See VHL, Mas E, Prescott SL, Beilin LJ, Burrows S, Barden AE, Huang RC, and Mori TA. "Effects of prenatal n-3 fatty acid supplementation on offspring resolvins at birth and 12 years of age: A double-blind, randomised controlled clinical trial." Br J Nutr 118: 971–980 (2017)

Serhan CN. "Lipoxins and novel aspirin-triggered 15-epi-lipoxins (ATL): A jungle of cell-cell interactions or a therapeutic opportunity?" Prostaglandins 53: 107–137 (1997)

Serhan CN, Brain SD, Buckley CD, Gilroy DW, Haslett C, O'Neill LA, Perretti M, Rossi AG, and Wallace JL. "Resolution of inflammation: State of the art, definitions and terms." FASEB J 21: 325–332 (2007)

Serhan CN. "Treating inflammation and infection in the 21st century: New hints from decoding resolution mediators and mechanisms." FASEB 31: 1273–1288 (2017)

Serhan CN, Chiang N, and Dalli J. "The resolution code of acute inflammation: Novel pro-resolving lipid mediators in resolution." Semin Immunol 27: 200–215 (2015)

Serhan CN. "Discovery of specialized pro-resolving mediators marks the dawn of resolution physiology and pharmacology." Mol Aspects Med 58: 1–11 (2017)

Sorgi PJ, Hallowell EM, Hutchins HL, and Sears B. "Effects of an open-label pilot study with high-dose EPA/DHA concentrates on plasma phospholipids and behavior in children with attention deficit hyperactivity disorder." Nutr J 6: 16 (2007)

Spite M, Claria J, and Serhan CN. "Resolvins, specialized proresolving lipid mediators, and their potential roles in metabolic diseases." Cell Metab 19:21–36 (2014)

Spite M and Serhan CN. "Novel lipid mediators promote resolution of acute inflammation: Impact of aspirin and statins." Circ Res 107: 1170–84 (2010)

Stark KD, Van Elswyk ME, Higgins MR, Weatherford CA, and Salem N. "Global survey of the omega-3 fatty acids, docosahexaenoic acid and eicosapentaenoic acid in the blood stream of healthy adults." Prog Lipid Res 63: 132–152 (2016)

Umhau JC, Zhou W, Carson RE, Rapoport SI, Polozova A, Demar J, Hussein N, Bhattacharjee AK, Ma K, Esposito G, Majchrzak S, Herscovitch P, Eckelman WC, Kurdziel KA, and Salem N. "Imaging incorporation of circulating docosahexaenoic acid into the human brain using positron emission tomography." J Lipid Res 50: 1259–1268 (2009)

Visser MJ. *Cold, Clear, and Deadly.* Michigan State University Press. East Lansing, MI (2007)

Willis AL. *Handbook of Eicosanoids.* CRC Press. Boca Raton, FL (1987)

Wu K, Gao X, Shi B, Chen S, Zhou X, Li Z, Gan Y, Cui L, Kang JX, Li W, and Huang R. "Enriched endogenous n-3 polyunsaturated fatty acids alleviate cognitive and behavioral deficits in a mice model of Alzheimer's disease." Neuroscience 333: 345–355 (2016)

Yokoyama M, Origasa H, Matsuzaki M, Matsuzawa Y, Saito Y, Ishikawa Y, Oikawa S, Sasaki J, Hishida H, Itakura H, Kita T, Kitabatake A, Nakaya N, Sakata T, Shimada K, and Shirato K. "Effects of eicosapentaenoic acid on major coronary events in hypercholesterolaemic patients (JELIS): A randomised open-label, blinded endpoint analysis." Lancet 369: 1090–1098 (2007)

Yurko-Mauro K, Kralovec J, Bailey-Hall E, Smeberg V, Stark JG, and Salem N. "Similar eicosapentaenoic acid and docosahexaenoic acid plasma levels achieved with fish oil or krill oil in a randomized double-blind four-week bioavailability study." Lipids Health Dis 14: 99 (2015)

Zhang Z, Fulgoni VL, Kris-Etherton PM, and Mitmesser SH. "Dietary intakes of EPA and DHA omega-3 fatty acids among US childbearing-age and pregnant women: An analysis of NHANES 2001–2014." Nutrients 10: E416 (2018)

CHAPTER 11: POLYPHENOLS: ACTIVATORS OF OUR GENES, GUARDIANS OF OUR GUT

Alvarado J, Schoenlau F, Leschot A, Salgad AM, and Vigil Portales P. "Standardized maqui berry extract significantly lowers blood glucose and improves blood lipid profile in prediabetic individuals in three-month clinical trial." Panminerva Med 58 (3 Suppl 1):1–6 (2016)

Alvarado JL, Leschot A, Olivera-Nappa Á, Salgado AM, Rioseco H, Lyon C, and Vigil P. "Delphinidin-rich maqui berry extract lowers fasting and postprandial glycemia and insulinemia in prediabetic individuals during oral glucose tolerance tests." Biomed Res Int 2016: 9070537 (2016)

Anhe FF, Pilon G, Roy D, Desjardins Y, Levy E, and Marette A. "Triggering *Akkermansia* with dietary polyphenols: A new weapon to combat the metabolic syndrome?" Gut Microbes 7:146–153 (2016)

Aragonès G, Suárez M, Ardid-Ruiz A, Vinaixa M, Rodríguez MA, Correig X, Arola L, and Bladé C. "Dietary proanthocyanidins boost hepatic NAD(+) metabolism and SIRT1 expression and activity in a dose-dependent manner in healthy rats." Sci Rep 6: 24977 (2016)

Aune D, Giovannucci E, Boffetta P, Fadnes LT, Keum N, Norat T, Greenwood DC, Riboli E, Vatten LJ, and Tonstad S. "Fruit and vegetable intake and the risk of cardiovascular disease, total cancer and all-cause mortality-a systematic review and dose-response meta-analysis of prospective studies." Int J Epidemiol 46: 1029–1056 (2017)

Ayissi VB, Ebrahimi A, and Schluesenner H. "Epigenetic effects of natural polyphenols: A focus on SIRT1-mediated mechanisms." Mol Nutr Food Res 58: 22–32 (2014)

Bao Y, Han J, Hu FB, Giovannucci EL, Stampfer MJ, Willett WC, and Fuchs SC. "Association of nut consumption with total and cause-specific mortality." N Engl J Med 369: 2001–2011 (2013)

Basu A, Du M, Leyva MJ, Sanchez K, Betts NM, Wu M, Aston CE, and Lyons TJ. "Blueberries decrease cardiovascular risk factors in obese men and women with metabolic syndrome." J Nutr 140: 1582–1587 (2010)

Brickman AM, Khan UA, Provenzano FA, Yeung LK, Suzuki W, Schroeter H, Wall M, Sloan RP, and Small SA. "Enhancing dentate gyrus function with dietary flavanols improves cognition in older adults." Nat Neurosci 17: 1798–1803 (2014)

Cani PD, Bibiloni R, Knauf C, Waget A, Neyrinck AM, Delzenne NM, and Burcelin R. "Changes in gut microbiota control metabolic endotoxemia-induced inflammation in high-fat diet-induced obesity and diabetes in mice." Diabetes 57:1470–1881(2008)

Cardona F, Andres-Lacueva C, Tulipani S, Tinahones FJ, and Queipo-Ortuno MI. "Benefits of polyphenols on gut microbiota and implications in human health." J Nutr Biochem 24: 1415–1422 (2013)

Cárdeno A, Sánchez-Hidalgo M, Aparicio-Soto M, Sánchez-Fidalgo S, and Alarcón-de-la-Lastra C. "Extra virgin olive oil polyphenolic extracts downregulate inflammatory responses in LPS-activated murine peritoneal macrophages suppressing NF-κB and MAPK signalling pathways." Food Funct 5: 1270–1277 (2014)

Cassidy A, Mukamal KJ, Liu L, Franz M, Eliassen AH and EB. "High anthocyanin intake is associated with a reduced risk of myocardial infarction in young and middle-aged women." Circulation 127: 188–196 (2013)

Cheng A, Han C, Fang X, Sun J, Chen X, and Wan F. "Extractable and non-extractable polyphenols from blueberries modulate LPS-induced expression of iNOS and COX-2 in RAW264.7 macrophages via the NF-κB signalling pathway." J Sci Food Agric 96: 3393–3400 (2016)

Chu AJ. "Antagonism by bioactive polyphenols against inflammation: A systematic view." Inflamm Allergy Drug Targets 13: 34–64 (2014)

Chung S, Yao H, Caito S, Hwang JW, Arunachalam G, and Rahman I. "Regulation of SIRT1 in cellular functions: Role of polyphenols." Arch Biochem Biophys 501: 79–90 (2010)

Coughlan KA, Balon TW, Valentine RJ, Petrocelli R, Schultz V, Brandon A, Cooney GJ, Kraegen EW, Ruderman NB, and Saha AK. "Nutrient excess and AMPK downregulation in incubated skeletal muscle and muscle of gluose-infused rats." PLOS One 10: e012388 (2015)

Dasguta B and Mibrandt J. "Resveratrol stimulates AMP kinase activity in neurons." Proc Nat Acad Sci USA 104: 7217–7222 (2007)

Davinelli S, Sapere N, Visentin M, Zella D, and Scapagnini G. "Enhancement of mitochondrial biogenesis with polyphenols: Combined effects of resveratrol and equol in human endothelial cells." Immun Ageing 10: 28 (2013)

Davinelli S, Bertoglio JC, Zarrelli A, Pina R, and Scapagnini G. "A randomized clinical trial evaluating the efficacy of an anthocyanin-maqui berry extract on oxidative stress biomarkers." J Am Coll Nutr 34 Suppl 1:28–33 (2015)

Davinelli S, Corbi G, Righetti S, Sears B, Olarte HH, Grassi D, and Scapagnini G. "Cardioprotection by cocoa polyphenols and omega-3 fatty acids: A disease-prevention perspective on aging-associated cardiovascular risk." J Med Food 21: 1–10 (2018)

Davison K, Coates AM, Buckley JD, and Howe PR. "Effect of cocoa flavanols and exercise on cardiometabolic risk factors in overweight and obese subjects." Int J Obesity 32: 1289–1296 (2008)

Donaldson IJ and Göttgens B. "Evolution of candidate transcriptional regulatory motifs since the human-chimpanzee divergence." Genome Biol 7: R52 (2006)

Erlank H, Elmann A, Kohen R, and Kanner J. "Polyphenols activate Nrf2 in astrocytes via H2O2, semiquinones, and quinones." Free Radic Biol Med 51: 2319–27 (2011)

Ford RJ, Desjardins EM, and Steinberg GR. "Are SIRTI activators another indirect method to increase AMPK for beneficial effects on aging and metabolic syndrome?" EBioMedicine 19: 16–17 (2017)

Gambelli L and Santaroni GP. "Polyphenols content in some Italian red wines of different geographical origins." Journal of Food Composition and Analysis. 17: 613–618 (2004)

Gijsbers L, van Eekelen HD, de Haan LH, Swier JM, Heijink NL, Kloet SK, Man HY, Bovy AG, Keijer J, Aarts JM, van der Burg B, and Rietjens IM. "Induction of peroxisome proliferator-activated receptor ɣ (PPARɣ)-mediated gene expression by tomato (Solanum lycopersicum L.) extracts." J Agric Food Chem 61: 3419–3427 (2013)

Gilad Y, Oshlack A, Smyth GK, Speed TP, and White KP. "Expression profiling in primates reveals a rapid evolution of human transcription factors." Nature 440: 242–245 (2006)

Hardie DG, Ross FA, and Hawley SA. "AMPK: A nutrient and energy sensor that maintains energy homeostasis." Nat Rev Mol Cell Biol 13: 251–262 (2012)

Hardie DG. "Keeping the home fires burning: AMP-activated protein kinase." J Royal Society Interface. 15: 20170774 (2018)

Herman WH, Pan Q, Edelstein SL, Mather KJ, Perreault L, Barrett-Connor E, Dabelea DM, Horton E, Kahn SE, Knowler WC, Lorenzo C, Pi-Sunyer X, Venditti E, and Ye W. "Impact of lifestyle and metformin interventions on the risk of progression to diabetes and regression to normal glucose regulation in overweight or obese people with impaired glucose regulation." Diabetes Care 40: 1668–1677 (2017)

Hidalgo J, Flores C, Hidalgo MA, Perez M, Yanez A, Quinones L, Caceres DD, and Burgos RA. "Delphinol standardized maqui berry extract reduces postprandial blood glucose increase in individuals with impaired glucose regulation by novel mechanism of sodium glucose cotransporter inhibition." Panminerva Med 56:1–7 (2014)

Huber B, Eberl L, Feucht W, and Polster J. "Influence of polyphenols on bacterial biofilm formation and quorum-sensing." Z Naturforsch C 58: 879–884 (2003)

Hwang JT, Kwon DY, and Yoon SH. "AMP-activated protein kinase: A potential target for the diseases prevention by natural occurring polyphenols." N Biotechnol 26: 17–22 (2009)

Hybertson BM, Gao B, Bose SK, and McCord JM. "Oxidative stress in health and disease: The therapeutic potential of Nrf2 activation." Mol Aspects Med 32: 234–246 (2011)

Know, L. *Life: The Epic Story of Our Mitochondria.* Friesen Press. Victoria, BC, Canada. (2014)

Knowler WC, Barrett-Connor E, Fowler SE, Hamman RF, Lachin JM, Walker EA, and Nathan DM. "Reduction in the incidence of type 2 diabetes with lifestyle intervention or metformin." N Engl J Med 346: 393–403 (2002)

Krikorian R, Shidler MD, Nash TA, Kalt W, Vinqvist-Tymchuk MR, Shukitt-Hale B, and Joseph JA. "Blueberry supplementation improves memory in older adults." J Agric Food Chem 58:3996–4000 (2010)

Kulkari SS and Canto C. "The molecular targets of resveratrol." Biochim Biophys Acta 1852: 1114–1123 (2015)

Lambert K, Hokayem M, Thomas C, Fabre O, Cassan C, Bourret A, Bernex F, Feuillet-Coudray C, Notarnicola C, Mercier J, Avignon A, and Bisbal C. "Combination of nutritional polyphenols supplementation with exercise training counteracts insulin resistance and improve endurance in high-fat diet-induced obese rats." Sci Rep 8: 2885 (2018)

Landete JM. "Updated knowledge about polyphenols: Functions, bioavailability, metabolism, and health." Crit Rev Food Sci Nutr 52: 936–948 (2012)

Lane N. *Power, Sex, and Suicide: Mitochondria and the Meaning of Life.* Oxford University Press. Oxford, UK (2005)

Lewis KN, Wason E, Edrey YH, Kristan DM, Nevo E, and Buffenstein R. "Regulation of Nrf2 signaling and longevity in naturally long-lived rodents." Proc Natl Acad Sci U S A 112: 3722–3727 (2015)

Li W, Khor TO, Xu C, Shen G, Jeong WS, Yu S, and Kong AN. "Activation of Nrf2-antioxidant signaling attenuates NF-κB-inflammatory response and elicits apoptosis." Biochem Pharmacol 76: 1485–1489 (2008)

Manoharan I, Suryawanshi A, Hong Y, Ranganathan P, Shanmugam A, Ahmad S, Swafford D, Manicassamy B, Ramesh G, Koni PA, Thangaraju M, and Manicassamy S. "Homeostatic PPARγ signaling limits inflammatory responses to commensal microbiota in the intestine." J Immunol 196: 4739–4749 (2016)

Matsumoto H, Inaba H, Kishi M, Tominaga S, Hirayama M, and Tsuda T. "Orally administered delphinidin 3-rutinoside and cyanidin 3-rutinoside are directly absorbed in rats and humans and appear in the blood as the intact forms." J Agric Food Chem 49: 1546–1551 (2001)

Menzies KJ, Singh K, Saleem A, and Hood DA. "Sirtuin 1-mediated effects of exercise and resveratrol on mitochondrial biogenesis." J Biol Chem 288: 6968–6979 (2013)

Nowick K, Gernat T, Almaas E, and Stubbs L. "Differences in human and chimpanzee gene expression patterns define an evolving network of transcription factors in brain." Proc Natl Acad Sci U S A 106: 22358–22363 (2009)

Ozdal T, Sela DA, Xiao J, Boyacioglu D, Chen F, and Capanoglu E. "The reciprocal interactions between polyphenols and gut microbiota and effects on bioaccessibility." Nutrients 8:2-36 (2016)

Perdomo-Sabogal A, Kanton S, Walter MB, and Nowick K. "The role of gene regulatory factors in the evolutionary history of humans." Curr Opin Genet Dev 29: 60–67 (2014)

Rabassa M, Zamora-Ros R, Andres-Lacueva C, Urpi-Sarda M, Bandinelli S, Ferrucci L and Cherubini A. "Association between both total baseline urinary and dietary polyphenols and substantial physical performance decline risk in older adults: A 9-year follow-up of the InCHIANTI Study." J Nutr Health Aging 20: 478–485 (2016)

Rivera-Chávez F, Zhang LF, Faber F, Lopez CA, Byndloss MX, Olsan EE, Xu G, Velazquez EM, Lebrilla CB, Winter SE, and Bäumler AJ. "Depletion of butyrate-producing clostridia from the gut microbiota drives an aerobic luminal expansion of Salmonella." Cell Host Microbe 19: 443–454 (2016)

Roopchand DE, Carmody RN, Kuhn P, Moskal K, Rojas-Silva P, Turnbaugh PJ, and Raskin I. "Dietary polyphenols promote growth of the gut bacterium *Akkermansia muciniphila* and attenuate high-fat diet-induced metabolic syndrome." Diabetes 64: 2847–2858 (2015)

Scalbert A, Johnson IT, and Saltmarsh M. "Polyphenols: Antioxidants and beyond." Am J Clin Nutr 81: 215S–217S (2005)

Scapagnini G, Vasto S, Abraham NG, Caruso C, Zella D, and Fabio G. "Modulation of Nrf2/ARE pathway by food polyphenols: A nutritional neuroprotective strategy for cognitive and neurodegenerative disorders." Mol Neurobiol 44: 192–201 (2011)

Scazzocchio B, Varì R, Filesi C, D'Archivio M, Santangelo C, Giovannini C, Iacovelli A, Silecchia G, Li Volti G, Galvano F, and Masella R. "Cyanidin-3-O-β-glucoside and protocatechuic acid exert insulin-like effects by upregulating PPARγ activity in human omental adipocytes." Diabetes 60: 2234–2244 (2011)

Schneeberger M, Everard A, Gómez-Valadés AG, Matamoros S, Ramírez S, Delzenne NM, Gomis R, Claret M, and Cani PD. "*Akkermansia muciniphila* inversely correlates with the onset of inflammation, altered adipose tissue metabolism and metabolic disorders during obesity in mice." Sci Rep 13: 16643 (2015)

Schottker B, Saum KU, Jansen EH, Boffetta P, Trichopoulou A, Holleczek B, Dieffenbach AK, and Brenner H. "Oxidative stress markers and all-cause mortality at older age: A population-based cohort study." J Gerontol A Biol Sci Med Sci 70: 518–24 (2015)

Sears B and Ricordi C. "Role of fatty acids and polyphenols in inflammatory gene transcription and their impact on obesity, metabolic syndrome, and diabetes." Eur Rev Med Pharmacol Sci 16: 1137–1154 (2012)

Sears B. *The Mediterranean Zone.* Ballantine Books. New York, NY (2014)

Sears B. "Polyphenols: Novel applications in human health." CellR4 5: e2437 (2017)

Serra D, Almeida LM, and Dinis TC. "Anti-inflammatory protection afforded by cyanidin-3-glucoside and resveratrol in human intestinal cells via Nrf2 and PPAR-γ: Comparison with 5-aminosalicylic acid." Chem Biol Interact 260: 102–109 (2016)

Slobodníková L, Fialova S, Rendekova K, Kovac, and Mucaji P. "Antibiofilm activity of plant polyphenols." Molecules 21: E1717 (2016)

Smith BK and Steinberg GR. "AMP-activated protein kinase, fatty acid, metabolism, and insulin sensitivity." Curr Opin Clin Nutr Metab Care 20: 248–253 (2017)

Solano C, Echeverz M, and Lasa I. "Biofilm dispersion and quorum sensing." Curr Opin Microbiol 18: 96–104 (2014)

Urpi-Sarda M, Andres-Lacueva C, Rabassa M, Ruggiero C, Zamora-Ros R, Bandinelli S, Ferrucci L, and Cherubini A. "The relationship between urinary total polyphenols and the frailty phenotype in a community-dwelling older population: The InCHIANTI study." J Gerontol A Biol Sci Med Sci 70: 1141–1147 (2015)

Zamora-Ros R, Rabassa M, Cherubini A, Urpí-Sardà M, Bandinelli S, Ferrucci L, and Andres-Lacueva C. "High concentrations of a urinary biomarker of polyphenol intake are associated with decreased mortality in older adults." J Nutr 143: 1445–1450 (2013)

Zang M, Xu S, Maitland-Toolan KA, Zuccollo A, Hou X, Jiang B, Wierzbicki M, Verbeuren TJ, and Cohen RA. "Polyphenols stimulate AMP-activated protein kinase, lower lipids, and inhibit accelerated atherosclerosis in diabetic LDL-receptor-deficient mice." Diabetes 55: 2180–2191 (2006)

CHAPTER 12: PERSONALIZING THE ZONE PRO-RESOLUTION NUTRITION SYSTEM

Beglinger C, and Degen L. "Fat in the intestine as a regulator of appetite—role of CCK." Physiol Behav 83: 617–621 (2004)

Cai Z, Xiao M, Chang L, and Yan LJ. "Role of insulin resistance in Alzheimer's disease." Metab Brain Dis 30: 839–851 (2015)

De Silva A and Bloom SR. "Gut hormones and appetite control: A focus on PYY and GLP-1 as therapeutic targets in obesity." Gut Liver 6: 10–20 (2012)

Duda-Chodak A, Tarko T, Satora P, and Sroka P. "Interaction of dietary compounds, especially polyphenols, with the intestinal microbiota." Eur J Nutr 54: 325–341 (2015)

Holst JJ. "Peptide YY and glucagon-like peptide-1 contribute to decreased food intake after Roux-en-Y gastric bypass surgery." Int J Obes 40:1699–1706 (2016)

Johnson CS, Sears B, Perry M, and Knurick JR. "Use of novel high-protein functional food products as part of a calorie-restricted diet to reduce insulin resistance and increase lean body mass in adults: A randomized controlled trial." Nutrients 9: 1182 (2017)

Kim J, Chae YK, and Chernoff A. "The risk for coronary heart disease according to insulin resistance with and without type 2 diabetes." Endocr Res 38: 195–205 (2013)

le Roux CW, Welbourn R, Werling M, Osborne A, Kokkinos A, Laurenius A, Lönroth H, Fändriks L, Ghatei MA, Bloom SR, and Olbers T. "Gut hormones as mediators of appetite and weight loss after Roux-en-Y gastric bypass." Ann Surg 246: 780–785 (2007)

Léveillé P, Chouinard-Watkins R, Windust A, Lawrence P, Cunnane SC, Brenna JT, and Plourde M. "Metabolism of uniformly labeled 13C-eicosapentaenoic acid and 13C-arachidonic acid in young and old men." Am J Clin Nutr 106: 467–474 (2017)

Ludwig DS, Majzoub JA, Al-Zahrani A, Dallal GE, Blanco I, and Roberts SB. "High glycemic index foods, overeating, and obesity." Pediatrics 103: E26 (1999)

Markovic TP, Jenkins AB, Campbell LV, Furler SM, Kraegen EW, and Chisholm DJ. "The determinants of glycemic responses to diet restriction and weight loss in obesity and NIDDM." Diabetes Care 21: 687–694 (1998)

McLaughlin T, Allison G, Abbasi F, Lamendola C, and Reaven G. "Prevalence of insulin resistance and associated cardiovascular disease risk factors among normal weight, overweight, and obese individuals." Metabolism 53: 495–499 (2004)

Ostman EM, Liljeberg Elmståhl HG, and Björck IM. "Inconsistency between glycemic and insulinemic responses to regular and fermented milk products." Am J Clin Nutr 74: 96–100 (2001)

Reaven GM. "Relationships among insulin resistance, type 2 diabetes, essential hypertension, and cardiovascular disease: similarities and differences." J Clin Hypertens 13: 238–243 (2011)

Reaven G. "Insulin resistance and coronary heart disease in nondiabetic individuals." Arterioscler Thromb Vasc Biol 32: 1754–1759 (2012)

Rubio L, Macia A, and Motilva MJ. "Impact of various factors on pharmacokinetics of bioactive polyphenols: An overview." Curr Drug Metab 5: 62–76 (2014)

Sears B. *The Zone*. Regan Books. New York, NY (1995)

Sears B. *Mastering the Zone*. Regan Books. New York, NY (1997)

Sears B. *Zone Perfect Meals in Minutes*. Regan Books. New York, NY (1997)

Sears B. *Zone Food Blocks*. Regan Books. New York, NY (1998)

Sears B. *100 Great Zone Foods*. Regan Books. New York, NY (2001)

Sears B. *What to Eat in the Zone*. Regan Books. New York, NY (2003)

Sears L and Sears B. *Zone Meals in Seconds*. Regan Books. New York, NY (2004)

Sears B and Perry M. "The role of fatty acids in insulin resistance." Lipids Health Disease 14: 121 (2015)

Sharon G, Garg N, Debelius J, Knight R, Dorrestein PC, and Mazmanian SK. "Specialized metabolites from the microbiome in health and disease." Cell Metab 20: 719–730 (2014)

Svane MS, Jørgensen NB, Bojsen-Møller KN, Dirksen C, Nielsen S, Kristiansen VB, Toräng S, Wewer Albrechtsen N, Rehfeld JF, Hartmann B, Madsbad S, Talbot K, Wang HY, Kazi H, Han LY, Bakshi KP, Stucky A, Fuino RL, Kawaguchi KR, Samoyedny AJ, Wilson RS, Arvanitakis Z, Schneider JA, Wolf BA, Bennett DA, Trojanowski JQ, and Arnold SE. "Demonstrated brain insulin resistance in Alzheimer's disease patients is associated with IGF-1 resistance, IRS-1 dysregulation, and cognitive decline." J Clin Invest 122: 1316–1338 (2012)

Umhau JC, Zhou W, Carson RE, Rapoport SI, Polozova A, Demar J, Hussein N, Bhattacharjee AK, Ma K, Esposito G, Majchrzak S, Herscovitch P, Eckelman WC, Kurdziel KA, and Salem N Jr. "Imaging incorporation of circulating docosahexaenoic acid into the human brain using positron emission tomography." J Lipid Res 50: 1259–1268 (2009)

Verdile G, Keane KN, Cruzat VF, Medic S, Sabale M, Rowles J, Wijesekara N, Martins RN, Fraser PE, and Newsholme P. "Inflammation and oxidative stress: The molecular connectivity between insulin resistance, obesity, and Alzheimer's disease." Mediators Inflamm 2015: 105828 (2015)

Wickremesekera K, Miller G, Naotunne TD, Knowles G, and Stubbs RS. "Loss of insulin resistance after Roux-en-Y gastric bypass surgery: A time course study." Obes Surg 15: 474–481 (2005)

Yee LD, Lester JL, Cole RM, Richardson JR, Hsu JC, Li Y, Lehman A, Belury MA, and Clinton SK. "Omega-3 fatty acid supplements in women at high risk of breast cancer have dose-dependent effects on breast adipose tissue fatty acid composition." Am J Clin Nutr 91: 1185–1194 (2010)

CHAPTER 13: DIET FACTS AND FALLACIES

Appleby PN, Crowe FL, Bradbury KE, Tavis RC, and Key TJ. "Mortality in vegetarians and comparable nonvegetarians in the United Kingdom." Am J Clin Nutr 103: 218–230 (2016)

Arnardottir H, Orr SK, Dalli J, and Serhan CN. "Human milk proresolving mediators stimulate resolution of acute inflammation." Mucosal Immunol 9: 757-766 (2016)

Bao J, de Jong V, Atkinson F, Petocz P, and Brand-Miller JC. "Food insulin index: Physiologic basis for predicting insulin demand evoked by composite meals." Am J Clin Nutr 90: 986–992 (2009)

Biesiekierski JR, Peters SL, Newnham ED, Rosella O, Muir JG, and Gibson PR. "No effects of gluten in patients with self-reported non-celiac gluten sensitivity after dietary reduction of fermentable, poorly absorbed, short-chain carbohydrates." Gastroenterology 145: 320–328 (2013)

Blaser MJ. "The theory of disappearing microbiota and the epidemics of chronic disease." Nat Rev 17: 461–463 (2017)

Boudry G, Hamilton MK, Chicholwski M, Wichramasinghe S, Barile D, Kalaneta KM, Mills DA, and Raybould HE. "Bovine milk oligosaccharides decrease gut permeability and improve inflammation and microbial dysbosis in diet-induced obese mice." J Dairy Sci 100:2471–2481 (2017)

Burger J, Kirchner M, Bramanti B, Haak W, and Thomas MG. "Absence of the lactase-persistence-associated allele in early Neolithic Europeans." Proc Nat Acad Sci USA 104: 3736–3741 (2007)

Cabrera G, Fernández-Brando RJ, Mejías MP, Ramos MV, Abrey-Recalde MJ, Vanzulli S, Vermeulen M, and Palermo MS. "Leukotriene C4 increases the susceptibility of adult mice to Shiga toxin-producing Escherichia coli infection." Int J Med Microbiol 305: 910–917 (2015)

Carden TJ and Carr TP. "Food availability of glucose and fat, but not fructose, increased in the U.S. between 1970 and 2009: Analysis of the USDA food availability data system." Nutr J 12: 130 (2013)

Cargnello M, Tcherkezian J, and Roux PP. "The expanding role of mTOR in cancer cell growth and proliferation." Mutagenesis 30: 169–176 (2015)

Chiarini F, Evangelisti C, McCubrey JA, and Martelli AM. "Current treatment strategies for inhibiting mTOR in cancer." Trends Pharmacol Sci 36: 124–135 (2015).

Cohen DH and LeRoith D. "Obesity, type 2 diabetes, and cancer: The insulin and IGF connection." Endocr Relat Cancer 19: F27–45 (2012)

Cozma AI, Sievenpiper JL, de Souza RJ, Chiavaroli L, Ha V, Wang DD, Mirrahimi A, Yu ME, Carleton AJ, Di Buono M, Jenkins AL, Leiter LA, Wolever TM, Beyene J, Kendall CW, and Jenkins DJ. "Effect of fructose on glycemic control in diabetes: A systematic review and meta-analysis of controlled feeding trials." Diabetes Care 35: 1611–1620 (2012)

Dong Z, Zhou S, and Mechef Y. "LC-MS/MS analysis of permethylated free oligosaccharides and N-glycans derived from human, bovine, and goat milk samples." Electrophoresis 37: 1532–1548 (2016)

Drago S, El Asmar R, Di Pierro M, Grazia Clemente M, Tripathi A, Sapone A, Thakar M, Iacono G, Carroccio A, D'Agate C, Not T, Zampini L, Catassi C, and Fasano A. "Gliadin, zonulin and gut permeability: Effects on celiac and non-celiac intestinal mucosa and intestinal cell lines." Scand J Gastroenterol 41: 408–419 (2006)

GBD 2016 Alcohol Collaborators. "Alcohol use and burden for 195 countries and territories, 1990-2016: A systematic analysis for the Global Burden of Disease study 2016." Lancet 392: 1015–1035 (2018)

Gerbault P, Libert A, Itan Y, Powell A, Currat M, and Burger J. "Evolution of lactose persistence: An example of human niche construction." Phil Trans Royal Soc B 366: 863–877 (2011)

Hamilton MK, Ronveaux CC, Rust BM, Newman JW, Hawley M, Barile D, and Raybould HE. "Prebiotic milk oligosaccharides prevent the development of obese phenotype, impairment of gut permeability, and microbial dysbiosis in high-fat fed mice." Am J Physiol Gastrointest Liver Physiol 312: G474–G487 (2017)

Hardie DG, Ross FA, and Hawley SA. "AMP-activate protein kinase: A target for drugs both ancient and modern." Chem Bio 19: 1222–1236 (2012)

Hokayem M, Blond E, Vidal H, Lambert K, Meugnier E, Feillet-Coudray C, Coudray C, Pesenti S, Luyton C, Lambert-Porcheron S, Sauvinet V, Fedou C, Brun JF, Rieusset J, Bisbal C, Sultan A, Mercier J, Goudable J, Dupuy AM, Cristol JP, Laville M, and Avignon A. "Grape polyphenols prevent fructose-induced oxidative stress and insulin resistance in first-degree relatives of type 2 diabetic patients." Diabetes Care 36: 1454–1461 (2013)

Hwang DH, Kim JA, and Lee JY. "Mechanisms for the activation of Toll-like receptor 2/4 by saturated fatty acids and inhibition by docosahexaenoic acid." Eur J Pharmacol 785: 24–35 (2016)

Institute of Medicine: *Dietary Reference Intakes: Energy, Carbohydrate, Fiber, Fat, Fatty Acids, Cholesterol, Protein, and Amino Acids.* Washington, DC, National Academies Press. (2002)

Itan Y, Powell A, Beaumont MA, Burger J, and Thomas MG. "The origin of lactase persistence in the Europe." PLoS Comput Biol 5: e1000491 (2009)

Jang C, Hui S, Lu W, Cowan AJ, Morscher RJ, Lee G, Liu W, Tesz GJ, Birnbaum MJ, and Rabinowitz JD. "The small intestine converts dietary fructose into glucose and organic acids." Cell Metab 27: 351–361 (2018)

Kendall CW, and Jenkins DJ. "Effect of fructose on postprandial triglycerides: A systematic review and meta-analysis of controlled feeding trials." Atherosclerosis 232: 125–133 (2014)

Kolberg J and Sollid L. "Lectin activity of gluten identified as wheat germ agglutinin." Biochem Biophys Res Commun 130: 867–872 (1985)

Kretchmer N. "Expression of lactase during development." Am J Human Genet 45: 487–488 (1989)

Kunz C and Rudloff S. "Potential anti-inflammatory and anti-infectious effects of human milk oligosaccharides." Adv Exp Med Bio 606: 455–465 (2006)

Levinovitz A. *The Gluten Lie.* Regan Arts. New York, NY (2015)

Li F, Yin Y, Tan B, Kong X, and Wu G. "Leucine nutrition in animals and humans: mTOR signaling and beyond." Amino Acids 41: 1185–1193 (2011)

Lowndes J, Kawiecki D, Pardo S, Nguyen V, Melanson KJ, Yu Z, and Rippe JM. "The effects of four hypocaloric diets containing different levels of sucrose or high fructose corn syrup on weight loss and related parameters." Nutr J 11: 55 (2012)

Marriott BP, Cole N, and Lee E. "National estimates of dietary fructose intake from 1977 to 2004 in the United States." J Nutrition 139: 1228S–1235S (2009)

Mehra R, Sarie D, Marotta M, Lebrille CB, Chu C, and German JB. "Novel high-molecular weight fucosylated milk oligosaccharides identified in dairy streams." PLoS One 9: e96040 (2014)

Mihrshahi S, Ding D, Gale J, Allman-Farinelli M, Banks E, and Bauman AE. "Vegetarian diet and all-cause mortality: Evidence from a large population-based Australian cohort-the 45 and Up Study." Preventive Medicine 97: 1–7 (2017)

Murry RD, Ailaboui AH, Powers PA McClung HJ, Li Bu, Heitlinger LA, and Sloan HR. "Absorption of lactose from the colon of the newborn piglet." Am J Physiol 261: G1–8 (1991)

Orlich MJ, Singh PN, Sabate J, Kaceido-Siegl K, Fan J, Knutsen S Beeson L, and Fraser GE. "Vegetarian dietary plans and mortality in Adventist Health Study 2." JAMA Intern Med 173: 1230–1238 (2013)

Ostman EM, Liljeberg Elmståhl HG, and Björck IM. "Inconsistency between glycemic and insulinemic responses to regular and fermented milk products." Am J Clin Nutr 74: 96–100 (2001)

Owen OE, Felig P, Morgan AP, Wahren J, and Cahill GF. "Liver and kidney metabolism during prolonged starvation." J Clin Invest 48: 574–583 (1969)

Peng L, Li ZR, Green RS, Holzman IR, and Lin J. "Butyrate enhances the intestinal barrier by facilitating tight junction assembly via activation of AMP-activated protein kinase in Caco-2 cell monolayers." J Nutr 139: 1619–1625 (2009)

Plöger S, Stumpff F, Penner GB, Schulzke JD, Gäbel G, Martens H, Shen Z, Günzel D, and Aschenbach JR. "Microbial butyrate and its role for barrier function in the gastrointestinal tract." Ann N Y Acad Sci 1258: 52–59 (2012)

Qin LQ, He K, and Xu JY. "Milk consumption and circulating insulin-like growth factor-I level: A systematic literature review." Int J Food Sci Nutr 60 (Suppl 7): 330–340 (2009)

Sears B. *The Anti-Aging Zone*. Regan Books. New York, NY (1999)

Sears B. *Toxic Fat*. Thomas Nelson. Nashville, TN (2008)

Sievenpiper JL, de Souza RJ, Mirrahimi A, Yu ME, Carleton AJ, Beyene J, Chiavaroli L, Di Buono M, Jenkins AL, Leiter LA, Wolever TM, Kendall CW, and Jenkins DJ. "Effect of fructose on body weight in controlled feeding trials: A systematic review and meta-analysis." Ann Intern Med 156: 291–304 (2012)

Siri-Tarino PW, Sun Q, Hu FB, and Krauss RM. "Meta-analysis of prospective cohort studies evaluating the association of saturated fat with cardiovascular disease." Am J Clin Nutr 91: 535–546 (2010)

Stahel P, Kim JJ, Xiao C, and Cant JP. "Of milk the sugars, galactose, but not prebiotic galacto-oligoscaccharide, improves insulin sensitivity in male Sprague-Dawley rats." PLoS 12: e0172260 (2017)

Suez J, Korem T, Zeevi D, Zilberman-Schapira G, Thaiss CA, Maza O, Israeli D, Zmora N, Gilad S, Weinberger A, Kuperman Y, Harmelin A, Kolodkin-Gal I, Shapiro H, Halpern Z, Segal E, and Elinav E. "Artificial sweeteners induce glucose intolerance by altering the gut microbiota." Nature 514: 181–186 (2014)

Tome D. "Criteria and markers for protein quality assessment - a review." Br J Nutr 108 (Suppl 2): S222–229 (2012)

Troelsen JT. "Adult-type hypolactasia and regulation of lactase expression." Biochim Biophys Acta 1723: 19–32 (2005)

Topiwala A, All CL, Valkanova V, Zsoldos E, Filippini N, Sexton C, Mahmood A, Fooks P, Signh-Manoux A, Mackay CE, Kivimaki M, and Ebeier KP. "Moderate alcohol consumption as risk factor for adverse brain outcomes and cognitive decline." BMJ 357: 2353 (2017)

Wang DD, Sievenpiper JL, de Souza RJ, Chiavaroli L, Ha V, Cozma AI, Mirrahimi A, Yu ME, Carleton AJ, Di Buono M, Jenkins AL, Leiter LA, Wolever TM, Beyene J, Kendall CW, and Jenkins DJ. "The effects of fructose intake on serum uric acid vary among controlled dietary trials." J Nutr 42: 916–923 (2012)

Wang DD, Sievenpiper JL, de Souza RJ, Cozma AI, Chiavaroli L, Ha V, Mirrahimi A, Carleton AJ, Di Buono M, Jenkins AL, Leiter LA, Wolever TM, Beyene J, Kendall CW, and Jenkins DJ. "Effect of fructose on postprandial triglycerides: A systematic review and meta-analysis of controlled feeding trials." Atherosclerosis 232: 125–133 (2014)

Zhao J, Stockwell T, Boemer A, Naimi T, and Chikritzhs T. "Alcohol consumption and morality from coronary heart disease." J Stud Alcohol Drugs 78: 375–386 (2017)

Zhou BR, Zhang JA, Zhang Q, Permatasari F, Xu Y, Wu D, Yin ZQ, and Luo D. "Palmitic acid induces production of proinflammatory cytokines interleukin-6, interleukin-1β, and tumor necrosis factor-αvia a NF-κB-dependent mechanism in HaCaT keratinocytes." Mediators Inflamm 2013: 530429 (2013)

Zong G, Li Y, Wanders AJ, Alssema M, Zock PL, Willett WC, Hu FB, and Sun Q. "Intake of individual saturated fatty acids and risk of coronary heart disease in US men and women: Two prospective longitudinal cohort studies." BMJ 355: i5796 (2016)

CHAPTER 14: DIET WARS: COMPARISON OF THE ZONE DIET TO OTHER DIETS

Andrews RC and Walker BR. "Glucocorticoids and insulin resistance: Old hormones, new targets." Clin Sci 96: 513–523 (1999)

Appel LJ, Moore TJ, Obarzanek E, Vollmer WM, Svetkey LP, Sacks FM, Bray GA, Vogt TM, Cutler JA, Windhauser MM, Lin PH, and Karanja N. "A clinical trial of the effects of dietary patterns on blood pressure. DASH Collaborative Research Group." N Engl J Med 336: 1117–1124 (1997)

Barnosky AR, Hoddy KK, Unterman TG, and Varady KA. "Intermittent fasting vs daily calorie restriction for type 2 diabetes prevention: A review of human findings." Transl Res 164: 302–311 (2014)

Carter S, Clifton PM, and Keogh JB. "Effect of intermittent compared with continuous energy restricted diet on glycemic control in patients with type

2 diabetes: A randomized noninferiority trial." JAMA Netw Open 1: e180756 (2018)

Eaton SB and Konner M. "Paleolithic nutrition. A consideration of its nature and current implications." N Engl J Med 312: 283–289 (1985)

Ebbeling CB, Swain JF, Feldman HA, Wong WW, Hachey DL, Garcia-Lago E, and Ludwig DS. "Effects of dietary composition on energy expenditure during weight-loss maintenance." JAMA 307: 2627–2634 (2012)

Estruch R, Ros E, Salas-Salvadó J, Covas MI, Corella D, Arós F, Gómez-Gracia E, Ruiz-Gutiérrez V, Fiol M, Lapetra J, Lamuela-Raventos RM, Serra-Majem L, Pintó X, Basora J, Muñoz MA, Sorlí JV, Martínez JA, and Martínez-González MA. "Primary prevention of cardiovascular disease with a Mediterranean diet." N Engl J Med 368: 1279–1290 (2013)

Estruch R, Ros E, Salas-Salvadó J, Covas MI, Corella D, Arós F, Gómez-Gracia E, Ruiz-Gutiérrez V, Fiol M, Lapetra J, Lamuela-Raventos RM, Serra-Majem L, Pintó X, Basora J, Muñoz MA, Sorlí JV, Martínez JA, and Martínez-González MA. "Retraction and republication: Primary prevention of cardiovascular disease with a Mediterranean diet." N Engl J Med 378: 2441–2442 (2018)

Estruch R, Ros E, Salas-Salvadó J, Covas MI, Corella D, Arós F, Gómez-Gracia E, Ruiz-Gutiérrez V, Fiol M, Lapetra J, Lamuela-Raventos RM, Serra-Majem L, Pintó X, Basora J, Muñoz MA, Sorlí JV, Martínez JA, Fitó M, Gea A, Hernán MA, and Martínez-González MA. "Primary prevention of cardiovascular disease with a Mediterranean diet supplemented with extra-virgin olive oil or nuts." N Engl J Med 378:e34 (2018)

Geer EB, Islam J, and Buettner C. "Mechanisms of glucocorticoid-induced insulin resistance: Focus on adipose tissue function and lipid metabolism." Endocrinol Metab Clin North Am 43: 75–102 (2014)

Giusti J and Rizzott J. "Interpreting the Joslin Diabetes Center and Joslin Clinic clinical guideline for overweight and obese adults with type 2 diabetes." Curr Diab Report 6: 405–408 (2006)

Hall KD, Bemis T, Brychta R, Chen KY, Courville A, Crayner EJ, Goodwin S, Guo J, Howard L, Knuth ND, Miller BV 3rd, Prado CM, Siervo M, Skarulis MC, Walter M, Walter PJ, and Yannai L. "Calorie for calorie, dietary fat restriction results in more body fat loss than carbohydrate restriction in people with obesity." Cell Metab 22: 427–436 (2015)

Hamdy O. "Diabetes weight management in clinical practice—the Why Wait model," US Endocrinology 4: 49–54 (2008)

Hamdy O and Carver C. "The Why WAIT program: Improving clinical outcomes through weight management in type 2 diabetes." Curr Diab Rep 8: 413–420 (2008)

Hamdy O, Mottalib A, Morsi A, El-Sayed N, Goebel-Fabbri A, Arathuzik G, Shahar J, Kirpitch A, and Zrebiec J. "Long-term effect of intensive lifestyle intervention on cardiovascular risk factors in patients with diabetes in real-world clinical practice: A 5-year longitudinal study." BMJ Open Diabetes Res Care 5: e000259 (2017)

Harris L, McGarty A, Hutchison L, Ells L, and Hankey C. "Short-term intermittent energy restriction interventions for weight management: A systematic review and meta-analysis." Obes Rev 19: 1–13 (2018)

Johnston CS, Tjonn SL, Swan PD, White A, Hutchins H, and Sears B. "Ketogenic low-carbohydrate diets have no metabolic advantage over non-ketogenic low-carbohydrate diets." Am J Clin Nutr 83: 1055–1061 (2006)

Johnston CS, Tjonn SL, Swan PD, White A, and Sears B. "Low-carbohydrate, high-protein diets that restrict potassium-rich fruits and vegetables promote calciuria." Osteoporos Int 17: 1820–1821 (2006)

Jornayvaz FR, Jurczak MJ, Lee HY, Birkenfeld AL, Frederick DW, Zhang D, Zhang XM, Samuel VT, and Shulman GI. "A high-fat, ketogenic diet causes hepatic insulin resistance in mice, despite increasing energy expenditure and preventing weight gain." Am J Physiol Endocrinol Metab 299: E808–815 (2010)

Khani S and Tayek JA. "Cortisol increases gluconeogenesis in humans: Its role in the metabolic syndrome." Clin Sci 101: 739–747 (2001)

Kuipers RS, Luxwolda MF, Dijck-Brouwer DA, Eaton SB, Crawford MA, Cordain L, and Muskiet FA. "Estimated macronutrient and fatty acid intakes from an East African Paleolithic diet." Br J Nutr 104: 1666–1687 (2010)

Morris MC, Tangney CC, Wang Y, Sacks FM, Bennett DA, and Aggarwal NT. "MIND diet associated with reduced incidence of Alzheimer's disease." Alzheimers Dement 11: 1007–1014 (2015)

Morris MC, Tangney CC, Wang Y, Sacks FM, Barnes LL, Bennett DA, and Aggarwal NT. "MIND diet slows cognitive decline with aging." Alzheimers Dement 11: 1015–1022 (2015)

Mosley M and Spencer M. *The Fast Diet*. Simon and Shuster. New York, NY (2013)

Nishihira J, Tokashiki T, Higashiuesato Y, Willcox DC, Mattek N, Shinto L, Ohya Y, and Dodge HH. "Associations between serum omega-3 fatty acid levels and cognitive functions among community-dwelling octogenarians in Okinawa, Japan: The KOCOA study." J Alzheimers Dis 51:857–866 (2016)

Sacks FM, Svetkey LP, Vollmer WM, Appel LJ, Bray GA, Harsha D, Obarzanek E, Conlin PR, Miller ER, Simons-Morton DG, Karanja N, and Lin PH. "Effects on blood pressure of reduced dietary sodium and the Dietary Approaches to Stop Hypertension (DASH) diet." N Engl J Med 344: 3–10 (2001)

Schübel R, Nattenmüller, Sookthai D, Nonnenmacher T, Graf ME, Riedl L, Schlett CL, von Stackelberg O, Johnson T, Nabers D, Kirsten R, Kratz M, Kauczor HU, Ulrich CM, Kaaks R, and Kühn T. "Effects of intermittent and continuous calorie restriction on body weight and metabolism over 50 wk: A randomized controlled trial." Am J Clin Nutr 108: 933–945 (2018)

Suzuki M, Willcox DC, Rosenbaum MW, and Willcox BJ. "Oxidative stress and longevity in Okinawa: An investigation of blood lipid peroxidation and tocopherol in Okinawan centenarians." Curr Gerontol Geriatr Res. 2010:380460 (2010)

Trepanowski JF, Kroeger CM, Barnosky A, Klempel MC, Bhutani S, Hoddy KK, Gabel K, Freels S, Rigdon J, Rood J, Ravussin E, and Varady KA. "Effect of alternate-day fasting on weight loss, weight maintenance, and cardioprotection among metabolically healthy obese adults: A randomized clinical trial." JAMA Intern Med 177: 930–938 (2017)

White AM, Johnston CS, Swan PD, Tjonn SL, and Sears B. "Blood ketones are directly related to fatigue and perceived effort during exercise in overweight adults adhering to low-carbohydrate diets for weight loss: A Pilot study." J Am Diet Assoc 107: 1792–1796 (2007)

Willcox BJ and Willcox DG. *The Okinawa Program: How the World's Longest-Lived People Achieve Everlasting Health—And How You Can Too.* Three Rivers Press. New York, NY (2001)

Willcox DC, Willcox BJ, Todoriki H, and Suzuki M. "The Okinawan diet: Health implications of a low-calorie, nutrient-dense, antioxidant-rich dietary pattern low in glycemic load." J Am Coll Nutr 28: 500S–516S (2009)

Willcox BJ and Willcox DC. "Caloric restriction, caloric restriction mimetics, and healthy aging in Okinawa: Controversies and clinical implications." Curr Opin Clin Nutr Metab Care17: 51–58 (2014)

Willcox DC, Scapagnini G, and Willcox BJ. "Healthy aging diets other than the Mediterranean: A focus on the Okinawan diet." Mech Ageing Dev 136-137: 148–162 (2014)

CHAPTER 15: ZONE PROTEIN: MAKING THE ZONE DIET EVEN EASIER TO FOLLOW

Chan JL, Mun EC, Stoyneva V, Mantzoros CS, and Goldfine AB. "Peptide YY levels are elevated after gastric bypass surgery." Obesity 14: 194–198 (2006)

De Silva A and Bloom SR. "Gut hormones and appetite control: A focus on PYY and GLP-1 as therapeutic targets in obesity." Gut Liver 6: 10–20 (2012)

Johnson CS, Sears B, Perry M, and Knurick JR. "Use of novel high-protein functional food products as part of a calorie-restricted diet to reduce insulin resistance and increase lean body mass in adults: A randomized controlled trial." Nutrients 9:1182 (2017)

Khalaf KH and Taegtmeyer H. "Clues from bariatric surgery: Reversing insulin resistance to heal the heart." Curr Diab Rep 13: 245–251 (2013)

Salehi M, Prigeon RL, and D'Alessio DA, "Gastric bypass surgery enhances glucagon-like peptide 1–stimulated postprandial insulin secretion in humans." Diabetes 60: 2308–2314 (2011)

Wickremesekera K, Miller G, Naotunne TD, Knowles G, and Stubbs RS. "Loss of insulin resistance after Roux-en-Y gastric bypass surgery: A time course study." Obes Surg 15: 474–48 (2005)

CHAPTER 16: YOUR FIRST 1,000 DAYS AND BEYOND

Ailhaud G, Guesnet P, and Cunnane SC. "An emerging risk factor for obesity: Does disequilibrium of polyunsaturated fatty acid metabolism contribute to excessive adipose tissue development?" Br J Nutr 100: 461–470 (2008)

Allis CD, Caparros M-L, Jenuwein T, and Reinberg D. *Epigenetics*. Cold Spring Harbor Laboratory Press. Cold Springs, NY (2007)

Alvheim AR, Malde MK, Osei-Hyiaman D, Lin YH, Pawlosky RJ, Madsen L, Kristiansen K, Frøyland L, and Hibbeln JR. "Dietary linoleic acid elevates endogenous 2-AG and anandamide and induces obesity." Obesity 20: 1984–1994 (2012)

Alvheim AR, Torstensen BE, Lin YH, Lillefosse HH, Lock EJ, Madsen L, Frøyland L, Hibbeln JR, and Malde MK. "Dietary linoleic acid elevates the endocannabinoids 2-AG and anandamide and promotes weight gain in mice fed a low-fat diet." Lipids 49: 59–69 (2014)

Bode L. "The functional biology of human milk oligosaccharides." Early Hum Dev 91: 619–622 (2015)

Calvani R, Picca A, Lo Monaco MR, Landi F, Bernabei R, and Marzetti E. "Of microbes and minds: A narrative review on the second brain aging." Front Med 5: 53 (2018)

Casey BJ, Jones RM, and Hare TA. "The adolescent brain." Ann N Y Acad Sci 1124: 111–126 (2008)

Catalano PM. "Trying to understand gestational diabetes." Diabet Med 31: 273–281 (2014)

Chalon S. "Omega-3 fatty acids and monoamine neurotransmission." Prostaglandins Leukot Essent Fatty Acids 75: 259–69 (2006)

Dabelea D, Mayer-Davis EJ, Saydah S, Imperatore G, Linder B, Divers J, Bell R, Badaru A, Talton JW, Crume T, Liese AD, Merchant AT, Lawrence JM, Reynolds K, Dolan L, Liu LL, and Hamman RF. "Prevalence of type 1 and type 2 diabetes among children and adolescents from 2001 to 2009." JAMA 311: 1778–1786 (2014)

Dominguez-Bello MG, Costello EK, Contreras M, Magris M, Hidalgo G, Fierer N, and Knight R. "Delivery mode shapes the acquisition and structure of the initial microbiota across multiple body habitats in newborns." Proc Natl Acad Sci U S A 107: 11971–11975 (2010)

el Hajj N, Schneider E, Lehnen H, and Haaf T. "Epigenetics and life-long consequences of an adverse nutritional and diabetic intrauterine environment." Reproduction 148: R111–20 (2014)

Evrensel A and Ceylan ME. "The gut-brain axis: The missing link in depression." Clin Psychopharmacol Neurosci 13: 239–244 (2015)

Ferrazzi E and Sears B eds. *Metabolic Syndrome and Complications of Pregnancy*. Springer. Heidelburg, Germany (2015)

Frye RE, Rose S, Chacko J, Wynne R, Bennuri SC, Slattery JC, Tippett M, Delhey L, Melnyk S, Kahler SG, and MacFabe DF. "Modulation of mitochondrial function by the microbiome metabolite propionic acid in autism and control cell lines." Transl Psychiatry 6: e927 (2016)

Germano M, Meleleo D, Montorfano G, Adorni L, Negroni M, Berra B, and Rizzo AM. "Plasma, red blood cells phospholipids and clinical evaluation after long chain omega-3 supplementation in children with attention deficit hyperactivity disorder (ADHD)." Nutr Neurosci 10: 1–9 (2007)

Hanbauer I, Rivero-Covelo I, Maloku E, Baca A, Hu Q, Hibbeln JR, and Davis JM. "The decrease of n-3 fatty acid energy percentage in an equicaloric diet fed to B6C3Fe mice for three generations elicits obesity." Cardiovasc Psychiatry Neurol 2009: 867041 (2009)

Jensen FE. *The Teenage Brain*. Harper Collins. New York, NY (2015)

Kodas E, Vancassel S, Lejeune B, Guilloteau D, and Chalon S. "Reversibility of n-3 fatty acid deficiency-induced changes in dopaminergic neurotransmission in rats: Critical role of developmental stage." J Lipid Res 43: 1209–1219 (2002)

Lacroix M, Kina E, and Hivert MF. "Maternal/fetal determinants of insulin resistance in women during pregnancy and in offspring over life." Curr Diab Rep 13: 238–244 (2013)

MacFabe DF. "Short-chain fatty acid fermentation products of the gut microbiome: Implications in autism spectrum disorders." Microb Ecol Health Dis 2012: 23 (2012)

Maftei O, Whitrow MJ, Davies MJ, Giles LC, Owens JA, and Moore VM. "Maternal body size prior to pregnancy, gestational diabetes and weight gain: Associations with insulin resistance in children at 9-10 years." Diabet Med 32: 174–180 (2015)

Massiera F, Saint-Marc P, Seydoux J, Murata T, Kobayashi T, Narumiya S, Guesnet P, Amri EZ, Negrel R, and Ailhaud G. "Arachidonic acid and prostacyclin signaling promote adipose tissue development: A human health concern?" J Lipid Res 44: 271–279 (2003)

Massiera F, Guesnet P, and Ailhaud G. "The crucial role of dietary n-6 polyunsaturated fatty acids in excessive adipose tissue development: Relationship to childhood obesity." Nestle Nutr Workshop Ser Pediatr Program 57: 235–242 (2006)

Massiera F, Barbry P, Guesnet P, Joly A, Luquet S, Moreilhon-Brest C, Mohsen-Kanson T, Amri EZ, and Ailhaud G. "A Western-like fat diet is sufficient to induce a gradual enhancement in fat mass over generations." J Lipid Res51: 2352–2361 (2010)

Mastrogiannis DS, Spiliopoulos M, Mulla W, and Homko CJ. "Insulin resistance: The possible link between gestational diabetes mellitus and hypertensive disorders of pregnancy." Curr Diab Rep 9: 296–302 (2009)

Möhler H. "The GABA system in anxiety and depression and its therapeutic potential." Neuropharmacology 62: 42–53 (2012)

Mojtabai R, Olfson M, and Han B. "National trends in the prevalence and treatment of depression in adolescents and young adults." Pediatrics 138: e20161878 (2016)

Morrison JL, Duffield JA, Muhlhausler BS, Gentili S, and McMillen IC. "Fetal growth restriction, catch-up growth and the early origins of insulin resistance and visceral obesity." Pediatr Nephrol 25: 669–677 (2010)

Mühlhäusler BS. "Programming of the appetite-regulating neural network: A link between maternal overnutrition and the programming of obesity?" J Neuroendocrinol 19: 67–72 (2007)

Muhlhausler BS and Ong ZY. "The fetal origins of obesity: Early origins of altered food intake." Endocr Metab Immune Disord Drug Targets11: 189–197 (2011)

Muhlhausler BS and Ailhaud GP. "Omega-6 polyunsaturated fatty acids and the early origins of obesity." Curr Opin Endocrinol Diabetes Obes 20: 56–61 (2013)

Munyaka PM, Khafipour E, and Ghia JE. "External influence of early childhood establishment of gut microbiota and subsequent health implications." Front Pediatr 2:109 (2014)

Nordgren TM, Lyden E. Anderson-Berry A, and and Hanson C. "Omega-3 fatty acid intake of pregnant women and women of childbearing age in the United States: Potential for deficiency?" Nutrients 9: 197 (2017)

Ong ZY and Muhlhausler BS. "Maternal "junk-food" feeding of rat dams alters food choices and development of the mesolimbic reward pathway in the offspring." FASEB J 25: 2167–2179 (2011)

Painter RC, de Rooij SR, Bossuyt PM, Simmers TA, Osmond C, Barker DJ, Bleker OP, and Roseboom TJ. "Early onset of coronary artery disease after prenatal exposure to the Dutch famine." Am J Clin Nutr 84: 322–327 (2006)

Pantham P, Aye IL, and Powell TL. "Inflammation in maternal obesity and gestational diabetes mellitus." Placenta 36: 709–715 (2015)

Poston L. "Intergenerational transmission of insulin resistance and type 2 diabetes." Prog Biophys Mol Biol 106: 315–322 (2011)

Ravelli AC, van Der Meulen JH, Osmond C, Barker DJ, and Bleker OP. "Obesity at the age of 50 y in men and women exposed to famine prenatally." Am J Clin Nutr 70: 811–816 (1999)

Roseboom TJ, van der Meulen JH, Ravelli AC, Osmond C, Barker DJ, and Bleker OP. "Effects of prenatal exposure to the Dutch famine on adult disease in later life: An overview." Mol Cell Endocrinol 185: 93–98 (2001)

Shultz SR, MacFabe DF, Ossenkopp KP, Scratch S, Whelan J, Taylor R, and Cain DP. "Intracerebroventricular injection of propionic acid, an enteric bacterial metabolic end-product, impairs social behavior in the rat: Implications for an animal model of autism." Neuropharmacology 54: 901–911 (2008)

See VHL, Mas E, Prescott SL, Beilin LJ, Burrows S, Barden AE, Huang RC, and Mori TA. "Effects of prenatal n-3 fatty acid supplementation on offspring resolvins at birth and 12 years of age: A double-blind, randomised controlled clinical trial." Br J Nutr 118:971–980 (2017)

Segovia SA, Vickers MH, Gray C, and Reynolds CM. "Maternal obesity, inflammation, and developmental programming." Biomed Res Int. 2014: 418975 (2014)

Singer K and Lumeng CN. "The initiation of metabolic inflammation in childhood obesity." J Clin Invest 127: 65–73 (2017)

Sorgi PJ, Hallowell EM, Hutchins HL, and Sears B. "Effects of an open-label pilot study with high-dose EPA/DHA concentrates on plasma phospholipids and behavior in children with attention deficit hyperactivity disorder." Nutr J 6: 16 (2007)

Stewart CJ, Ajami AJ, O'Brien JL, Hutchinson DS, Smith DP, Wong MC, Ross MC, Lloyd RE, Doddapaneni HV, Metcalf GA, Muzny D, Gibbs RA, Vatanen T, Huttenhower C, Xavier RJ, Rewers M, Hagopian W, Toppari J, Ziegler A-G, She J-X, Akolkar B, Lernmark A, Hyoty H, Vehik K, Krischer JP, and Petrosino JF. "Temporal development of the gut microbiome in early childhood from the TEDDY study." Nature 562: 583–588 (2018)

Strandwitz P. "Neurotransmitter modulation by the gut microbiota." Brain Res 1693(Pt B):128–133 (2018)

Tollesbol T. *Transgenerational Epigenetics.* Academic Press. London, UK (2014)

van Dijk SJ, Peters TJ, Buckley M, Zhou J, Jones PA, Gibson RA, Makrides M, Muhlhausler BS, and Molloy PL. "DNA methylation in blood from neonatal screening cards and the association with BMI and insulin sensitivity in early childhood." Int J Obes 42: 28–35 (2018)

Vickers MH. "Early life nutrition, epigenetics and programming of later life disease." Nutrients 6: 2165–2178 (2014)

Weinberger AH, Gbedemah M, Martinez AM, Nash D, Galea S, and Goodwin RD. "Trends in depression prevalence in the USA from 2005 to 2015: Widening disparities in vulnerable groups." Psychol Med 48: 1308–1315 (2018)

CHAPTER 17: REACHING PEAK PERFORMANCE

Anzalone A, Carbuhn A, Jones L, Gallop A, Smith A, Johnson P, Swearingen L, Moore C, Rimer E, McBeth J, Harris W, Kirk KM, Gable D, Askow A, Jennings W, and Oliver JM. "The omega-3 index in National Collegiate Athletic Association Division I collegiate football athletes." J Athl Train 54: 7–11 (2019)

Bergmann O, Zdunek S, Felker A, Salehpour M, Alkass K, Bernard S, Sjostrom SL, Szewczykowska M, Jackowska T, Dos Remedios C, Malm T, Andrä M, Jashari R, Nyengaard JR, Possnert G, Jovinge S, Druid H, and Frisén J. "Dynamics of cell generation and turnover in the human heart." Cell 61: 1566–1575 (2015)

Bloomer RJ, Larson DE, Fisher-Wellman KH, Galpin AJ, and Schilling BK. "Effect of eicosapentaenoic and docosahexaenoic acid on resting and exercise-induced inflammatory and oxidative stress biomarkers." Lipids Health Dis. 8: 36 (2009)

Bruckner G, Webb P, Greenwell L, Chow C, and Richardson D. "Fish oil increase peripheral capillary blood cell velocity in humans." Atherosclerosis 66: 237–245 (1987)

Budgett R. "Overtraining syndrome." Br J Sports Med 24: 231–236 (1990)

Burns TW, Terry BE, Langley PE, and Robison GA. "Insulin inhibition of lipolysis of human adipocytes: The role of cyclic adenosine monophosphate." Diabetes 28: 957–961 (1979)

Cantó C and Auwerx J. "Calorie restriction: Is AMPK a key sensor and effector?" Physiology 26: 214–224 (2011)

Casanova E, Baselga-Escudero L, Ribas-Latre A, Cedó L, Arola-Arnal A, Pinent M, Bladé C, Arola L, and Salvadó MJ. "Chronic intake of proanthocyanidins and docosahexaenoic acid improves skeletal muscle oxidative capacity in diet-obese rats." J Nutr Biochem 25: 1003–1010 (2014)

Clark A and Mach N. "The crosstalk between the gut microbiota and mitochondria during exercise." Front Physiol 8: 319 (2017)

Clarke SD and Jump D. "Polyunsaturated fatty acids regulate lipogenic and peroxisomal gene expression by independent mechanisms." Prostaglandins, Leukotrienes, and Essential Fatty Acids 57: 65–69 (1997)

Clavel S, Farout L, Briand M, Briand Y, and Jouanel P. "Effect of endurance training and/or fish oil supplemented diet on cytoplasmic fatty acid binding protein in rat skeletal muscles and heart." Eur J Appl Physiol 87: 193–201 (2002)

Constanti N and Hackney AC eds. *Endocrinology of Physical Activity and Sport.* Humana Press. New York, NY. (2013)

Dubé JJ, Broskey NT, Despines AA, Stefanovic-Racic M, Toledo FG, Goodpaster BH, and Amati F. "Muscle characteristics and substrate energetics in lifelong endurance athletes." Med Sci Sports Exerc 48: 472–480 (2016)

Eguchi T, Kumagai C, Fujihara T, Takemasa T, Ozawa T, and Numata O. "Black tea high-molecular-weight polyphenol stimulates exercise training-induced improvement of endurance capacity in mouse via the link between AMPK and GLUT4." PLoS One 8: e69480 (2013)

Ernst E, Saradeth T, and Achhammer G. "n-3 fatty acids and acute-phase proteins." Eur J Clin Invest 21: 77–82 (1991)

Fontani G, Corradeschi F, Felici A, Alfatti F, Bugarini R, Fiaschi AI, Cerretani D, Montorfano G, Rizzo AM, and Berra B. "Blood profiles, body fat and mood state in healthy subjects on different diets supplemented by omega-3 polyunsaturated fatty acids." Eur J Clin Invest 35: 499–507 (2005)

Fontani G, Corradeschi F, Felici A, Alfatti F, Migliorini S, and Lodi L. "Cognitive and physiological effects of omega-3 polyunsaturated fatty acid supplementation in healthy subjects." Eur J Clin Invest 35: 691–699 (2005)

Ghigo E, Miola C, Aimaretti G, Valente F, Procopio M, Arvat E, Yin-Zhang W, and Camanni F. "Arginine abolishes the inhibitory effect of glucose on the growth hormone response to growth hormone-releasing hormone in man." Metabolism 41:1000–1003 (1992)

Giampieri F, Alvarez-Suarez JM, Cordero MD, Gasparrini M, Forbes-Hernandez TY, Afrin S, Santos-Buelga C, González-Paramás AM, Astolfi P, Rubini C, Zizzi A, Tulipani S, Quiles JL, Mezzetti B, and Battino M. "Strawberry consumption improves aging-associated impairments, mitochondrial biogenesis and functionality through the AMP-activated protein kinase signaling cascade." Food Chem 234: 464–471 (2017)

Gibala M. "Molecular responses to high-intensity interval exercise." Appl Physiol Nutr Metab 34: 428–432 (2009)

Grassi D, Desideri G, Necozione S, di Giosia P, Barnabei R, Allegaert L, Bernaert H, and Ferri C. "Cocoa consumption dose-dependently improves flow-mediated dilation and arterial stiffness decreasing blood pressure in healthy individuals." J Hypertens 33: 294–303 (2015)

Guglielmo CG, Haunerland NH, Hochachka PW, and Williams TD. "Seasonal dynamics of flight muscle fatty acid binding proteins and catabolic enzymes in a migratory shorebird." Amer J Physiol 282: R1405–R1413 (2002)

Guglielmo CG. "Move that fatty acid: Fuel selection and transport in migratory birds and bats." Integr Comp Biol 50:336–345 (2010)

Guimarães-Ferreira L, Cholewa JM, Naimo MA, Zhi XI, Magagnin D, de Sá RB, Streck EL, Teixeira Tda S, and Zanchi NE. "Synergistic effects of resistance training and protein intake: Practical aspects." Nutrition 30: 1097–1103 (2014)

Guzmán JF, Esteve H, Pablos C, Pablos A, Blasco C, and Villegas JA. "DHA-rich fish oil improves complex reaction time in female elite soccer players." J Sports Sci Med 10:301–305 (2011)

Hardie DG. "AMP-activated protein kinase: A key system mediating metabolic responses to exercise." Med Sci Sports Exerc 36: 28–34 (2004)

Hardie DG, Ross FA, and Hawley SA. "AMP-activate protein kinase: A target for drugs both ancient and modern." Chem Bio 19: 1222–1236 (2012)

Hardie DG. "Keeping the home fires burning: AMP-activated protein kinase." J Royal Society Interface 15: 20170774 (2018)

Hezel MP and Weitzberg E. "The oral microbiome and nitric oxide homoeostasis." Oral Dis 21: 7–16 (2015)

Hostetler HA, Petrescu AD, Kier AB, and Schroeder F. "Peroxisome proliferator-activated receptor alpha interacts with high affinity and is conformationally responsive to endogenous ligands." J Biol Chem 280: 18667–18682 (2005)

Huffman DM, Altena TS, Mawhinney TP, and Thomas TR. "Effect of n-3 fatty acids on free tryptophan and exercise fatigue." Eur J Appl Physiol 92: 584–591 (2004)

Hwang JT, Kwon DY, and Yoon SH. "AMP-activated protein kinase: A potential target for disease prevention by natural occurring polyphenols." N Biotechnol 26: 17–22 (2009)

Jessen N, Sundelin EI, and Møller AB. "AMP kinase in exercise adaptation of skeletal muscle." Drug Discov Today 19: 999–1002 (2014)

Jouris KB, McDaniel JL, and Weiss EP. "The effect of omega-3 fatty acid supplementation on the inflammatory response to eccentric strength exercise." J Sports Sci Med 10:432–438 (2011)

Kane MO, Sene M, Anselm E, Dal S, Schini-Kerth VB, and Augier C. "Role of AMP-activated protein kinase in NO- and EDHF-mediated endothelium-dependent relaxations to red wine polyphenols." Indian J Physiol Pharmacol 59: 369–379 (2015)

Kawabata F, Neya M, Hamazaki K, Watanabe Y, Kobayashi S, and Tsuji T. "Supplementation with eicosapentaenoic acid-rich fish oil improves exercise economy and reduces perceived exertion during submaximal steady-state exercise in normal healthy untrained men." Biosci Biotechnol Biochem 78: 2081–2028 (2014)

Know, L. *Life: The epic story of our mitochondria.* Friesen Press. Victoria, BC, Canada (2014)

Lane N. *Power, Sex, and Suicide: Mitochondria and the meaning of life.* Oxford University Press. Oxford, UK (2005)

Lantier L, Fentz J, Mounier R, Leclerc J, Treebak JT, Pehmøller C, Sanz N, Sakakibara I, Saint-Amand E, Rimbaud S, Maire P, Marette A, Ventura-Clapier R, Ferry A, Wojtaszewski JF, Foretz M, and Viollet B. "AMPK controls exercise endurance, mitochondrial oxidative capacity, and skeletal muscle integrity." FASEB J 28: 3211–3224 (2014)

Layman DK and Baum JI. "Dietary protein impact on glycemic control during weight loss." J Nutr 134: 968S–973S (2004)

Layman DK, Anthony TG, Rasmussen BB, Adams SH, Lynch CJ, Brinkworth GD, and Davis TA. "Defining meal requirements for protein to optimize metabolic roles of amino acids." Am J Clin Nutr 101: 1330S–1338S (2015)

Lewis EJ, Radonic PW, Wolever TM, and Wells GD. "21 days of mammalian omega-3 fatty acid supplementation improves aspects of neuromuscular function and performance in male athletes compared to olive oil placebo." J Int Soc Sports Nutr 12: 28 (2015)

Lembke P, Capodice J, Hebert K, and Swenson T. "Influence of omega-3 index on performance and wellbeing in young adults after heavy eccentric exercise." J Sports Sci Med 13: 151–156 (2014).

LeMond G and Hom M. *The Science of Fitness.* Academic Press. Waltham, MA (2015)

Maillet D and Weber JM. "Performance enhancing role of dietary fatty acids in a long-distance migrant shorebird." J Exp Bio 209: 2686–2695 (2006)

Maillet D and Weber JM. "Relationship between n-3 PUFA content and energy metabolism in the flight muscles of a migrating shorebird." J Exp Biol 210: 413–420 (2007)

Marcinko K and Steinberg GR. "The role of AMPK in controlling metabolism and mitochondrial biogenesis during exercise. Exp Physiol 99: 158–1585 (2014)

Marsh CE, Carter HH, Guelfi KJ, Smith KJ, Pike KE, Naylor LH, and Green DJ. "Brachial and cerebrovascular functions are enhanced in postmenopausal women after ingestion of chocolate with a high concentration of cocoa." J Nutr 147:1686–1692 (2017)

Mickelborough TD. "Omega-3 polyunsaturated fatty acids in physical performance optimization." Int J Sport Nutr Exec Metab 23: 83–96 (2013)

Mills JD, Bailes JE, Sedney CL, Hutchins H, and Sears B. "Omega-3 dietary supplementation reduces traumatic axonal injury in a rodent head injury model." J Neurosurgery 114: 77–84 (2011)

Mounier R, Théret M, Lantier L, Foretz M, and Viollet B. "Expanding roles for AMPK in skeletal muscle plasticity." Trends Endocrinol Metab 26: 275–286 (2015)

Niederberger E, King TS, Russe OQ, and Geisslinger G. "Activation of AMPK and its impact on exercise capacity." Sports Med 45: 1497–1509 (2015)

Norton LE and Layman DK. "Leucine regulates translation initiation of protein synthesis in skeletal muscle after exercise." J Nutr 136: 533S–537S (2006)

O'Brien RJ and Wong PC. "Amyloid precursor protein processing and Alzheimer's disease." Annu Rev Neurosci 34: 185–204 (2011)

Phillips SM. "A brief review of critical processes in exercise-induced muscular hypertrophy." Sports Med 44 (Suppl 1): S71–77 (2014)

Phillips T, Childs AC, Dreon DM, Phinney S, and Leeuwenburgh C. "A dietary supplement attenuates IL-6 and CRP after eccentric exercise in untrained males." Med Sci Sports Exerc 35: 2032–2037 (2003)

Pons V, Riera J, Capó X, Martorell M, Sureda A, Tur JA, Drobnic F, and Pons A. "Calorie restriction regime enhances physical performance of trained athletes." J Int Soc Sports Nutr. 2018 Mar 9;15:12.

Poprzecki S, Zajac A, Chalimoniuk M, Waskiewicz Z, and Langfort J. "Modification of blood antioxidant status and lipid profile in response to high-intensity endurance exercise after low doses of omega-3 polyunsaturated fatty acid supplementation in healthy volunteers." Int J Food Sci Nutr 60: 67–79 (2009)

Reznick RM and Shulman GI. "The role of AMP-activated protein kinase in mitochondrial biogenesis." J Physiol 574(Pt 1): 33–39 (2006)

Richter EA and Ruderman NB. "AMPK and the biochemistry of exercise: Implications for human health and disease." Biochem J 418: 261–275 (2009)

Rodacki CL, Rodacki AL, Pereira G, Naliwaiko K, Coelho I, Pequito D, and Fernandes LC. "Fish oil supplementation enhances the effects of strength training in elderly women." Am J Clin Nutr 95: 428–436 (2012)

Rodriguez-Mateos A, Hezel M, Aydin H, Kelm M, Lundberg JO, Weitzberg E, Spencer JP, and Heiss C. "Interactions between cocoa flavanols and inorganic nitrate: Additive effects on endothelial function at achievable dietary amounts." Free Radic Biol Med 80: 121–128 (2015)

Ruderman NB, Xu XJ, Nelson L, Cacicedo JM, Saha AK, Lan F, and Ido Y. "AMPK and SIRT1: A long-standing partnership?" Am J Physiol Endocrinol Metabl 298: E751–E760 (2010)

Spalding KL, Bhardwaj RD, Buchholz BA, Druid H, and Frisén J. "Retrospective birth dating of cells in humans." Cell 122: 133–143 (2005)

Su W and Jones PJ. "Dietary fatty acid composition influences energy accretion in rats." J Nutr 123: 2109–2114 (1993)

Tartibian B, Maleki BH, and Abbasi A. "The effects of ingestion of omega-3 fatty acids on perceived pain and external symptoms of delayed onset muscle soreness in untrained men." Clin J Sport Med 19: 115–119 (2009)

Tartibian B, Maleki BH, and Abbasi A. "The effects of omega-3 supplementation on pulmonary function of young wrestlers during intensive training." J Sci Med Sport 13: 281–286 (2010)

Tartibian B, Maleki BH, and Abbasi A. "Omega-3 fatty acids supplementation attenuates inflammatory markers after eccentric exercise in untrained men." Clin J Sport Med 21: 131–137 (2011)

Tinsley GM, Gann JJ, Huber SR, Andre TL, La Bounty PM, Bowden RG, Gordon PM, and Grandjean PW. "Effects of fish oil supplementation on post resistance exercise muscle soreness." J Diet Suppl 21: 1–12 (2016)

van Loon LJ and Goodpaster BH. "Increased intramuscular lipid storage in the insulin-resistant and endurance-trained state." Pflugers Arch 451:606–616 (2006)

Viru A. *Hormones in Muscular Activity*. CRC Press. Boca Raton, FL (1985)

von Schacky C, Kemper M, Haslbauer R, and Halle M. "Low omega-3 index in 106 German elite winter endurance athletes: A pilot study." Int J Sport Nutr Exerc Metab 24: 559–564 (2014)

Weber JM "Metabolic fuels: Regulating fluxes to select mix." J Exp Biol 214: 286–294 (2011)

White AM, Johnston CS, Swan PD, Tjonn SL, and Sears B. "Blood ketones are directly related to fatigue and perceived effort during exercise in overweight adults adhering to low-carbohydrate diets for weight loss: A Pilot study." J Am Diet Assoc 107: 1792–1796 (2007)

Whitten P. "Stanford's secret weapon." Swimming World. March/April (1993)

Williams M, Raven PB, Fogt DL, and Ivy JL. "Effects of recovery beverages on glycogen restoration and endurance exercise performance." J Strength Cond Res. 2003 Feb;17(1):12–9.

Wilson PB and Madrigal LA. "Associations between whole blood and dietary omega-3 polyunsaturated fatty acid levels in collegiate athletes." Int J Sport Nutr Exerc Metab 26: 497–505 (2016)

Winder WW, Taylor EB, and Thomson DM. "Role of AMP-activated protein kinase in the molecular adaptation to endurance exercise." Med Sci Sports Exerc 38: 1945–1949 (2006)

Wroble K, Trott MN, Schweitzer GG, Rahman RS, Kelly PV, and Weiss EP. "Low-carbohydrate, ketogenic diet impairs anaerobic exercise performance in exercise-trained women and men: a randomized-sequence crossover trial." J Sports Med Phys Fitness 59: 600–607 (2019)

Xu ZR, Tan ZJ, Zhang Q, Gui QF, and Yang YM. "The effectiveness of leucine on muscle protein synthesis, lean body mass and leg lean mass accretion in older people: Systematic review and meta-analysis." Br J Nutr 113: 25–34 (2015)

Đebrowska A, Mizia-Stec K, Mizia M, GĐsior Z, and PoprzĐcki S. "Omega-3 fatty acids supplementation improves endothelial function and maximal oxygen uptake in endurance-trained athletes." Eur J Sport Sci 15: 305–314 (2015)

Zhao L, Zou T, Gomez NA, Wang B, Zhu MJ, and Du M. "Raspberry alleviates obesity-induced inflammation and insulin resistance in skeletal muscle through activation of AMP-activated protein kinase (AMPK)" Nutr Diabetes 8: 39 (2018)

Zoladz JA, Koziel A, Woyda-Ploszczyca A, Celichowski J, and Jarmuszkiewicz W. "Endurance training increases the efficiency of rat skeletal muscle mitochondria." Pflugers Arch 468: 1709–1724 (2016)

CHAPTER 18: WHY DO WE GET FAT?

Arentson-Lantz E, Clairmont S, Paddon-Jones D, Tremblay A, and Elango R. "Protein: A nutrient in focus." Appl Physiol Nutr Metab 40: 755–761 (2015)

Avena NM, Bocarsly ME, and Hoebel BG. "Animal models of sugar and fat bingeing: Relationship to food addiction and increased body weight." Methods Mol Biol 829: 351–65 (2012)

Cai D. "Neuroinflammation and neurodegeneration in overnutrition-induced diseases." Trends Endocrinol Metab 24: 40–47 (2013)

Cani PD, Amar J, Iglesias MA, Poggi M, Knauf C, Bastelica D, Neyrinck AM, Fava F, Tuohy KM, Chabo C, Waget A, Delmée E, Cousin B, Sulpice T, Chamontin B, Ferrières J, Tanti JF, Gibson GR, Casteilla L, Delzenne NM, Alessi MC, and Burcelin R. "Metabolic endotoxemia initiates obesity and insulin resistance." Diabetes 56: 1761–1772 (2007)

Crewe C, An YA, and Scherer PE. "The ominous triad of adipose tissue dysfunction: Inflammation, fibrosis, and impaired angiogenesis." J Clin Invest 127: 74–82 (2017)

Fildes A, Charlton J, Rudisill C, Littlejohns P, Prevost AT, and Gulliford MC. "Probability of an obese person attaining normal body weight: Cohort study using electronic health records". Am J Public Health 105: e54–59 (2015)

Fothergill E, Guo J, Howard L, Kerns JC, Knuth ND, Brychta R, Chen KY, Skarulis MC, Walter M, Walter PJ, and Hall KD. "Persistent metabolic adaptation 6 years after "The Biggest Loser" competition." Obesity 24: 1612–1619 (2016)

Gray B, Steyn F, Davies PS, and Vitetta L. "Omega-3 fatty acids: A review of the effects on adiponectin and leptin and potential implications for obesity management." Eur J Clin Nutr 67: 1234–1242 (2013)

Gregor MF and Hotamisligil GS. "Inflammatory mechanisms in obesity." Annu Rev Immunol 29: 415–445 (2011)

Guyenet SJ. *The Hungry Brain*. Flatiron Books. New York, NY (2017)

Haghiac M, Yang XH, Presley L, Smith S, Dettelback S, Minium J, Belury MA, Catalano PM, and Hauguel-de Mouzon S. "Dietary omega-3 fatty acid supplementation reduces inflammation in obese pregnant women: A randomized double-blind controlled clinical trial." PLoS One 10: e0137309 (2015)

Hall KD, Chen KY, Guo J, Lam YY, Leibel RL, Mayer LE, Reitman ML, Rosenbaum M, Smith SR, Walsh BT, and Ravussin E. "Energy expenditure and body composition changes after an isocaloric ketogenic diet in overweight and obese men." Am J Clin Nutr 104: 324–333 (2016)

Hellström PM. "Satiety signals and obesity." Curr Opin Gastroenterol 29: 222–227 (2013)

Hernandez TL, Kittelson JM, Law CK, Ketch LL, Stob NR, Lindstrom RC, Scherzinger A, Stamm ER, and Eckel RH. "Fat redistribution following suction lipectomy: Defense of body fat and patterns of restoration." Obesity 19: 1388–1395 (2011)

Johnson C, Day CS, and Swan PD. "Postprandial thermogenesis is increased 100% on a high-protein, low-fat diet versus a high-carbohydrate, low-fat diet in healthy, young women." J Amer Coll Nutr 21: 55–61 (2002)

Kaliannan K, Wang B, Li XY, Kim KJ, and Kang JX. "A host-microbiome interaction mediates the opposing effects of omega-6 and omega-3 fatty acids on metabolic endotoxemia." Sci Rep 5:11276 (2015)

Keith SW, Redden DT, Katzmarzyk PT, Boggiano MM, Hanlon EC, Benca RM, Ruden D, Pietrobelli A, Barger JL, Fontaine KR, Wang C, Aronne LJ, Wright SM, Baskin M, Dhurandhar NV, Lijoi MC, Grilo CM, DeLuca M, Westfall AO, and Allison DB. "Putative contributors to the secular increase in obesity: Exploring the roads less traveled." Int J Obes 30: 1585–1594 (2006)

Kim J, Li Y, and Watkins BA. "Fat to treat fat: Emerging relationship between dietary PUFA, endocannabinoids, and obesity." Prostaglandins Other Lipid Mediat 104-105: 32–41 (2013)

Kraemer FB, Takeda D, Natu V, and Sztalryd C. "Insulin regulates lipoprotein lipase activity in rat adipose cells via wortmannin- and rapamycin-sensitive pathways." Metabolism 47: 555–559 (1998)

le Roux CW, Welbourn R, Werling M, Osborne A, Kokkinos A, Laurenius A, Lönroth H, Fändriks L, Ghatei MA, Bloom SR, and Olbers T. "Gut hormones as mediators of appetite and weight loss after Roux-en-Y gastric bypass." Ann Surg 246: 780–785 (2007)

Li C, Ford ES, Zhao G, Balluz LS, and Giles WH. "Estimates of body composition with dual-energy X-ray absorptiometry in adults." Am J Clin Nutr 90: 1457–1465 (2009)

Lustig RH. "Childhood obesity: Behavioral aberration or biochemical drive? Reinterpreting the first law of thermodynamics." Nat Clin Pract Endocrinol Metab 2: 447–458 (2006)

Maric T, Woodside B, and Luheshi GN. "The effects of dietary saturated fat on basal hypothalamic neuroinflammation in rats." Brain Behav Immun 36: 35–45 (2014)

McGuire MT, Wing RR, Klem ML, Seagle HM, and Hill JO. "Long-term maintenance of weight loss: Do people who lose weight through various weight loss methods use different behaviors to maintain their weight?" Int J Obes Relat Metab Disord 22: 572–577 (1998)

Morris MJ, Beilharz JE, Maniam J, Reichelt AC, and Westbrook RF. "Why is obesity such a problem in the 21st century? The intersection of palatable food, cues and reward pathways, stress, and cognition." Neurosci Biobehav Rev 58: 36–45 (2015)

Muhammad HFL, Vink RG, Roumans NJT, Arkenbosch LAJ, Mariman EC, and van Baak MA. "Dietary intake after weight loss and the risk of weight regain: Macronutrient composition and inflammatory properties of the diet." Nutrients 9: 11 (2017)

Murray S, Tulloch A, Gold MS, and Avena NM. "Hormonal and neural mechanisms of food reward, eating behaviour and obesity." Nat Rev Endocrinol 10: 540–552 (2014)

Psichas A, Sleeth ML, Murphy KG, Brooks L, Bewick GA, Hanyaloglu AC, Ghatei MA, Bloom SR, and Frost G. "The short chain fatty acid propionate stimulates GLP-1 and PYY secretion via free fatty acid receptor 2 in rodents." Int J Obes 39: 424–429 (2015)

Raynor HA, Jeffery RW, Phelan S, Hill JO, and Wing RR. "Amount of food group variety consumed in the diet and long-term weight loss maintenance." Obes Res 13: 883–890 (2005)

Ruderman NB, Carling D, Prentki M, and Cacicedo JM. "AMPK, insulin resistance, and the metabolic syndrome." J Clin Invest 123: 2764–2772 (2013)

Sáinz N, González-Navarro CJ, Martínez JA, and Moreno-Aliaga MJ. "Leptin signaling as a therapeutic target of obesity." Expert Opin Ther Targets 19: 893–909 (2015)

Sears B. *Toxic Fat*. Thomas Nelson. Nashville, TN (2008)

Sears B. *The Mediterranean Zone*. Ballantine Books. New York, NY (2014)

Sears B and Perry M. "The role of fatty acids in insulin resistance." Lipids Health Disease 14: 121 (2015)

Shick SM, Wing RR, Klem ML, McGuire MT, Hill JO, and Seagle H. "Persons successful at long-term weight loss and maintenance continue to consume a low-energy, low-fat diet." J Am Diet Assoc 98: 408–413 (1998)

Sun K, Kusminski CM, and Scherer PE. "Adipose tissue remodeling and obesity." J Clin Invest 121: 2094–2101 (2011) van der Klaauw AA, Keogh JM, Henning E, Trowse VM, Dhillo WS, Ghatei MA, and Farooqi IS. "High protein intake stimulates postprandial GLP-1 and PYY release." Obesity 21: 1602–1607 (2013)

van devijvere S, Chow CC, Hall KD, Umali E, and Swinburn BA. "Increased food energy supply as a major driver of the obesity epidemic: A global analysis." Bull World Heath Organ 93: 446–456 (2015)

Vink RG, Roumans NJ, Arkenbosch LA, Mariman EC, and van Baak MA. "The effect of rate of weight loss on long-term weight regain in adults with overweight and obesity." Obesity 24: 321–327 (2016)

Weisberg SP, McCann D, Desai M, Rosenbaum M, Leibel RL, and Ferrante AW. "Obesity is associated with macrophage accumulation in adipose tissue." J Clin Invest 112: 1796–1808 (2003)

Zhou QY and Palmiter RD. "Dopamine-deficient mice are severely hypoactive, adipsic, and aphagic." Cell 83: 1197–1209 (1995)

CHAPTER 19: WHY DO WE GET SICK?

Ahmed S, Mahmood Z, and Zahid S. "Linking insulin with Alzheimer's disease: Emergence as type III diabetes." Neurol Sci 36: 1763–1769 (2015)

Amminger GP, Schäfer MR, Schlögelhofer M, Klier CM, and McGorry PD. "Longer-term outcome in the prevention of psychotic disorders by the Vienna omega-3 study." Nat Commun 6: 7934 (2015)

Baidal DA, Ricordi C, Garcia-Contreras M, Sonnino A, and Fabbri A. "Combination high-dose omega-3 fatty acids and high-dose cholecalciferol in new onset type 1 diabetes: A potential role in preservation of beta-cell mass." Eur Rev Med Pharmacol Sci 20: 3313–3318 (2016)

Bellamkonda K, Chandrashekar NK, Osman J, Selvanesan BC, Savari S, and Sjölander A. "The eicosanoids leukotriene D4 and prostaglandin E2 promote the tumorigenicity of colon cancer-initiating cells in a xenograft mouse model." BMC Cancer 16: 425 (2016)

Berk M, Williams LJ, Jacka FN, O'Neil A, Pasco JA, Moylan S, Allen NB, Stuart AL, Hayley AC, Byrne ML, and Maes M. "So depression is an inflammatory disease, but where does the inflammation come from?" BMC Med 11: 200 (2013)

Bienenstock J, Kunze W, and Forsythe P. "Microbiota and the gut-brain axis." Nutr Rev 73 (Suppl 1): 28–31 (2015)

Bos DJ, Oranje B, Veerhoek ES, Van Diepen RM, Weusten JM, Demmelmair H, Koletzko B, de Sain-van der Velden MG, Eilander A, Hoeksma M, and Durston S. "Reduced symptoms of inattention after dietary omega-3 fatty acid supplementation in boys with and without attention deficit/hyperactivity disorder." Neuropsychopharmacology 40: 2298–2306 (2015)

Burrell RA, McGranahan N, Bartek J, and Swanton C. "The causes and consequences of genetic heterogeneity in cancer evolution." Nature 501: 338–345 (2013)

Buydens-Branchey L and Branchey M. "n-3 polyunsaturated fatty acids decrease anxiety feelings in a population of substance abusers." J Clin Psychopharmacol 26: 661–665 (2006)

Buydens-Branchey L, Branchey M, and Hibbeln JR. "Associations between increases in plasma n-3 polyunsaturated fatty acids following supplementation and decreases in anger and anxiety in substance abusers." Prog Neuropsychopharmacol Biol Psychiatry 32: 568–575 (2008)

Cadario F, Savastio S, Rizzo AM, Carrera D, Bona G, and Ricordi C. "Can Type 1 diabetes progression be halted? Possible role of high dose vitamin D and omega 3 fatty acids." Eur Rev Med Pharmacol Sci 21: 1604–1609 (2017)

Chanock SJ. "The paradox of mutations and cancer." Science 362: 893–894 (2018)

Chatterjee S, Peters SA, Woodward M, Mejia Arango S, Batty GD, Beckett N, Beiser A, Borenstein AR, Crane PK, Haan M, Hassing LB, Hayden KM, Kiyohara Y, Larson EB, Li CY, Ninomiya T, Ohara T, Peters R, Russ TC, Seshadri S, Strand BH, Walker R, Xu W, and Huxley RR. "Type 2 diabetes as a risk factor for dementia in women compared with men." Diabetes Care 39: 300–307 (2016)

Catry E, Bindels LB, Tailleux A, Lestavel S, Neyrinck AM, Goossens JF, Lobysheva I, Plovier H, Essaghir A, Demoulin JB, Bouzin C, Pachikian BD, Cani PD, Staels B, Dessy C, and Delzenne NM. "Targeting the gut microbiota with insulin-type fructans: Preclinical demonstration of a novel approach in the management of endothelial dysfunction." Gut 67: 271–283 (2018)

Centers for Disease Control. "More than 100 million Americans have diabetes or prediabetes." Press Release July 18, 2017

Chiarini F, Evangelisti C, McCubrey JA, and Martelli AM. "Current treatment strategies for inhibiting mTOR in cancer." Trends Pharmacol Sci 36: 124–135 (2015)

Conquer JA, Tierney MC, Zecevic J, Bettger WJ, and Fisher RH. "Fatty acid analysis of blood plasma of patients with Alzheimer's disease, other types of dementia, and cognitive impairment." Lipids 35: 1305–1312 (2000)

Crewe C, An YA, and Scherer PE. "The ominous triad of adipose tissue dysfunction: Inflammation, fibrosis, and impaired angiogenesis." J Clin Invest 127: 74–82 (2017)

Das UN. "Is multiple sclerosis a proresolution deficiency disorder?" Nutrition 28: 951–958 (2012)

DiDonato JA, Mercurio F, and Karin M. "NF-κB and the link between inflammation and cancer." Immunol Rev 246:3 79–400 (2012)

Dinan TG and Cryan JF. "The microbiome-gut-brain axis in health and disease." Gastroenterol Clin North Am 46: 77–89 (2017)

Eming SA, Wynn TA, and Martin P. "Inflammation and metabolism in tissue repair and regeneration." Science 356: 1026–1030 (2017)

Endres S, Ghorbani R, Kelley VE, Georgilis K, Lonnemann G, van der Meer JW, Cannon JG, Rogers TS, Klempner MS, Weber PC, Schaeffer EJ, Wolff SM, and

Dinarello CA. "The effect of dietary supplementation with n-3 polyunsaturated fatty acids on the synthesis of interleukin-1 and tumor necrosis factor by mononuclear cells." N Engl J Med 320: 265–271 (1989)

Fontani G, Corradeschi F, Felici A, Alfatti F, Migliorini S, and Lodi L. "Cognitive and physiological effects of omega-3 polyunsaturated fatty acid supplementation in healthy subjects." Eur J Clin Invest 35: 691–699 (2005)

Frye RE, Rose S, Chacko J, Wynne R, Bennuri SC, Slattery JC, Tippett M, Delhey L, Melnyk S, Kahler SG, and MacFabe DF. "Modulation of mitochondrial function by the microbiome metabolite propionic acid in autism and control cell lines." Transl Psychiatry 6: e927 (2016)

Geovanini GR and Libby P. "Atherosclerosis and inflammation: Overview and updates." Clin Sci 132: 1243–1252 (2018)

Germano M, Meleleo D, Montorfano G, Adorni L, Negroni M, Berra B, and Rizzo AM. "Plasma, red blood cells phospholipids and clinical evaluation after long chain omega-3 supplementation in children with attention deficit hyperactivity disorder (ADHD)." Nutr Neurosci 10: 1–9 (2007)

Gustafsson PA, Birberg-Thornberg U, Duchen K, Landgren M, Malmberg K, Pelling H, Strandvik B, and Karlsson T. "EPA supplementation improves teacher-rated behaviour and oppositional symptoms in children with ADHD." Acta Paediatr 99: 1540–1549 (2010)

Han QQ and Yu J. "Inflammation: A mechanism of depression?" Neurosci Bull 30:515–523 (2014)

Hardie DG. "AMPK: A target for drugs and natural products with effects on both diabetes and cancer." Diabetes 62: 2164–2172 (2013)

Heydari B, Abdullah S, Pottala JV, Shah R, Abbasi S, Mandry D, Francis SA, Lumish H, Ghoshhajra BB, Hoffmann U, Appelbaum E, Feng JH, Blankstein R, Steigner M, McConnell JP, Harris W, Antman EM, Jerosch-Herold M, and Kwong RY. "Effect of omega-3 acid ethyl esters on left ventricular remodeling after acute myocardial infarction: The OMEGA-REMODEL randomized clinical trial." Circulation 134: 378–391 (2016)

Huang CC, Chung CM, Leu HB, Lin LY, Chiu CC, Hsu CY, Chiang CH, Huang PH, Chen TJ, Lin SJ, Chen JW, and Chan WL. "Diabetes mellitus and the risk of Alzheimer's disease: A nationwide population-based study." PLoS One 9: e87095 (2014)

Itakura H, Yokoyama M, Matsuzaki M, Saito Y, Origasa H, Ishikawa Y, Oikawa S, Sasaki J, Hishida H, Kita T, Kitabatake A, Nakaya N, Sakata T, Shimada K, Shirato K, and Matsuzawa Y. "Relationships between plasma fatty acid composition and coronary artery disease." J Atheroscler Thromb 18: 99–107 (2011)

Jelinek GA, Hadgkiss EJ, Weiland TJ, Pereira NG, Marck CH, and van der Meer DM. "Association of fish consumption and n-3 supplementation with quality of life, disability and disease activity in an international cohort of people with multiple sclerosis." Int J Neurosci 123: 792–800 (2013)

Kelly CT, Mansoor J, Dohm GL, Chapman WH, Pender JR, and Pories WJ. "Hyperinsulinemic syndrome: The metabolic syndrome is broader than you think." Surgery 156: 405–411 (2014)

Khan A and Brown WA. "Antidepressants versus placebo in major depression: Overview." World Psychiatry 14: 294–300 (2015)

Kiecolt-Glaser JK, Belury MA, Andridge R, Malarkey WB, and Glaser R. "Omega-3 supplementation lowers inflammation and anxiety in medical students: Randomized controlled trial." Brain Behav Immun 25: 1725–1734 (2011)

Kiecolt-Glaser JK, Derry HM, and Fagundes CP. "Inflammation: Depression fans the flames and feasts on the heat." Am J Psychiatry 172: 1075–1091 (2015)

Klein CP, Sperotto ND, Maciel IS, Leite CE, Souza AH, and Campos MM. "Effects of D-series resolvins on behavioral and neurochemical changes in a fibromyalgia-like model in mice." Neuropharmacology 86: 57–66 (2014)

Kromann N and Green A. "Epidemiological studies in the Upernavik district, Greenland: Incidence of some chronic diseases 1950–1974." Acta Med Scand 208: 401–406 (1980)

Laakso M. "Cardiovascular disease in type 2 diabetes from population to man to mechanisms." Diabetes Care 33: 442–449 (2010)

La Chance L, McKenzie K, Taylor VH, and Vigod SN. "Omega-6 to omega-3 fatty acid ratio in patients with ADHD: A meta-analysis." J Can Acad Adoles Psychiarty 25: 87–96 (2016)

Lazic M, Inzaugarat ME, Povero D, Zhao IC, Chen M, Nalbandian M, Miller YI, Cherñavsky AC, Feldstein AE, and Sears DD. "Reduced dietary omega-6 to omega-3 fatty acid ratio and 12/15-lipoxygenase deficiency are protective against chronic high fat diet-induced steatohepatitis." PLoS One 9: e107658 (2014)

Lesperance F, Frasure-Smith N, St-Andre E, Turecki G, Lesperance P, and Wisniewski SR. "The efficacy of omega-3 supplementation for major depression: Randomized controlled trial." J Clin Psychiatry 72: 1054–1062 (2011)

Li YC, Chen Y, and Du J. "Critical roles of intestinal epithelial vitamin D receptor signaling in controlling gut mucosal inflammation." J Steroid Biochem Mol Biol 148: 179–183 (2015)

Li W, Saud SM, Young MR, Chen G, and Hua B. "Targeting AMPK for cancer prevention and treatment." Oncotarget 6: 7365–7378 (2015)

Libby P, Ridker PM, and Maseri A. "Inflammation and atherosclerosis." Circulation 105: 1135–1143 (2002)

Libby P. "Inflammation in atherosclerosis." Arterio Thromb Vasc Biol 32: 2045–2051 (2012)

Libby P, Tabas I, Fredman G, and Fisher EA. "Inflammation and its resolution as determinants of acute coronary syndromes." Circ Res 114: 1867–1879 (2014)

Lim EL, Hollingsworth KG, Aribisala BS, Chen MJ, Mathers JC, and Taylor R. "Reversal of type 2 diabetes: Normalisation of beta cell function in association with decreased pancreas and liver triacylglycerol." Diabetologia 54: 2506–2514 (2011)

Lotrich, FE, Sears, B, and McNamara RK. "Elevated ratio of arachidonic acid to long-chain omega-3 fatty acids predicts depression development following interferon-alpha treatment: Relationship with interleukin-6." Brain, Behavior, and Immunity 31: 48–53 (2013)

Lotrich FE, Sears B, and McNamara R.K. "Anger induced by interferon-alpha is moderated by ratio of arachidonic acid to omega-3 fatty acids." J Psychosomatic Res 75: 475–483 (2013)

Ma K, Nunemaker CS, Wu R, Chakrabarti SK, Taylor-Fishwick DA, and Nadler JL. "12-lipoxygenase products reduce insulin secretion and beta-cell viability in human islets." J Clin Endocrinol Metab 95: 887–893 (2010)

MacFabe DF, Cain DP, Rodriguez-Capote K, Franklin AE, Hoffman JE, Boon F, Taylor AR, Kavaliers M, and Ossenkopp KP. "Neurobiological effects of intraventricular propionic acid in rats: Possible role of short chain fatty acids on the pathogenesis and characteristics of autism spectrum disorders." Behav Brain Res 176: 149–169 (2007)

Martincornea I, Folwer JC, Wabik A. Lawson ARJ, Abascal F, Hall MWJ, Cagan A, Murai K, Mahbubani K, Stratton MR, Fitzgerald RC, Handford PA, Campbell PJ, Saeb-Parsy K, and Jones PH. "Somatic mutant clones colonize the human esophagus with age." Science 362: 911–917 (2018)

Martinez KE, Tucker LA, Bailey BW, and LeCheminant JD. "Expanded normal weight obesity and insulin resistance in US adults of the National Health and Nutrition Examination Survey." J Diabetes Res 2017: 9502643 (2017)

Markovic TP, Jenkins AB, Campbell LV, Furler SM, Kraegen EW, and Chisholm DJ. "The determinants of glycemic responses to diet restriction and weight loss in obesity and NIDDM." Diabetes Care 21: 687–694 (1998)

Martins JG. "EPA but not DHA appears to be responsible for the efficacy of omega-3 long chain polyunsaturated fatty acid supplementation in depression: Evidence from a meta-analysis of randomized controlled trials." J Am Coll Nutr 28:525–542 (2009)

Mazza M, Marano G, Traversi G, Di Nicola M, Catalano V, and Janiri L. "The complex interplay of depression, inflammation and omega-3: State of the art and progresses in research." Clin Ter 166: e242–247 (2015)

McNamara RK, Perry M, and Sears, B. "Dissociation of C-reactive protein levels from long-chain omega-3 fatty acid status and anti-depressant response in adolescents with major depressive disorder: An open-label dose-ranging trial." J Nutr Therapeutics 2:235–243 (2013)

Miller AH and Raison CL. "The role of inflammation in depression: From evolutionary imperative to modern treatment target." Nat Rev Immunology 16: 22–34 (2016)

Miller PE, Van Elswyk M, and Alexander DD. "Long-chain omega-3 fatty acids eicosapentaenoic acid and docosahexaenoic acid and blood pressure: A meta-analysis of randomized controlled trials." Am J Hypertens 27: 885–96 (2014)

Mills JD, Bailes JE, Sedney CL, Hutchins H, and Sears B. "Omega-3 dietary supplementation reduces traumatic axonal injury in a rodent head injury model." J Neurosurgery 114: 77–84 (2011)

Milte CM, Parletta N, Buckley JD, Coates AM, Young RM, and Howe PR. "Increased erythrocyte eicosapentaenoic acid and docosahexaenoic acid are associated with improved attention and behavior in children with ADHD in a randomized controlled three-way crossover trial." J Atten Disord 19: 954–964 (2015)

Möhler H. "The GABA system in anxiety and depression and its therapeutic potential." Neuropharmacology 62: 42–53 (2016)

Mozaffari-Khosravi H, Yassini-Ardakani M, Karamati M, and Shariati-Bafghi SE. "Eicosapentaenoic acid versus docosahexaenoic acid in mild-to-moderate depression: A randomized, double-blind, placebo-controlled trial." Eur Neuropsychopharmacol 23: 636–644 (2013)

Naviaux RK, Naviaux JC, Li K, Bright AT, Alaynick WA, Wang L, Baxter A, Nathan N, Anderson W, and Gordon E. "Metabolic features of chronic fatigue syndrome." Proc Natl Acad Sci U S A 113: E5472–5480 (2016)

Nemets H, Nemets B, Apter A, Bracha Z, and Belmaker RH. "Omega-3 treatment of childhood depression: A controlled, double-blind pilot study." Am J Psychiatry 163: 1098–1100 (2006)

Nordvik I, Myhr KM, Nyland H, and Bjerve KS. "Effect of dietary advice and n-3 supplementation in newly diagnosed MS patients." Acta Neurol Scand 102: 143–149 (2000)

Oshima H and Oshima M. "The role of PGE2-associated inflammatory responses in gastric cancer development." Semin Immunopathol 35: 139–150 (2013)

Rehman G, Shehzad A, Khan AL, and Hamayun M. "Role of AMP-activated protein kinase in cancer therapy." Arch Pharm 347: 457–468 (2014)

Ruderman NB, Carling D, Prentki M, and Cacicedo JM. "AMPK, insulin resistance, and the metabolic syndrome." J Clin Invest 123: 2764–2772 (2013)

Sears B. *Toxic Fat*. Thomas Nelson. Nashville, TN (2008)

Sears B, Bailes J, and Asselin B. "Therapeutic uses of high-dose omega-3 fatty acids to treat comatose patients with severe brain injury." PharmaNutrition 1: 86–89 (2013)

Sekikawa A, Steingrimsdottir L, Ueshima H, Shin C, Curb JD, Evans RW, Hauksdottir AM, Kadota A, Choo J, Masaki K, Thorsson B, Launer LJ, Garcia

ME, Maegawa H, Willcox BJ, Eiriksdottir G, Fujiyoshi A, Miura K, Harris TB, Kuller LH, and Gudnason V. "Serum levels of marine-derived n-3 fatty acids in Icelanders, Japanese, Koreans, and Americans—a descriptive epidemiologic study." Prostaglandins Leukot Essent Fatty Acids 87: 11–16 (2012)

Seyfried TN. *Cancer as a Metabolic Disease.* Wiley and Sons. Hoboken, NJ (2012)

Seyfried TN, Flores RE, Poff AM, and D'Agostino DP. "Cancer as a metabolic disease: Implications for novel therapeutics." Carcinogenesis 35: 515–527 (2014)

Shattuck EC and Muehlenbein MP. "Towards an integrative picture of human sickness behavior." Brain Behav Immun 57: 255–262 (2016)

Solano C, Echeverz M, and Lasa I. "Biofilm dispersion and quorum sensing." Curr Opin Microbiol 18: 96–104 (2014)

Sorgi PJ, Hallowell EM, Hutchins HL, and Sears B. "Effects of an open-label pilot study with high-dose EPA/DHA concentrates on plasma phospholipids and behavior in children with attention deficit hyperactivity disorder." Nutr J 13: 16 (2007)

Spalding KL, Bhardwaj RD, Buchholz BA, Druid H, and Frisén J. "Retrospective birth dating of cells in humans." Cell 122: 133–143 (2005)

Spalding KL, Bergmann O, Alkass K, Bernard S, Salehpour M, Huttner HB, Boström E, Westerlund I, Vial C, Buchholz BA, Possnert G, Mash DC, Druid H, and Frisén J. "Dynamics of hippocampal neurogenesis in adult humans." Cell 153: 1219–1227 (2013)

Stene LC and Joner G. "Use of cod liver oil during the first year of life is associated with lower risk of childhood-onset type 1 diabetes: A large, population-based, case-control study." Am J Clin Nutr 78: 1128–1134 (2003)

Stoll AL, Severus WE, Freeman MP, Rueter S, Zboyan HA, Diamond E, Cress KK, and Marangell LB. "Omega 3 fatty acids in bipolar disorder: A preliminary double-blind, placebo-controlled trial." Arch Gen Psychiatry 56: 407–412 (1999)

Su KP, Huang SY, Chiu CC, and Shen WW. "Omega-3 fatty acids in major depressive disorder. A preliminary double-blind, placebo-controlled trial." Eur Neuropsychopharmacol 13: 267–271 (2003)

Su D, Nie Y, Zhu A, Chen Z, Wu P, Zhang L, Luo M, Sun Q, Cai L, Lai Y, Xiao Z, Duan Z, Zheng S, Wu G, Hu R, Tsukamoto H, Lugea A, Liu Z, Pandol SJ, and Han YP. "Vitamin D signaling through induction of Paneth cell defensins maintains gut microbiota and improves metabolic disorders and hepatic steatosis in animal models." Front Physiol 7: 498 (2016)

Sulciner ML, Serhan CN, Gilligan MM, Mudge DK, Chang J, Gartung A, Lehner KA, Bielenberg DR, Schmidt B, Dalli J, Greene ER, Gus-Brautbar Y, Piwowarski J, Mammoto T, Zurakowski D, Perretti M, Sukhatme VP, Kaipainen A, Kieran MW, Huang S, and Panigrahy D. "Resolvins suppress tumor growth and enhance cancer therapy." J Exp Med 215: 115–140 (2018)

Taylor-Fishwick DA, Weaver J, Glenn L, Kuhn N, Rai G, Jadhav A, Simeonov A, Dudda A, Schmoll D, Holman TR, Maloney DJ, and Nadler JL. "Selective inhibition of 12-lipoxygenase protects islets and beta cells from inflammatory cytokine-mediated beta cell dysfunction." Diabetologia 58: 549–57 (2015)

Tessaro FH, Ayala TS, and Martins JO. "Lipid mediators are critical in resolving inflammation: A review of the emerging roles of eicosanoids in diabetes mellitus." Biomed Res Int 2015: 568408 (2015)

Wang X, Zhu M, Hjorth E, Cortés-Toro V, Eyjolfsdottir H, Graff C, Nennesmo I, Palmblad J, Eriksdotter M, Sambamurti K, Fitzgerald JM, Serhan CN, Granholm AC, and Schultzberg M. "Resolution of inflammation is altered in Alzheimer's disease." Alzheimers Dement 11: 40–50 (2015)

Weisberg SP, McCann D, Desai M, Rosenbaum M, Leibel RL, and Ferrante AW. "Obesity is associated with macrophage accumulation in adipose tissue." J Clin Invest 112: 1796–1808 (2003)

Wenzlau JM and Hutton JC. "Novel diabetes autoantibodies and prediction of type 1 diabetes." Curr Diab Rep 13: 608–615 (2013)

Wick G, Grundtman C, Mayerl C, Wimpissinger TF, Feichtinger J, Zelger B, Sgonc R, and Wolfram D. "The immunology of fibrosis." Annu Rev Immunol 31: 107–135 (2013)

Wynn TA. "Cellular and molecular mechanisms of fibrosis." J Pathol 214: 199–210 (2008)

Yokoyama M, Origasa H, Matsuzaki M, Matsuzawa Y, Saito Y, Ishikawa Y, Oikawa S, Sasaki J, Hishida H, Itakura H, Kita T, Kitabatake A, Nakaya N, Sakata T, Shimada K, and Shirato K. "Effects of eicosapentaenoic acid on major coronary events in hypercholesterolaemic patients (JELIS): A randomised open-label, blinded endpoint analysis." Lancet 369: 1090–1098 (2007)

CHAPTER 20: WHY DO WE AGE?

Allan CA, Strauss BJ, Burger HG, Forbes EA, and McLachlan RI. "Testosterone therapy prevents gain in visceral adipose tissue and loss of skeletal muscle in nonobese aging men." J Clin Endocrinol Metab 93: 139–46 (2008)

Arai Y, Martin-Ruiz CM, Takayama M, Abe Y, Takebayashi T, Koyasu S, Suematsu M, Hirose N, and von Zglinicki T. "Inflammation, but not telomere length, predicts successful ageing at extreme old age: A longitudinal study of semi-supercentenarians." EBioMedicine 2: 1549–1558 (2015)

Barzilai N, Cuervo AM, and Austad S. "Aging as a biological target for prevention and therapy." JAMA 320: 1321–1322 (2018)

Brattbakk HR, Arbo I, Aagaard S, Lindseth I, de Soysa AK, Langaas M, Kulseng B, Lindberg F, and Johansen B. "Balanced caloric macronutrient composition downregulates immunological gene expression in human blood cells-adipose tissue diverges." OMICS 17: 41–52 (2013)

Calder PC, Bosco N, Bourdet-Sicard R, Capuron L, Delzenne N, Doré J, Franceschi C, Lehtinen MJ, Recker T, Salvioli S, and Visioli F. "Health relevance of the modification of low-grade inflammation in ageing (inflammageing) and the role of nutrition." Ageing Res Rev 40: 95–119 (2017)

Cardel M, Jensen SM, Pottegård A, Jørgensen TL, and Hallas J. "Long-term use of metformin and colorectal cancer risk in type II diabetics: A population-based case-control study." Cancer Med 3: 1458–1466 (2014)

Das SK, Gilhooly CH, Golden JK, Pittas AG, Fuss PJ, Cheatham RA, Tyler S, Tsay M, McCrory MA, Lichtenstein AH, Dallal GE, Dutta C, Bhapkar MV, Delany JP, Saltzman E, and Roberts SB. "Long-term effects of 2 energy-restricted diets differing in glycemic load on dietary adherence, body composition, and metabolism in CALERIE: A 1-y randomized controlled trial." Am J Clin Nutr. 85: 1023–1030 (2007)

Das SK, Roberts SB, Bhapkar MV, Villareal DT, Fontana L, Martin CK, Racette SB, Fuss PJ, Kraus WE, Wong WW, Saltzman E, Pieper CF, Fielding RA, Schwartz AV, Ravussin E, and Redman LM. "Body-composition changes in the comprehensive assessment of long-term effects of reducing intake of energy (CALERIE)-2 study: A 2-y randomized controlled trial of calorie restriction in nonobese humans." Am J Clin Nutr 105: 913–927 (2017)

Fishman JR, Flatt MA, and Settersten RA. "Bioidentical hormones, menopausal women, and the lure of the 'natural' in U.S. anti-aging medicine." Soc Sci Med 132: 79–87 (2015)

Fontana L, Klein S, and Holloszy JO. "Effects of long-term calorie restriction and endurance exercise on glucose tolerance, insulin action, and adipokine production." Age 32: 97–108 (2010)

Fontana L, Kennedy BK, Longo VD, Seals D, and Melov S. "Medical research: Treat ageing." Nature 511: 405–407 (2014)

Fontana L, Villareal DT, Das SK, Smith SR, Meydani SN, Pittas AG, Klein S, Bhapkar M, Rochon J, Ravussin E, and Holloszy JO. "Effects of 2-year calorie restriction on circulating levels of IGF-1, IGF-binding proteins and cortisol in nonobese men and women: A randomized clinical trial." Aging Cell 15: 22–27 (2016)

Franceschi C and Campisi J. "Chronic inflammation (inflammaging) and its potential contribution to age-associated diseases." J Gerontol A Biol Sci Med Sci 69 (Suppl 1): S4–9 (2014)

Giampieri F, Alvarez-Suarez JM, Cordero MD, Gasparrini M, Forbes-Hernandez TY, Afrin S, Santos-Buelga C, González-Paramás AM, Astolfi P, Rubini C, Zizzi A, Tulipani S, Quiles JL, Mezzetti B, and Battino M. "Strawberry consumption improves aging-associated impairments, mitochondrial biogenesis and functionality through the AMP-activated protein kinase signaling cascade." Food Chem 234: 464–471 (2017)

Gottlieb RA and Gustafsson AB. "Mitochondrial turnover in the heart." Biochim Biophys Acta 1813: 1295–1301 (2011)

Gottlieb RA and Stotland A. "MitoTimer: A novel protein for monitoring mitochondrial turnover in the heart." J Mol Med 93: 271–278 (2015)

Heilbronn LK, de Jonge L, Frisard MI, DeLany JP, Larson-Meyer DE, Rood J, Nguyen T, Martin CK, Volaufova J, Most MM, Greenway FL, Smith SR, Deutsch WA, Williamson DA, and Ravussin E. "Effect of 6-month calorie restriction on biomarkers of longevity, metabolic adaptation, and oxidative stress in overweight individuals: A randomized controlled trial." JAMA 295: 1539–1548 (2006)

Hung WW, Ross JS, Boockvar KS, and Siu AL. "Recent trends in chronic disease, impairment and disability among older adults in the United States." BMC Geriatrics 11: 47 (2011)

Kaeberlein M, Rabinovitch PS, and Martin GM. "Healthy aging: The ultimate preventative medicine." Science 350: 1191–1193 (2015)

Kain V, Ingle KA, Kachman M, Baum H, Shanmugam G, Rajasekaran NS, Young ME, and Halade GV. "Excess n-6 fatty acids influx in aging drives metabolic dysregulation, electrocardiographic alterations, and low-grade chronic inflammation." Am J Physiol Heart Circ Physiol 314: H160–H169 (2018)

Kiecolt-Glaser JK, Epel ES, Belury MA, Andridge R, Lin J, Glaser R, Malarkey WB, Hwang BS, and Blackburn E. "Omega-3 fatty acids, oxidative stress, and leukocyte telomere length: A randomized controlled trial." Brain Behav Immun 28: 16–24 (2013)

Lewis KN, Wason E, Edrey YH, Kristan DM, Nevo E, and Buffenstein R. "Regulation of Nrf2 signaling and longevity in naturally long-lived rodents." Proc Natl Acad Sci U S A. 112: 3722–3727 (2015)

Liang J and Shang Y. "Estrogen and cancer." Annu Rev Physiol 75: 225–240 (2013)

Longo VD, Antebi A, Bartke A, Barzilai N, Brown-Borg HM, Caruso C, Curiel TJ, de Cabo R, Franceschi C, Gems D, Ingram DK, Johnson TE, Kennedy BK, Kenyon C, Klein S, Kopchick JJ, Lepperdinger G, Madeo F, Mirisola MG, Mitchell JR, Passarino G, Rudolph KL, Sedivy JM, Shadel GS, Sinclair DA, Spindler SR, Suh Y, Vijg J, Vinciguerra M, and Fontana L. "Interventions to slow aging in humans: Are we ready?" Aging Cell 14: 497–510 (2015)

Marin P, Holmang S, Jonsson L, Sjostrom L, Kvist H, Holm G, Lindstedt G, and Bjorntorp P. "The effects of testosterone treatment on body composition and metabolism in middle-aged obese men." Int J Obes Relat Metab Disord 16: 991–997 (1992)

Martin-Montalvo A, Mercken EM, Mitchell SJ, Palacios HH, Mote PL, Scheibye-Knudsen M, Gomes AP, Ward TM, Minor RK, Blouin MJ, Schwab M, Pollak M, Zhang Y, Yu Y, Becker KG, Bohr VA, Ingram DK, Sinclair DA, Wolf NS, Spindler SR, Bernier M, and de Cabo R. "Metformin improves healthspan and lifespan in mice." Nat Commun 4: 2192 (2013)

McCay CM and Crowell MF. "Prolonging the life span." Scientific Monthly 39: 405–414 (1934)

Mendelsohn AR and Larrick JW. "Inflammation, stem cells, and the aging hypothalamus." Rejuvenation Res 20: 346–349 (2017)

Meydani SN, Das SK, Pieper CF, Lewis MR, Klein S, Dixit VD, Gupta AK, Villareal DT, Bhapkar M, Huang M, Fuss PJ, Roberts SB, Holloszy JO, and Fontana L. "Long-term moderate calorie restriction inhibits inflammation without impairing cell-mediated immunity: A randomized controlled trial in non-obese humans." Aging 8: 1416–1431 (2016)

Olshansky SJ, Passaro DJ, Hershow RC, Layden J, Carnes BA, Brody J, Hayflick L, Butler RN, Allison DB, and Ludwig DS. "A potential decline in life expectancy in the United States in the 21st century." N Engl J Med 352: 1138–1145 (2005)

Olshansky SJ. "From lifespan to healthspan." JAMA 320: 1323–1324 (2018)

Owen MR, Doran E, and Halestrap AP. "Evidence that metformin exerts its anti-diabetic effects through inhibition of complex 1 of the mitochondrial respiratory chain." Biochem J 348 (Pt 3): 607–614 (2000)

Pandey MK, Gupta SC, Nabavizadeh A, and Aggarwal BB. "Regulation of cell signaling pathways by dietary agents for cancer prevention and treatment." Semin Cancer Biol 46: 158–181 (2017)

Pittas AG, Das SK, Hajduk CL, Golden J, Saltzman E, Stark PC, Greenberg AS, and Roberts SB. "A low-glycemic load diet facilitates greater weight loss in overweight adults with high insulin secretion but not in overweight adults with low insulin secretion in the CALERIE Trial." Diabetes Care 28: 2939–2941 (2005)

Prattichizzo F, De Nigris V, Spiga R, Mancuso E, La Sala L, Antonicelli R, Testa R, Procopio AD, Olivieri F, and Ceriello A. "Inflammageing and metaflammation: The yin and yang of type 2 diabetes." Ageing Res Rev 41: 1–17 (2018)

Rabassa M, Cherubini A, Zamora-Ros R, Urpi-Sarda M, Bandinelli S, Ferrucci L, and Andres-Lacueva C. "Low levels of a urinary biomarker of dietary polyphenol are associated with substantial cognitive decline over a 3-year period in older adults: The Invecchiare in Chianti study." J Am Geriatr Soc 63: 938–946 (2015)

Rabassa M, Zamora-Ros R, Andres-Lacueva C, Urpi-Sarda M, Bandinelli S, Ferrucci L, and Cherubini A. "Association between both total baseline urinary and dietary polyphenols and substantial physical performance decline risk in older adults: A 9-year follow-up of the InCHIANTI study." J Nutr Health Aging 20: 478–485 (2016)

Racette SB, Weiss EP, Villareal DT, Arif H, Steger-May K, Schechtman KB, Fontana L, Klein S, and Holloszy JO. "One year of caloric restriction in humans: Feasibility and effects on body composition and abdominal adipose tissue." J Gerontol A Biol Sci Med Sci 61: 943–950 (2006)

Rea IM, Gibson DS, McGilligan V, McNerlan SE, Alexander HD, and Ross OA. "Age and age-related diseases: Role of inflammation triggers and cytokines." Front Immunol 9: 586 (2018)

Reubinoff BE, Wurtman J, Rojansky N, Adler D, Stein P, Schenker JG, and Brzezinski A. "Effects of hormone replacement therapy on weight, body composition, fat distribution, and food intake in early postmenopausal women: A prospective study." Fertil Steril 64: 963–968 (1995)

Salminen A and Kaarniranta K. "AMP-activated protein kinase (AMPK) controls the aging process via an integrated signaling network." Ageing Res Rev 11: 230–241 (2012)

Sears B. *The Zone*. Regan Books. New York, NY (1995)

Sears B. *The Anti-Aging Zone*. Regan Books. New York, NY (1999)

Sears B. *Toxic Fat*. Thomas Nelson. Nashville, TN (2008)

Sears B. "Delaying adverse health consequences of aging: The role of omega-3 fatty acids on inflammation and resoleomics." CellR4 4: e2111 (2016)

Spalding KL, Bhardwaj RD, Buchholz BA, Druid and H, and Frisén J. "Retrospective birth dating of cells in humans." Cell 122: 133–143 (2005)

Spalding KL, Arner E, Westermark PO, Bernard S, Buchholz BA, Bergmann O, Blomqvist L, Hoffstedt J, Näslund E, Britton T, Concha H, Hassan M, Rydén M, Frisén J, and Arner P. "Dynamics of fat cell turnover in humans." Nature 453: 783–787 (2008)

Spalding KL, Bergmann O, Alkass K, Bernard S, Salehpour M, Huttner HB, Boström E, Westerlund I, Vial C, Buchholz BA, Possnert G, Mash DC, Druid H, and Frisén J. "Dynamics of hippocampal neurogenesis in adult humans." 153: 1219–1227 (2013)

Stephenne X, Foretz M, Taleux N, van der Zon GC, Sokal E, Hue L, Viollet B, and Guigas B. "Metformin activates AMP-activated protein kinase in primary human hepatocytes by decreasing cellular energy status." Diabetologia 54: 3101–3110 (2011)

Sun N, Youle RJ, and Finkel T. "The mitochondrial basis of aging." Mol Cell 61: 654–666 (2016)

Szklarczyk R, Nooteboom M, and Osiewacz HD. "Control of mitochondrial integrity in ageing and disease." Philos Trans R Soc Lond B Biol Sci 369: 20130439 (2014)

Urpi-Sarda M, Andres-Lacueva C, Rabassa M, Ruggiero C, Zamora-Ros R, Bandinelli S, Ferrucci L, and Cherubini A. "The relationship between urinary total polyphenols and the frailty phenotype in a community-dwelling older population: The InCHIANTI study." J Gerontol A Biol Sci Med Sci 70: 1141–1147 (2015)

Ward BW, Schiller JS, and Goodman RA. "Multiple chronic conditions among US adults: A 2012 update." Prev Chronic Dis 11: E62 (2014)

Welsh JA. *Sharks Get Cancer, Mole Rats Don't: How Animals Could Hold the Key to Unlocking Cancer Immunity in Humans*. Prometheus Books, New York, NY (2016)

Zamora-Ros R, Rabassa M, Cherubini A, Urpí-Sardà M, Bandinelli S, Ferrucci L, and Andres-Lacueva C. "High concentrations of a urinary biomarker of polyphenol intake are associated with decreased mortality in older adults." J Nutr 143: 1445–1450 (2013)

CHAPTER 21: THE FUTURE OF MEDICINE

Arai Y, Martin-Ruiz CM, Takayama M, Abe Y, Takebayashi T, Koyasu S, Suematsu M, Hirose N, and von Zglinicki T. "Inflammation, but not telomere length, predicts successful ageing at extreme old age." EBioMedicine 2: 1549–1558 (2015)

Baidal DA, Ricordi C, Garcia-Contreras M, Sonnino A, and Fabbri A. "Combination high-dose omega-3 fatty acids and high-dose cholecalciferol in new onset type 1 diabetes: A potential role in preservation of beta-cell mass." Eur Rev Med Pharmacol Sci 20: 3313–3318 (2016)

Brand S, Holsboer-Trachsler E, Naranjo JR, and Schmidt S. "Influence of mindfulness practice on cortisol and sleep in long-term and short-term meditators." Neuropsychobiology 65: 109–118 (2012)

Bowden Davies KA, Sprung VS, Norman JA, Thompson A, Mitchell KL, Halford JCG, Harrold JA, Wilding JPH, Kemp GJ, and Cuthbertson DJ. "Short-term decreased physical activity with increased sedentary behaviour causes metabolic derangements and altered body composition: effects in individuals with and without a first-degree relative with type 2 diabetes." Diabetologia 61: 1282–1294 (2018)

Cadario F, Savastio S, Rizzo AM, Carrera D, Bona G, and Ricordi C. "Can Type 1 diabetes progression be halted? Possible role of high dose vitamin D and omega 3 fatty acids." Eur Rev Med Pharmacol Sci 21: 1604–1609 (2017)

Cadario F, Savastio S, Ricotti R, Rizzo AM, Carrera D, Maiuri L, and Ricordi C. "Administration of vitamin D and high dose of omega 3 to sustain remission of type 1 diabetes." Eur Rev Med Pharmacol Sci 22: 512–515 (2018)

Das SK, Gilhooly CH, Golden JK, Pittas AG, Fuss PJ, Cheatham RA, Tyler S, Tsay M, McCrory MA, Lichtenstein AH, Dallal GE, Dutta C, Bhapkar MV, Delany JP, Saltzman E, and Roberts SB. "Long-term effects of 2 energy-restricted diets differing in glycemic load on dietary adherence, body composition, and metabolism in CALERIE: A 1-y randomized controlled trial." Am J Clin Nutr 85: 1023–1030 (2007)

Day EA, Ford RJ, and Steinberg GR. "AMPK as a therapeutic target for treating metabolic diseases." Trends Endocrinol Metab 28: 545–560 (2017)

Dohrn IM, Kwak L, Oja P, Sjöström M, and Hagströmer M. "Replacing sedentary time with physical activity: A 15-year follow-up of mortality in a national cohort." Clin Epidemiol 10: 179–186 (2018)

Fontana L, Villareal DT, Das SK, Smith SR, Meydani SN, Pittas AG, Klein S, Bhapkar M, Rochon J, Ravussin E, and Holloszy JO. "Effects of 2-year calorie restriction on circulating levels of IGF-1, IGF-binding proteins and cortisol in nonobese men and women: A randomized clinical trial." Aging Cell 15: 22–27 (2016)

Gibala M. "Molecular responses to high-intensity interval exercise." Appl Physiol Nutr Metab 34: 428–432 (2009)

Hardie DG. "Keeping the home fires burning: AMP-activated protein kinase." J Royal Society Interface 15: 20170774 (2018)

Harris R. *Rigor Mortis*. Basic Books. New York, NY (2017)

Hotamisligil GS. "Inflammation and metabolic disorders." Nature 444: 860–867 (2006)

Hotamisligil GS. "Inflammation, metaflammation and immunometabolic disorders." Nature 542: 177–185 (2017)

Hotamisligil GS. "Foundations of immunometabolism and implications for metabolic health and disease." Immunity 47: 406–420 (2017)

Hua X, Carvalho N, Tew M, Huang ES, Herman WH, and Clarke P. "Expenditures and prices of antihyperglycemic medications in the United States: 2002-2013." JAMA 315: 1400–1402 (2016)

Ioannidis JP. "Why most published research findings are false." PLoS Med 2: e124 (2005)

Katsumata Y, Todoriki H, Higashiuesato Y, Yasura S, Willcox DC, Ohya Y, Willcox BJ, and Dodge HH. "Metabolic syndrome and cognitive decline among the oldest old in Okinawa: In search of a mechanism. The KOCOA project." J Gerontol A Biol Sci Med Sci 67: 126–134 (2012)

Katsumata Y, Todoriki H, Higashiuesato Y, Yasura S, Ohya Y, Willcox DC, and Dodge HH. "Very old adults with better memory function have higher low-density lipoprotein cholesterol levels and lower triglyceride to high-density lipoprotein cholesterol ratios: KOCOA project." J Alzheimers Dis 34: 273–279 (2013)

Kirwan AM, Lenighan YM, O'Reilly ME, McGillicuddy FC, and Roche HM. "Nutritional modulation of metabolic inflammation." Biochem Soc Trans 45: 979–985 (2017)

Kochanek KD, Murphy SL, Xu J, and Arias E. "Mortality in the United States, 2016." NCHS Data Brief No. 293 (2017)

Marcinko K and Steinberg GR. "The role of AMPK in controlling metabolism and mitochondrial biogenesis during exercise." Exp Physiol 99: 1581–1585 (2014)

Marcinko K, Sikkema SR, Samaan MC, Kemp BE, Fullerton MD, and Steinberg GR. "High intensity interval training improves liver and adipose tissue insulin sensitivity." Mol Metab 4: 903–915 (2015)

Martin CK, Bhapkar M, Pittas AG, Pieper CF, Das SK, Williamson DA, Scott T, Redman LM, Stein R, Gilhooly CH, Stewart T, Robinson L, and Roberts SB. "Effect of calorie restriction on mood, quality of life, sleep, and sexual function in healthy nonobese adults: The CALERIE 2 randomized clinical trial." JAMA Intern Med 176: 743–752 (2016)

Mattison JA, Colman RJ, Beasley TM, Allison DB, Kemnitz JW, Roth GS, Ingram DK, Weindruch R, de Cabo R, and Anderson RM. "Caloric restriction improves health and survival of rhesus monkeys." Nat Comm 8: 14063 (2017)

Naviaux RK. "Metabolic features and regulation of the healing cycle: A new model for chronic disease pathogenesis and treatment." Mitochondrion 43: S1567 (2018)

McGlory C, von Allmen MT, Stokes T, Morton RW, Hector AJ, Lago BA, Raphenya AR, Smith BK, McArthur AG, Steinberg GR, Baker SK, and Phillips SM. "Failed recovery of glycemic control and myofibrillar protein synthesis with 2 wk of physical inactivity in overweight, prediabetic older adults." J Gerontol A Biol Sci Med Sci 73: 1070–1077 (2018)

Meydani M, Das S, Band M, Epstein S, Roberts S. "The effect of caloric restriction and glycemic load on measures of oxidative stress and antioxidants in humans: Results from the CALERIE trial of human caloric restriction." J Nutr Health Aging 15:456–60 (2011)

Nishihira J, Tokashiki T, Higashiuesato Y, Willcox DC, Mattek N, Shinto L, Ohya Y, and Dodge HH. "Associations between serum omega-3 fatty acid levels and cognitive functions among community-dwelling octogenarians in Okinawa, Japan: The KOCOA study." J Alzheimers Dis 51: 857–866 (2016)

Prinz F, Schlange T, and Asadullah K. "Believe it or not: How much can we rely on published data on potential drug targets?" Nat Rev Drug Discov 10: 712 (2011)

Ravussin E, Redman LM, Rochon J, Das SK, Fontana L, Kraus WE, Romashkan S, Williamson DA, Meydani SN, Villareal DT, Smith SR, Stein RI, Scott TM, Stewart TM, Saltzman E, Klein S, Bhapkar M, Martin CK, Gilhooly CH, Holloszy JO, Hadley EC, and Roberts SB. "A 2-year randomized controlled trial of human caloric restriction: Feasibility and effects on predictors of healthspan and longevity." J Gerontol A Biol Sci Med Sci. 70: 1097–1104 (2015)

Redman LM, Smith SR, Burton JH, Martin CK, Il'yasova D, and Ravussin E. "Metabolic slowing and reduced oxidative damage with sustained caloric restriction support the rate of living and oxidative damage theories of aging." Cell Metab 27: 805–815 (2018)

Rezende LFM, Sá TH, Mielke GI, Viscondi JYK, Rey-López JP, and Garcia LMT. "All-cause mortality attributable to sitting time: Analysis of 54 countries worldwide." Am J Prev Med 51: 253–263 (2016)

Richter EA and Ruderman NB. "AMPK and the biochemistry of exercise: Implications for human health and disease." Biochem J 418: 261–275 (2009)

Romashkan SV, Das SK, Villareal DT, Ravussin E, Redman LM, Rochon J, Bhapkar M, and Kraus WE. "Safety of two-year caloric restriction in non-obese healthy individuals." Oncotarget 7: 19124–19133 (2016)

Scannell JW, Blanckley A, Boldon H, and Warrington B. "Diagnosing the decline in pharmaceutical R&D efficiency." Nat Rev Drug Discov 11: 191–200 (2012)

Sears B. "Synthetic phospholipid compounds." U.S. Patent No. 4,426,330 (1984)

Sears B. "Delaying adverse health consequences of aging: The role of omega-3 fatty acids on inflammation and resoleomics." CellR4 4: e2111 (2016)

Suzuki M, Willcox DC, Rosenbaum MW, and Willcox BJ. "Oxidative stress and longevity in Okinawa: An investigation of blood lipid peroxidation and tocopherol in Okinawan centenarians." Curr Gerontol Geriatr Res. 2010: 380460 (2010)

Szarc vel Szic K, Declerck K, Vidakovic M, and Vanden Berghe W. "From inflammaging to healthy aging by dietary lifestyle choices: Is epigenetics the key to personalized nutrition?" Clin Epigenetics 7: 33 (2015)

Taylor R, Al-Mrabeh A, Zhyzhneuskaya S, Peters C, Barnes AC, Aribisala BS, Hollingsworth KG, Mathers JC, Sattar N, and Lean MEJ. "Remission of human type 2 diabetes requires decrease in liver and pancreas fat content but is dependent upon capacity for beta cell recovery." Cell Metab 28: 667 (2018)

Wick G, Grundtman C, Mayerl C, Wimpissinger TF, Feichtinger J, Zelger B, Sgonc R, and Wolfram D. "The immunology of fibrosis." Annu Rev Immunol 31: 107–135 (2013)

Willcox DC, Willcox BJ, Todoriki H, Curb JD, and Suzuki M. "Caloric restriction and human longevity: What can we learn from the Okinawans?" Biogerontology 7: 173–177 (2006)

Willcox BJ, Willcox DC, Todoriki H, Fujiyoshi A, Yano K, He Q, Curb JD, and Suzuki M. "Caloric restriction, the traditional Okinawan diet, and healthy aging: The diet of the world's longest-lived people and its potential impact on morbidity and life span." Ann N Y Acad Sci 1114: 434–455 (2007)

Willcox DC, Willcox BJ, Todoriki H, and Suzuki M. "The Okinawan diet: Health implications of a low-calorie, nutrient-dense, antioxidant-rich dietary pattern low in glycemic load." J Am Coll Nutr 28: 500S–516S (2009)

Willcox DC, Scapagnini G, and Willcox BJ. "Healthy aging diets other than the Mediterranean: A focus on the Okinawan diet." Mech Ageing Dev 136-137: 148–162 (2014)

Willcox BJ and Willcox DC. "Caloric restriction, caloric restriction mimetics, and healthy aging in Okinawa: Controversies and clinical implications." Curr Opin Clin Nutr Metab Care 17: 51–58 (2014)

Xu J, Murphy SL, Kochanek KD, and Arias E. "Mortality in the United States, 2015." NCHS Data Brief No. 267 (2016)

APPENDIX C. INFLAMMATION: THE SLIGHTLY LONGER COURSE

Afonso PV, Janka-Junttila M, Lee YJ, McCann CP, Oliver CM, Aamer KA, Losert W, Cicerone MT, and Parent CA. "LTB4 is a signal-relay molecule during neutrophil chemotaxis." Dev Cell 22: 1079–1091 (2012)

Baker RG, Hayden MS, and Ghosh S. "NF-κB, inflammation, and metabolic disease." Cell Metab 13: 11–22 (2011)

Bierhaus A, Stern DM, and Nawroth PP. "RAGE in inflammation: a new therapeutic target?" Curr Opin Investig Drugs 7: 985–991 (2006)

Cai D. "Neuroinflammation and neurodegeneration in overnutrition-induced diseases." Trends Endocrinol Metab 24: 40–47 (2013)

Camandola S, Leonarduzzi G, Musso T, Varesio L, Carini R, Scavazza A, Chiarpotto E, Baeuerle PA, and Poli G. "Nuclear factor κB is activated by arachidonic acid but not by eicosapentaenoic acid." Biochem Biophys Res Commun 229: 643–647 (1996)

Canetti C, Silva JS, Ferreira SH, and Cunha FQ. "Tumour necrosis factor-alpha and leukotriene B(4) mediate the neutrophil migration in immune inflammation." Br J Pharmacol 134:1619–28 (2001)

Crofts CAP, Zinn C, Wheldon MC, and Schofield GM. "Hyperinsulinemia: A unifying theory of chronic disease?" Diabesity 1: 34–43 (2015)

Fielding CA, Jones GW, McLoughlin RM, McLeod L, Hammond VJ, Uceda J, Williams AS, Lambie M, Foster TL, Liao CT, Rice CM, Greenhill CJ, Colmont CS, Hams E, Coles B, Kift-Morgan A, Newton Z, Craig KJ, Williams JD, Williams GT, Davies SJ, Humphreys IR, O'Donnell VB, Taylor PR, Jenkins BJ, Topley N, and Jones SA. "Interleukin-6 signaling drives fibrosis in unresolved inflammation." Immunity 40: 40–50 (2014)

Gloire G, Legrand-Poels S, and Piette J. "NF-κB activation by reactive oxygen species: Fifteen years later." Biochem Pharmacol 72: 1493–1505 (2006)

Guo H, Callaway JB, and Ting J. "Inflammasomes: Mechanism of action, role in disease and therapeutics." Nat Med 21: 677–687 (2015)

Hardie DG. "Keeping the home fires burning: AMP-activated protein kinase." J Royal Society Interface 15:20170774 (2018)

Hardie DG, Ross FA, and Hawley SA. "AMP-activated protein kinase: A target for drugs both ancient and modern." Chem Bio 19: 1222–1236 (2012)

Huang S, Rutkowsky JM, Snodgrass RG, Ono-Moore KD, Schneider DA, Newman JW, Adams SH, and Hwang DH. "Saturated fatty acids activate TLR-mediated proinflammatory signaling pathways." J Lipid Res 53: 2002–2013 (2012)

Iwasaki A and Medzhitov R. "Control of adaptive immunity by the innate immune system." Nat Immunol 16: 343–353 (2015)

Kawai T and Akira S. "The role of pattern-recognition receptors in innate immunity: Update on toll-like receptors." Nat Immunol 11: 373–384 (2010)

Sánchez-Galán E, Gómez-Hernández A, Vidal C, Martín-Ventura JL, Blanco-Colio LM, Muñoz-García B, Ortega L, Egido J, and Tuñón J. "Leukotriene B4 enhances the activity of nuclear factor-kappaB pathway through BLT1 and BLT2 receptors in atherosclerosis." Cardiovasc Res 81: 216–225 (2009)

Sen R and Baltimore D. "Multiple nuclear factors interact with the immunoglobulin enhancer sequences." Cell 46: 705–716. (1986)

Serhan CN, Ward PA, Gilroy DW, and Samir S. *Fundamentals of Inflammation.* Cambridge University Press. Cambridge, UK (2010)

Serhan CN. "Pro-resolving lipid mediators are leads for resolution physiology." Nature 510: 92–101 (2014)

Tóbon-Velasco JC, Cuevas E, and Torres-Ramos MA. "Receptor for AGEs (RAGE) as mediator of NF-κB pathway activation in neuroinflammation and oxidative stress." CNS Neurol Disord Drug Targets 13: 1615–1626 (2014)

Trowbridge HO and Emling RC. *Inflammation: A Review of the Process.* Quintessence Publising. Chicago, IL (1997)

Volchenkov R, Sprater F, Vogelsang P, and Appel S. "The 2011 Nobel Prize in physiology or medicine." Scand J Immunol 75: 1–4 (2012)

Weisberg SP, McCann D, Desai M, Rosenbaum M, Leibel RL, and Ferrante AW. "Obesity is associated with macrophage accumulation in adipose tissue." J Clin Invest 112: 1796–1808 (2003)

Wick G, Grundtman C, Mayerl C, Wimpissinger TF, Feichtinger J, Zelger B, Sgonc R, and Wolfram D. "The immunology of fibrosis." Annu Rev Immunol 31: 107–135 (2013)

Yan SF, Ramasamy R, and Schmidt AM. "Mechanisms of disease: Advanced glycation end-products and their receptor in inflammation and diabetes complications." Nat Clin Pract Endocrinol Metab 4: 285–293 (2008)

Zang M, Xu S, Maitland-Toolan KA, Zuccollo A, Hou X, Jiang B, Wierzbicki M, Verbeuren TJ, and Cohen RA. "Polyphenols stimulate AMP-activated protein kinase, lower lipids, and inhibit accelerated atherosclerosis in diabetic LDL-receptor-deficient mice." Diabetes 55: 2180–2191 (2006)

Zhang Q, Lenardo MJ, and Baltimore D. "30 Years of NF-κB: A Blossoming of Relevance to Human Pathobiology." Cell 168: 37–57 (2017)

Zhang X, Zhang G, Zhang H, Karin M, Bai H, and Cai D. "Hypothalamic IKKbeta/NF-κB and ER stress link overnutrition to energy imbalance and obesity." Cell 135: 61–73 (2008)

APPENDIX D. METABOLISM OF ESSENTIAL FATTY ACIDS, EICOSANOIDS, AND RESOLVINS

Brenner RR. "Nutritional and hormonal factors influencing desaturation of essential fatty acids." Prog Lipid Res 20: 41–47 (1981)

Serhan CN. "Discovery of specialized pro-resolving mediators marks the dawn of resolution physiology and pharmacology." Mol Aspects Med 58: 1–11 (2017)

Serhan CN, Chiang N, and Dalli J. "The resolution code of acute inflammation: Novel pro-resolving lipid mediators in resolution." Semin Immunol 27: 200–215 (2015)

Spite M, Clària J, and Serhan CN. "Resolvins, specialized proresolving lipid mediators, and their potential roles in metabolic diseases." Cell Metab 19: 21–36 (2014)

Willis AL. *Handbook of Eicosanoids.* CRC Press. Boca Raton, FL (1987)

APPENDIX E. ENERGY-SENSING GENE TRANSCRIPTION FACTORS

Ford RJ Desjardins EM, and Steinberg GR. "Are SIRTI activators another indirect method to increase AMPK for beneficial effects on aging and metabolic syndrome?" EBioMedicine 19: 16–17 (2017)

Hardie DG, Ross FA, and Hawley SA. "AMP-activate protein kinase: A target for drugs both ancient and modern." Chem Bio 19: 1222–1236 (2012)

Hardie DG. "Keeping the home fires burning: AMP-activated protein kinase." J Royal Society Interface. 15: 20170774 (2018)

Park S-J, Ahmad F, Um JH, Brown AL, Xu X, Kang H, Ke H, Feng X, Ryall J, Philp A, Schenk S, Kim MK, Sartorelli V, and Chung JH. "Specific Sirt1 activator-mediated improvement in glucose homeostatsis requires Sirt 1-independent activation of AMPK." EBioMedicine 18: 128–138 (2017)

Peng L, Li ZR, Green RS, Holzman IR, Lin J. "Butyrate enhances the intestinal barrier by facilitating tight junction assembly via activation of AMP-activated protein kinase in Caco-2 cell monolayers." J Nutr 139: 1619–1625 (2009)

Price NL, Gomes AP, Ling AJ, Duarte FV, Martin-Montalvo A, North BJ, Agarwal B, Ye L, Ramadori G, Teodoro JS, Hubbard BP, Varela AT, Davis JG, Varamini B, Hafner A, Moaddel R, Rolo AP, Coppari R, Palmeira CM, de Cabo R, Baur JA, and Sinclair DA. "SIRT-1 is required for AMPK activation and the beneficial effects of resveratrol on mitochondrial function." Cell Metab 15: 675–690 (2012)

Rahnasto-Rilla M, Tyni J, Huovinen M, Jarho E, Kulikowicz T, Ravichandran S, A Bohr V, Ferrucci L, Lahtela-Kakkonen M, and Moaddel R. "Natural polyphenols as sirtuin 6 modulators." Sci Rep 8:4163 (2018)

Ruderman NB, Xu XJ, Nelson L, Cacicedo JM, Saha AK, Lan F, and Ido Y. "AMPK and SIRT1: A long-standing partnership?" Am J Physiol Endocrinol Metabol 298: E751–E760 (2010)

Sun X and Zhu MJ. "AMP-activated protein kinase: A therapeutic target in intestinal diseases. Open Biol 7: 170104 (2017)

Sun X, Yang Q, Rogers CJ, Du M, and Zhu MJ. "AMPK improves gut epithelial differentiation and barrier function via regulating Cdx2 expression." Cell Death Differ 24: 819–831 (2017)

Zhang L, Li J, Young LH, and Caplan MJ. "AMP-activated protein kinase regulates the assembly of epithelial tight junctions." Proc Natl Acad Sci U S A. 103:17272–17227 (2006)

APPENDIX F. AMP KINASE AND MITOCHONDRIA

Chan K, Truong D, Shangari N, and O'Brien PJ. "Drug-induced mitochondrial toxicity." Expert Opin Drug Metab Toxicol 1: 655–669 (2005)

Davinelli S, Corbi G, Righetti S, Sears B, Olarte HH, Grassi D, and Scapagnini G. "Cardioprotection by cocoa polyphenols and n-3 fatty acids: A disease-prevention perspective on aging-associated cardiovascular risk." J Med Food 21: 1060–1069 (2018)

Duarte DA, Rosales MA, Papadimitriou A, Silva KC, Amancio VH, Mendonça JN, Lopes NP, de Faria JB, and de Faria JM. "Polyphenol-enriched cocoa protects the diabetic retina from glial reaction through the sirtuin pathway." J Nutr Biochem 26: 64–74 (2015)

Herzig S and Shaw RJ. "AMPK: Guardian of metabolism and mitochondrial homeostasis." Nat Rev Mol Cell Biol 19: 121–135 (2018)

Hwang JT, Kwon DY, and Yoon SH. "AMP-activated protein kinase: A potential target for the diseases prevention by natural occurring polyphenols." N Biotechnol 26: 17–22 (2009)

Know, L. *Life: The Epic Story of Our Mitochondria*. Friesen Press. Victoria, BC, Canada. (2014)

Krishnamoorthy RM and Carani Venkatraman A. "Polyphenols activate energy sensing network in insulin resistant models." Chem Biol Interact 275: 95–107 (2017)

Laker RC, Drake JC, Wilson RJ, Lira VA, Lewellen BM, Ryall KA, Fisher CC, Zhang M, Saucerman JJ, Goodyear LJ, Kundu M, and Yan Z. "AMPK phosphorylation of ULK1 is required for targeting of mitochondria to lysosomes in exercise-induced mitophagy." Nat Commun 15: 548 (2017)

Lane N. *Power, Sex, and Suicide: Mitochondria and the Meaning of Life*. Oxford University Press. Oxford, UK (2005)

Rieusset J. "Role of endoplasmic reticulum-mitochondria communication in type 2 diabetes." Adv Exp Med Biol 997: 171–186 (2017)

Scatena R. "Mitochondria and drugs." Adv Exp Med Biol 942: 329–346 (2012)

Sears B and Ricordi C. "Role of fatty acids and polyphenols in inflammatory gene transcription and their impact on obesity, metabolic syndrome and diabetes." Eur Rev Med Pharmacol Sci 16: 1137–54 (2012)

Sears B. "Anti-inflammatory diets." J Am Coll Nutr 34 Suppl 1:14–21 (2015)

Tagaya M and Arasaki K. "Regulation of mitochondrial dynamics and autophagy by the mitochondria-associated membrane." Adv Exp Med Biol 997: 33–47 (2017)

Tang BL. "Sirt1 and the mitochondria." Mol Cells 39: 87–95 (2016)

Thoudam T, Jeon JH, Ha CM, and Lee IK. "Role of mitochondria-associated endoplasmic reticulum membrane in inflammation-mediated metabolic diseases." Mediators Inflamm 2016: 1851420 (2016)

Tubbs E, Theurey P, Vial G, Bendridi N, Bravard A, Chauvin MA, Ji-Cao J, Zoulim F, Bartosch B, Ovize M, Vidal H, and Rieusset J. "Mitochondria-associated endoplasmic reticulum membrane (MAM) integrity is required for insulin signaling and is implicated in hepatic insulin resistance." Diabetes 63: 3279–3294 (2014)

Varga ZV, Ferdinandy P, Liaudet L, and Pacher P. "Drug-induced mitochondrial dysfunction and cardiotoxicity." Am J Physiol Heart Circ Physiol 309: H1453–467 (2015)

Weir HJ, Yao P, Huynh FK, Escoubas CC, Goncalves RL, Burkewitz K, Laboy R, Hirschey MD, and Mair WB. "Dietary restriction and AMPK increase lifespan via mitochondrial network and peroxisome remodeling." Cell Metab 5: 884–896 (2017)

APPENDIX G. GUT PHYSIOLOGY

Anderson SC. *The Psychobitoic Revolution.* National Geographic Books. Washington DC (2017)

Anhê FF, Roy D, Pilon G, Dudonné S, Matamoros S, Varin TV, Garofalo C, Moine Q, Desjardins Y, Levy E, and Marette A. "A polyphenol-rich cranberry extract protects from diet-induced obesity, insulin resistance and intestinal inflammation in association with increased *Akkermansia* spp. population in gut microbiota of mice." Gut 64: 872–883 (2015)

Asarian L and Bächler T. "Neuroendocrine control of satiation." Horm Mol Biol Clin Investig 19: 163–192 (2014)

Bergmann O, Zdunek S, Felker A, Salehpour M, Alkass K, Bernard S, Sjostrom SL, Szewczykowska M, Jackowska T, Dos Remedios C, Malm T, Andrä M, Jashari R, Nyengaard JR, Possnert G, Jovinge S, Druid H, and Frisén J. "Dynamics of cell generation and turnover in the human heart." Cell 161: 1566–1575 (2015)

Blasser MJ. *Missing Microbes.* Henry Holt. New York, NY (2014)

Bliss ES and Whiteside E. "The gut-brain axis, the human gut microbiota and their integration in the development of obesity." Front Physiol 9: 900 (2018)

Cani PD, Amar J, Iglesias MA, Poggi M, Knauf C, Bastelica D, Neyrinck AM, Fava F, Tuohy KM, Chabo C, Waget A, Delmée E, Cousin B, Sulpice T, Chamontin B, Ferrières J, Tanti JF, Gibson GR, Casteilla L, Delzenne NM, Alessi MC, and Burcelin R. "Metabolic endotoxemia initiates obesity and insulin resistance." Diabetes 56: 1761–1772 (2007)

Caesasr R, Tremaroli V, Kovatcheva-Datchary P, Cani PD, and Backhed F. "Crosstalk between gut microbiota and dietary lipids aggravates WAT inflammation through TLR signaling." Cell Metabol 22: 1–11 (2015)

Chambers ES, Morrison DJ, and Frost G. "Control of appetite and energy intake by SCFA: What are the potential underlying mechanisms?" Proc Nutr Soc 74: 328–336 (2015)

Chio CC, Baba T, and Black KL. "Selective blood-tumor barrier disruption by leukotrienes." J Neurosurg 77: 407–410 (1992)

Christiansen CB, Gabe MBN, Svendsen B, Dragsted LO, Rosenkilde MM, and Holst JJ. "The impact of short-chain fatty acids on GLP-1 and PYY secretion from the isolated perfused rat colon." Am J Physiol Gastrointest Liver Physiol 315: G53–G65 (2018)

Chronaiou A, Tsoli M, Kehagias I, Leotsinidis M, Kalfarentzos F, and Alexandrides TK. "Lower ghrelin levels and exaggerated postprandial peptide-YY, glucagon-like peptide-1, and insulin responses, after gastric fundus resection, in patients undergoing Roux-en-Y gastric bypass: A randomized clinical trial." Obes Surg 22: 1761–1770 (2012)

Collen A. *10% Human*. Harper Collins. New York, NY (2015)

Cornick S, Tawiah A, and Chadee K. "Roles and regulation of the mucus barrier in the gut." Tissue Barriers 3: e982426 (2015)

Delcour JA, Aman P, Courtin CM, Hamaker BR, and Verbeke K. "Prebiotics, fermentable dietary fiber, and health claims." Adv Nutr 7: 1–4 (2016)

Derrien M. "*Akkermansia muciniphila*, a human intestinal mucin-degrading bacterium." Int J Systematic and Evolutionary Microbiology 54: 1469–1476 (2004)

Daud NM, Ismail NA, Thomas EL, Fitzpatrick JA, Bell JD, Swann JR, Costabile A, Childs CE, Pedersen C, Goldstone AP, and Frost GS. "The impact of oligofructose on stimulation of gut hormones, appetite regulation and adiposity." Obesity 22: 1430–1438 (2014)

de Vogel-van den Bosch HM, Bünger M, de Groot PJ, Bosch-Vermeulen H, Hooiveld GJ, and Müller M. "PPARγ-mediated effects of dietary lipids on intestinal barrier gene expression." BMC Genomics 9: 231 (2008)

Everard A and Cani PD. "Gut microbiota and GLP-1." Rev Endocr Metab Disord 15: 189–196 (2014)

Fasano A. "Zonulin and its regulation of intestinal barrier function: the biological door to inflammation, autoimmunity, and cancer." Physiol Rev 91: 151–175 (2011)

Fredricks D. *The Human Microbiota: How Microbial Communities Affect Health and Disease*. Wiley-Blackwell. New York, NY (2013)

Gershon MD. *The Second Brain*. Harper Collins. New York, NY (1999)

Goodman BE. "Insights into digestion and absorption of major nutrients in humans." Adv Physiol Educ 34: 44–53 (2010)

Greiner TU and Bäckhed F. "Microbial regulation of GLP-1 and L-cell biology." Mol Metab 5: 753–758 (2016)

Grossi E and Pace F eds. *Human Nutrition from the Gastroenterologist's Perspective*. Springer. New York, NY (2016)

Kaliannan K, Wang B, Xiang-Yong L, Kim K-J, and Kang JX. "A host-microbiome interaction mediates the opposing effects of omega-6 and omega-3 fatty acids on metabolic endotoxemia." Sci Reports 5: 112276 (2015)

Kimura R, Takahashi N, Lin S, Goto T, Murota K, Nakata R, Inoue H, and Kawada T. "DHA attenuates postprandial hyperlipidemia via activating PPARγ in intestinal epithelial cells." J Lipid Res 54: 3258–3268 (2013)

Konturek SJ and Brzozowski T. "Role of leukotrienes and platelet activating factor in gastric mucosal damage and repair." J Physiol Pharmacol 42:107–133 (1991)

Larraufie P, Martin-Gallausiaux C, Lapaque N, Dore J, Gribble FM, Reimann F, and Blottiere HM. "SCFAs strongly stimulate PYY production in human enteroendocrine cells." Sci Rep 8: 74 (2018)

Leclercq S, Matamoros S, Cani PD, Neyrinck AM, Jamar F, Stärkel P, Windey K, Tremaroli V, Bäckhed F, Verbeke K, de Timary P, and Delzenne NM. "Intestinal permeability, gut-bacterial dysbiosis, and behavioral markers of alcohol-dependence severity." Proc Natl Acad Sci U S A 111: E4485–4493 (2014)

López-Moreno J, García-Carpintero S, Jimenez-Lucena R, Haro C, Rangel-Zúñiga OA, Blanco-Rojo R, Yubero-Serrano EM, Tinahones FJ, Delgado-Lista J, Pérez-Martínez P, Roche HM, López-Miranda J, and Camargo A. "Effect of dietary lipids on endotoxemia influences postprandial inflammatory response." J Agric Food Chem 65: 7756–7763 (2017)

Lyte M and Cryan JF. *Microbial Endocrinology: The Microbiota-Gut-Brain Axis.* Springer. New York, NY (2014)

Masumoto S, Terao A, Yamamoto Y, Mukai T, Miura T, and Shoji T. "Non-absorbable apple procyandian prevent obesity associated with gut microbial and metabolomics changes." Sci Reports 6: 31208 (2016)

Mayer E. *The Mind-Gut Connection.* Harper Wave. New York, NY (2016)

Nettleton JE, Reimer RA, and Shearer J. "Reshaping the gut microbiota: Impact of low-calorie sweeteners and the link to insulin resistance?" Physiol Behav164 (Pt B): 488–493 (2016)

Pelaseyed T, Bergström JH, Gustafsson JK, Ermund A, Birchenough GM, Schütte A, van der Post S, Svensson F, Rodríguez-Piñeiro AM, Nyström EE, Wising C, Johansson ME, and Hansson GC. "The mucus and mucins of the goblet cells and enterocytes provide the first defense line of the gastrointestinal tract and interact with the immune system." Immunol Rev 260: 8–20 (2014)

Pepino MY, Tiemann CD, Patterson BW, Wice BM, and Klein S. "Sucralose affects glycemic and hormonal responses to an oral glucose load." Diabetes Care 36: 2530–2535 (2013)

Pepino MY. "Metabolic effects of non-nutritive sweeteners." Physiol Behav 152 (Pt B): 450–5 (2016)

Psichas A, Sleeth ML, Murphy KG, Brooks L, Bewick GA, Hanyaloglu AC, Ghatei MA, Bloom SR, and Frost G. "The short chain fatty acid propionate stimulates GLP-1 and PYY secretion via free fatty acid receptor 2 in rodents." Int J Obes 39: 424–429 (2015)

Roach M. *Gulp.* W.W. Norton and Company. New York, NY (2013)

Roopchand DE, Carmody RN, Kuhn P, Moskal K, Rojas-Silva, Turnbaugh PJ, and Raskin I. "Dietary polyphenols promote growth of gut bacterium *Akkermansia muninphila* and attenuate high-fat diet-induced metabolic syndrome." Diabetes 64: 2847–2858 (2015)

Schneeberger M, Everard A, Gómez-Valadés AG, Matamoros S, Ramírez S, Delzenne NM, Gomis R, Claret M, and Cani PD. "*Akkermansia muciniphila* inversely correlates with the onset of inflammation, altered adipose tissue metabolism and metabolic disorders in mice." Sci Reports 5: 16643 (2015)

Schroeder N, Marquart LF, and Gallaher DD. "The role of viscosity and fermentability of dietary fibers on satiety- and adiposity-related hormones in rats." Nutrients 5: 2093–2113 (2013)

Slavin J. "Fiber and prebiotics." Nutrients 5: 1417–1435 (2013)

Sonnenburg ED, Smits SA, Tikhonov M, Higginbottom SK, Wingreen NS, and Sonnenburg JL. "Diet-induced extinctions in the gut microbiota compound over generations." Nature 529: 212–215 (2016)

Sonneburg J and Sonnenburg E. *The Good Gut*. Penguin Books. New York, NY (2016)

Spalding KL, Bhardwaj RD, Buchholz BA, Druid H, and Frisén J. "Retrospective birth dating of cells in humans." Cell 122: 133–143 (2005)

Spalding KL, Arner E, Westermark PO, Bernard S, Buchholz BA, Bergmann O, Blomqvist L, Hoffstedt J, Näslund E, Britton T, Concha H, Hassan M, Rydén M, Frisén J, and Arner P. "Dynamics of fat cell turnover in humans." Nature 453: 783–787 (2008)

Spalding KL, Bergmann O, Alkass K, Bernard S, Salehpour M, Huttner HB, Boström E, Westerlund I, Vial C, Buchholz BA, Possnert G, Mash DC, Druid H, and Frisén J. "Dynamics of hippocampal neurogenesis in adult humans." Cell 153: 1219–1227 (2013)

Spreckley E and Murphy KG. "The L-cell in nutritional sensing and the regulation of appetite." Front Nutr 2: 23 (2015)

Suez J, Korem T, Zeevi D, Zilberman-Schapira G, Thaiss CA, Maza O, Israeli D, Zmora N, Gilad S, Weinberger A, Kuperman Y, Harmelin A, Kolodkin-Gal I, Shapiro H, Halpern Z, Segal E, and Elinav E. "Artificial sweeteners induce glucose intolerance by altering the gut microbiota." Nature 514: 181–186 (2014)

van der Klaauw AA, Keogh JM, Henning E, Trowse VM, Dhillo WS, Ghatei MA, and Farooqi IS. "High protein intake stimulates postprandial GLP-1 and PYY release." Obesity 21: 1602–1607 (2013)

Vanuytsel T, van Wanrooy S, Vanheel H, Vanormelingen C, Verschueren S, Houben E, Salim Rasoel S, Toth J, Holvoet L, Farré R, Van Oudenhove L, Boeckxstaens G, Verbeke K, and Tack J. "Psychological stress and corticotropin-releasing hormone increase intestinal permeability in humans by a mast cell-dependent mechanism." Gut 63: 1293–1299 (2014)

Tuohy K and Del Rio D. *Diet-Microbe Interactions in the Gut*. Academic Press. London, UK (2015)

Wrangham R. *Cooking with Fire*. Basic Books. New York, NY (2010)

Yeomans MR, Tepper BJ, Rietzschel J, and Prescott J. "Human hedonic responses to sweetness: Role of taste genetics and anatomy." Physiol Behav 91: 264–273 (2007)

Zanchi D, Depoorter A, Egloff L, Haller S, Mählmann L, Lang UE, Drewe J, Beglinger C, Schmidt A, and Borgwardt S. "The impact of gut hormones on the neural circuit of appetite and satiety: A systematic review." Neurosci Biobehav Rev 80: 457–475 (2017)

ACKNOWLEDGMENTS

I WOULD LIKE to greatly thank Kathy Huck for her excellent general editorial support, as well as my brother Doug Sears and Andy Yurcho for their critical reading and insightful suggestions for the final book. Finally, I also wish to thank Judith Regan for her continuing belief and support of the concept of the Zone.

DR. BARRY SEARS is a leading authority on the impact of diet on inflammation. He is a former research scientist at the Boston University School of Medicine and the Massachusetts Institute of Technology and founder of one of the first biotechnology companies in Massachusetts that has been in continuous operation since 1976. He is the author of more than 50 scientific publications and holds 14 U.S. patents in the areas of intravenous cancer drug delivery systems and the dietary regulation of hormonal responses for the treatment of cardiovascular disease.

The general awareness of Dr. Sears' research on the dietary control of hormonal and genetic responses began with the publication of his landmark book, *The Zone*, which became a #1 *New York Times* bestseller. The books he has written on his Zone technology have sold more than six million copies in the U.S. and have been a translated into 23 different languages. *The Resolution Zone* brings together his decades of research using the diet as a powerful "drug" to address the problem of unresolved inflammation that is the ultimate cause of chronic disease.

Dr. Sears continues his research as the president of the non-profit Inflammation Research Foundation in Peabody, Massachusetts. In addition to his research into the hormonal and genetic effects of the diet, he continues to develop innovative dietary technologies used in the management of diabetes and cardiovascular and neurological conditions.